Behavior and the Menstrual Cycle

SEXUAL BEHAVIOR

edited by

Richard C. Friedman

The New York Hospital-Cornell Medical Center, Westchester Division
White Plains, New York

1. Behavior and the Menstrual Cycle, edited by Richard C. Friedman

Additional Volumes in Preparation

Behavior and the Menstrual Cycle

edited by

RICHARD C. FRIEDMAN

The New York Hospital–Cornell Medical Center,
    Westchester Division
White Plains, New York

MARCEL DEKKER, INC.   New York and Basel

Library of Congress Cataloging in Publication Data

Main entry under title:

Behavior and the menstrual cycle.

    (Sexual behavior ; v. 1)
    Includes indexes.
    1. Menstrual cycle.   2. Menstrual cycle–Psychological aspects.
3. Premenstrual syndrome.   4. Women–Mental health.   5. Endocrine
gynecology.   I. Friedman, Richard C. [date]. II. Series: Sexual
behavior (Marcel Dekker, Inc.) ; v. 1. [DNLM: 1. Menstruation.
2. Menstruation disorders. 3. Premenstrual tension. 4. Sex
behavior. W1 SE99E v.1 / WP 540 B419]
RG163.B43 1982   618.1'72   82-17995
ISBN 0-8247-1852-6

Preface

The chapters in this book illustrate diverse ways of looking at the extremely complex relationships between behavior and the menstrual cycle. Despite the fact that this topic has generated great interest during the past 50 years, hard facts have been difficult to come by and remain relatively scant. Major studies carried out many years ago still await replication.

Some of the articles emphasize behavior in the general population; others are restricted to psychiatric patients. It is notable that, although symptoms of behavioral pathology may be associated with the cycle in many women, premenstrual tension is not identified as a specific syndrome of psychiatric illness in the most recent edition of the diagnostic nomenclature of the American Psychiatric Association (DSM-III). The criteria that would define such a syndrome had not been adequately established even as recently as 1980, the year the DSM-III was published.

The authors represented in this book come from different disciplines, each with its own methodology and point of view. Occasionally, authors directly contradict each other about data interpretation. Such contradictions, when they occur, would appear to reflect the state of the field at present.

This book was not intended to provide an encyclopedic overview. Important aspects of the general topic had to be omitted because of limitations of space. By providing a variety of approaches to associations between relevant biological, psychological, and social events, it is hoped that *Behavior and the Menstrual Cycle* stimulates interest and future research in this important area.

—Richard C. Friedman

Contributors

MICHAEL S. ARONOFF, The New York Hospital-Cornell Medical Center, Westchester Division, White Plains, New York

SUSAN E. BENNETT, Beth Israel Hospital, Boston, Massachusetts, and Harvard Medical School, Boston, Massachusetts

JEANNE BROOKS-GUNN, Institute for the Study of Exceptional Children, Educational Testing Service, Princeton, New Jersey, and Department of Pediatrics, College of Physicians and Surgeons, Columbia University, New York, New York

DONALD M. BROVERMAN, Department of Psychology, Worcester State Hospital, Worcester, Massachusetts

JOHN CLARKIN, The New York Hospital-Cornell Medical Center, Westchester Division, White Plains, New York

RUTH CORN, The New York Hospital-Cornell Medical Center, Westchester Division, White Plains, New York

KATHARINA DALTON, Premenstrual Syndrome Clinic, University College Hospital, London, England

PAULA G. DAVIS,* Department of Neuroendocrinology, The Rockefeller University, New York, New York

---

*Present affiliation: M.E.D. Communications, Hopelawn, New Jersey

CAROL A. DUDLEY, Department of Physiology, University of Texas Health Science Center, Dallas, Texas

JEAN ENDICOTT, Department of Psychiatry, College of Physicians and Surgeons, Columbia University, New York, New York, and New York State Psychiatric Institute, New York, New York

MICHEL FERIN, Departments of Obstetrics and Gynecology and Physiology, College of Physicians and Surgeons, Columbia University, New York, New York

RICHARD C. FRIEDMAN, The New York Hospital-Cornell Medical Center, Westchester Division, White Plains, New York

FRITZ FUCHS, Department of Obstetrics and Gynecology, The New York Hospital-Cornell Medical Center, New York, New York

IRA D. GLICK, Department of Psychiatry, Cornell University Medical College, New York, New York, and The Payne Whitney Clinic, The New York Hospital-Cornell Medical Center, New York, New York

JUDITH GREEN, Departments of Psychology and Biology, William Paterson College of New Jersey, Wayne, New Jersey

URIEL HALBREICH, Department of Psychiatry, Albert Einstein College of Medicine, Bronx, New York

KATHERINE A. HALMI, The New York Hospital-Cornell Medical Center, Westchester Division, White Plains, New York

STEPHEN W. HURT, The New York Hospital-Cornell Medical Center, Westchester Division, White Plains, New York

DAVID S. JANOWSKY, Department of Psychiatry, University of California, San Diego, La Jolla, California

JAMES A. KENNEDY, Department of Psychiatry, Worcester State Hospital, Worcester, Massachusetts

EDWARD L. KLAIBER, The Worcester Foundation for Experimental Biology, Shrewsbury, Massachusetts

DANIEL M. LINKIE,* Departments of Obstetrics and Gynecology and Anatomy and Cell Biology, College of Physicians and Surgeons, Columbia University, New York, New York

BRUCE S. McEWEN, Department of Neuroendocrinology, The Rockefeller University, New York, New York

*Present affiliation: Ferring Laboratories, Inc., Ridgewood, New Jersey

NAOMI M. MORRIS,* Department of Pediatrics, University of Health Sciences/ The Chicago Medical School, Chicago, Illinois

ROBERT L. MOSS, Department of Physiology, University of Texas Health Science Center, Dallas, Texas

CONRAD J. L. NADEAU, Department of Psychiatry, University of Massachusetts Medical Center, Worcester, Massachusetts

MARY BROWN PARLEE, Center for the Study of Women and Society, Graduate School and University Center, City University of New York, New York

JEFFREY L. RAUSCH, Department of Psychiatry, University of California, San Diego, La Jolla, California

DIANE N. RUBLE,† Department of Psychology, University of Toronto, Toronto, Ontario, Canada

BARBARA SOMMER, Department of Psychology, University of California, Davis, California

MICHAEL H. STONE, Department of Psychiatry, University of Connecticut Health Center, Farmington, Connecticut

J. RICHARD UDRY, Carolina Population Center, The University of North Carolina at Chapel Hill, Chapel Hill, North Carolina

WILLIAM VOGEL, Department of Psychology, Worcester State Hospital, Worcester, Massachusetts

ANN MARIE WILLIAMS, Marriage Council of Philadelphia, Inc., Philadelphia, Pennsylvania

GREGORY D. WILLIAMS, Department of Medicine, Presbyterian-University of Pennsylvania Medical Center, Philadelphia, Pennsylvania

---

*Present affiliation: Community Health Sciences Program, School of Public Health, University of Illinois at the Medical Center, Chicago, Illinois
†Present affiliation: Department of Psychology, New York University, New York, New York

Contents

Preface
Contributors

1. The Physiology of the Menstrual Cycle   1

    Daniel M. Linkie

2. The Neuroendocrinologic Control of the Menstrual Cycle   23

    Michel Ferin

3. Neuroendocrine Regulation of Sexual Behavior   43

    Paula G. Davis and Bruce S. McEwen

4. Hypothalamic Peptides and Sexual Behavior   65

    Robert L. Moss and Carol A. Dudley

5. The Psychology of the Menstrual Cycle: Biological and
    Psychological Perspectives   77

    Mary Brown Parlee

6.   Cognitive Behavior and the Menstrual Cycle   101

     Barbara Sommer

7.   Epidemiological Patterns of Sexual Behavior in the
     Menstrual Cycle   129

     Naomi M. Morris and J. Richard Udry

8.   Sexual Behavior and the Menstrual Cycle   155

     Gregory D. Williams and Ann Marie Williams

9.   A Developmental Analysis of Menstrual Distress in Asolescence   177

     Diane N. Ruble and Jeanne Brooks-Gunn

10. Dysmenorrhea and Dyspareunia   199

     Fritz Fuchs

11. Premenstrual Tension: An Overview   217

     Katharina Dalton

12. Classification of Premenstrual Syndromes   243

     Uriel Halbreich and Jean Endicott

13. Estrogens and Central Nervous System Function:
     Electroencephalography, Cognition, and Depression   267

     *Edward L. Klaiber, Donald M. Broverman, William Vogel,
     James A. Kennedy, and Conrad J. L. Nadeau*

14. The Menstrual Cycle in Anorexia Nervosa   291

     Katherine A. Halmi

15. Psychopathology and the Menstrual Cycle   299

     *Stephen W. Hurt, Richard C. Friedman, John Clarkin,
     Ruth Corn, and Michael S. Aronoff*

16. Premenstrual Tension in Borderline and Related Disorders   317

     Michael H. Stone

Contents

17. **Oral Contraceptives and the Menstrual Cycle** 345

    Ira Glick and Susan E. Bennett

18. **Recent Trends in the Treatment of Premenstrual Syndrome: A Critical Review** 367

    Judith Green

19. **Premenstrual Tension: Etiology** 397

    Jeffrey L. Rausch and David S. Janowsky

Author Index   *429*
Subject Index   *461*

1 The Physiology of the Menstrual Cycle

DANIEL M. LINKIE* College of Physicians and Surgeons, Columbia University, New York, New York

The menstrual cycle of the human female is characterized by a series of coordinated physiological events. Once these events are initiated, regular menstrual cyclicity may continue for nearly 40 consecutive years. This chapter presents the physiology of a normal menstrual cycle. Emphasis has been placed upon the endocrine role in these overt physiological events and the subtle covert biochemical interactions which underlie menstrual cyclicity.

I. The Menstrual Cycle: Descriptive Aspects

The human female spends approximately one-half of her life span in a reproductively competent state. The other years are spent in nonfertile growth and development (prepubertal) or atrophic stages (postmenopausal) (Fig. 1). The reproductively competent years are featured by the near-monthly repetition of menses. Menstruation, however, is only the outward manifestation of underlying cyclic endocrine changes. These hormonal changes were summarized by Corner in 1942 [1] and detailed more recently (1981) by Ross and Vande Wiele [2].

The menstrual cycle results from the actions of hypothalamic, pituitary, and ovarian hormones upon the components of the reproductive system. The central nervous system integrates the hormonal rhythms of the internal milieu with exteroceptive stimuli and regulates the synthesis and secretion of hypothalamic hormones which further direct the production and release of the pituitary gonadotropins. The gonadotropins in turn determine the activities of the ovaries including

*Present affiliation: Ferring Laboratories, Inc., Ridgewood, New Jersey

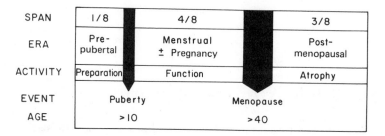

SPAN	1/8		4/8		3/8
ERA	Pre-pubertal		Menstrual ± Pregnancy		Post-menopausal
ACTIVITY	Preparation		Function		Atrophy
EVENT		Puberty		Menopause	
AGE		>10		>40	

Figure 1 The life cycle of the human female is unequally divided into three general reproductive eras. Approximately one-half of the life span is reproductively incompetent. Transition into (puberty) and out of (menopause) the reproductively competent era occurs at 10 to 15 and 40 to 50 years respectively.

the production of steroid hormones, follicle development, and gamete maturation. The ovarian steroid hormones act on the oviducts, uterus, vagina, and breasts, and feed back to modulate the central nervous system and pituitary. Such diverse factors as stress; nutrition; visual, olfactory, and auditory cues; altitude; and time zone changes are also known to influence the regulation of the reproductive system [3].

A. The Reproductive System

The female reproductive system consists of a pair of ovaries suspended in the abdominal cavity with each ovary closely apposed to the ipsilateral oviduct. Each oviduct is continuous with the common genital ducts of the uterus and vagina. The external genitalia and such nongenital organs as the pituitary, hypothalamus, brain, and mammary glands are essential members of this organ system. The changes occurring in these components during a menstrual cycle are described below. The primary function of the reproductive system in the mature female is the provision and nurture of the cytogenic products of the ovary. This function has underlying hormonal bases which vary during the menstrual cycle (Fig. 2). The menstrual cycle actually reflects uterine and ovarian cycles with concommitant pituitary gonadotropin cycles. Hence, the proliferative (uterine)-follicular (ovarian) phase precedes, whereas the secretory (uterine)-luteal (ovarian) phase follows the midcycle gonadotropin surge (pituitary) which is necessary for ovulation. The preovulatory ovarian estrogens are therefore joined by postovulatory luteal progestins. These steroid hormones are important at all levels of the reproductive system by effecting growth and maintenance of the reproductive organs, feedback regulation of the hypothalamus and pituitary, and related behavioral aspects of reproduction.

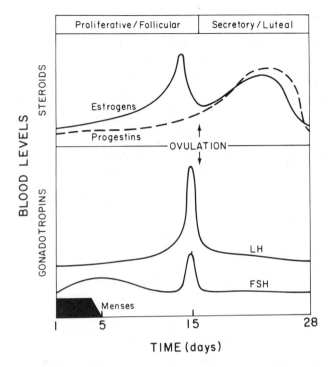

Figure 2 Hormone changes during a normal menstrual cycle. The two phases of the cycle, proliferative/follicular and secretory/luteal, reflect uterine and ovarian changes; blood levels of steroids and gonadotropins reflect ovarian and hypophyseal changes. Ovulation occurs approximately 1 day after the surge of the gonadotropins. The secretion of the ovulatory quota of LH and FSH is based upon prior sensitization of the pituitary by ovarian steroid to hypothalamic hormone.

B. Menstruation

The onset of a menstrual cycle may be taken to begin with the appearance of the menses. The menstrual discharge consists of the mucus glands and their secretions, intervening stromal tissue, and extravasated arterial and venous blood. Menses normally lasts 3 to 5 days during an average 28 day cycle. The daily discharge volume approximates 35 ml. Blood which has been in contact with this tissue does not clot and is rich in prostaglandins, locally produced lipid hormones with vasoactive properties. The psychological importance of menstruation during the reproductive years is reflected in the development of contraceptive methods which do not interfere with menses.

C. Vaginal Cytology and Endocervical Gland Activities

The vagina is a fibromuscular tube forming the opening of the reproductive tract. The anterior and posterior walls are ordinarily collapsed resulting in a potential space. The walls of the tube consist of three layers: mucous membrane, muscle, and adventitia. The inner mucous membrane layer of stratified squamous epithelium reflects cyclic changes in steroid hormones during the menstrual cycle. During the follicular phase the epithelial cells proliferate in response to estrogens and yield characteristic morphologic changes. As the epithelial cells migrate from their basal origin towards the luminal surface, glycogen accumulates and the nuclei become pyknotic. The surface cells desquamate continuously throughout the cycle, a process that can be hastened by progestin treatment. The progesterone-dominated luteal phase, therefore, is characterized by an increase in the number of desquamated cells. The leukocytes in the connective tissue underlying the mucous membrane show increased mobility during the luteal phase so that their presence among the exfoliated epithelial cells is characteristic for the approaching menses. Vaginal cytology can therefore be useful in monitoring the endocrine (ovarian) components of the reproductive system. In the absence of estrogenic stimulation, as during the prepubertal and postmenopausal states, the vaginal epithelium remains atrophic.

The vagina notably lacks any glandular elements. The lubrication for this region of the genital tract, therefore, must derive from a nonvaginal source. Lubrication is provided by the mucous secretions of the superior endocervical glands located in the cervix, the lowest and narrowest portion of the uterus. Significant differences in composition of the mucosa set the inferior cervical region apart from superior regions of the uterus. Thus, three regions of the cervix can be defined: a portion protruding into the vagina (portio vaginalis) and covered by stratified squamous epithelium similar to the vagina; an uppermost region facing the cervical canal continuous with the remainder of the uterus and containing columnar epithelium with branched (rather than tubular) glands reaching deep into the connective tissue; and an intervening transition region where the epithelium changes abruptly from squamous to collumnar. The glandular elements are the critical physiologic feature of the cervix because of their secretions; both mucus quantity and quality indicate the cyclic changes in ovarian steroidogenesis during a menstrual cycle. Small amounts of viscous mucus are produced during menses but soon thereafter copious quantities (30-fold increase) are made in response to estrogens. This latter material is watery, yet extremely viscous and elastic. Elasticity is maximal ("spinnbarkeit") just prior to ovulation. If a sample of stretched preovulatory mucous is cut, the division is not followed by retraction of the cut ends. In addition, a dried film of this material yields a fernlike pattern that results from crystallization of salts in the watery secretion. The luteal phase ovarian hormone, progesterone, diminishes all aspects of mucus secretion (decreased quantity, viscosity, and elasticity). Taken together, the assess-

ment of vaginal cytology and endocervical mucosal products offers simple and indirect measures of ovarian function during a menstrual cycle.

D. The Uterus and its Morphologic Changes

The uterus is that segment of the reproductive tract in which the cytogenic products of the ovary, if fertilized, can be nurtured until parturition. The organ is
pear-shaped, thick-walled ($7 \times 5 \times 3$ cm), protrudes into the vagina at one pole
(cervix) and extends towards the ovaries (oviducts) at the other. Two major regions are noted: the narrow neck or cervix already discussed and the enlarged
upper body portion (corpus uteri). The uterus is a muscular organ consisting of
an outer serosal cover or visceral peritoneum (perimetrium), a middle thickened
mass of interdigitating smooth muscle (myometrium), and an inner mucous membrane (endometrium). The entire organ (muscle and epithelium) responds to
changes in ovarian steroids but the endometrium yields menstrual products. If
fertilization followed by implantation does not occur the ovarian hormonal support for the uterus will be withdrawn and much of the endometrium shed. Like
the vagina, endometrial tissues respond to ovarian hormones by means of a unique
population of specific intracellular proteins (steroid receptors). The molecular
basis for steroid directed responses in the reproductive system will be described
below (Section II).

At the time of menstruation, numerous ovarian follicles have already begun
a series of developmental, morphologic, and endocrine activities that will culminate in the selection of one follicle and maturation of its ovum for ovulation.
The other cohort follicles will become atretic, a process of degradation. Until
atresia is signaled, however, these follicles participate by producing specific
steroids. The endometrial response to ovarian estrogen is repair, growth, and
reconstruction of the underlying basal layer of cells thereby constituting the onset of the proliferative phase of the cycle. Within 2 to 3 days a completely re-
newed surface epithelium of the endometrium is evident in marked contrast to
the previously disrupted and disorganized state, and the torn vasculature and
glandular elements are healed. The endometrial glands are characteristically nar-
now, tubular, and lined by cuboidal epithelium. Subsequently, the epithelium
becomes columnar, has basal nuclei, and conventional staining techniques yield
an eosinophilic cytoplasm indicating secretory activity. The stroma remains
compact in the basal region but becomes progressively less dense towards the epithelium. The endometrial glands increase in size and become convoluted as ovulation (midcycle) approaches. Vacuolation appears at the base of the cells lining
the glands and reflects glycogen accumulation. Enhanced enzyme activities are
also characteristic, e.g., alkaline phosphatase, ribonuclease; and the vasculature
becomes increasingly coiled. At the time of ovulation, 11 to 25 days after the
onset of menses, the thickness of the endometrium has increased by two- to
threefold from its initial depth of 1 mm. A change in the steroid environment

occurs following ovulation that is featured by progesterone. This luteal phase hormone enhances the growth, but especially the secretory activities, of the endometrial glands and is synonymous with the secretory phase. The luteal/secretory phase is more consistent in length (13 days) than the follicular/proliferative stages throughout the reproductive years. The convolutions of the glands become progressively more tortuous to yield characteristic luteal phase stages that are termed "corkscrew" and then "sawtooth" as the next menstrual cycle approaches. The increasing uterine glandular secretions during the early luteal phase yield a succulent endometrium favorable to implantation should a blastocyst arrive within the 7 days following ovulation. These secretions are rich in glycogen and lipids and are presumed to have a potential nutritive function. The mucosa of the uterus at this stage of the cycle consists of three distinct layers: (1) the superficial compacted vascular-rich region, (2) a central spongy zone of the dilated and convoluted glands, and (3) a deep basal layer with the inactive fundi of the glands. The underlying stroma becomes edematous in the basal layer as the demise of the corpus luteum proceeds and progesterone production declines. Prostaglandin secretion at the uterine level may be instrumental in the vasoconstriction that effects the penultimate ischemia and ultimate loss of support for the overlying mucosal layer. The mucosa becomes infiltrated with leukocytes, much like an inflammatory response, and shows a decrease in thickness, appears necrotic, and fragments. The result is the bloody discharge of menstrual flow and the beginning of a new reproductive cycle. The sloughing process will continue until the basal layer of the endometrium remains with its straight arteries, compact stroma, and simple glands. Myometrial dimensions are essentially unchanged, but evidence of altered irritability, especially at midcycle and the late luteal phase, is common.

E. The Oviducts and Gamete Transport

The bilaterally arranged oviducts are a critical link in reproductive processes. The oviducts function to: (1) actively capture the released ovum, (2) aid in the transit of migrating spermatozoa, (3) provide a hospitable site for fertilization, and (4) transport the products of conception to the uterus. During the follicular phase the mucosal cells undergo marked proliferation whereas in the luteal phase their secretions are dominant. The ciliary activity of the adluminal cells is regulated by the ovarian hormones and the irritability of the underlying musculature is pronounced near the time of ovulation. The importance of these structures in reproductive biology is best realized by recalling that the event of ovulation releases the ovum to the exterior, i.e., abdominal, cavity. Automatic transfer to the uterus does not occur, rather, properly functioning oviducts actively police the ovaries at midcycle to prevent potential retention of the ovum outside the reproductive tract. The effectiveness of the oviducts in this regard is demonstrated in the occurrence of pregnancy in hemiovariectomized animals lacking their contralateral oviduct.

F. The Ovaries and Ovulation

Approximately 400,000 primary follicles exist in each ovary of the human female at birth. This is a reduction from the nearly 7 million present at the sixth month *in utero* [4]. Nearly 400 ovulations can be anticipated in the course of a woman's normal life span and reproductive years. The movement of several primary follicles and their ova from a stage of inactivity to one of growth and future development coincides with the onset of a menstrual cycle. The underlying basis for this event is endocrine, both pituitary and ovarian. The result is provision of a single ovum 11 to 18 days later that is competent for ovulation in response to an ovulatory quota of gonadotropin. The sequence of follicle growth and development is basically an increased number of cells in the thecal layer, division of granulosa cells, and the production of an antrum. The antrum, which increases in volume during the follicular phase, is a product of secretion by both ovum and the surrounding granulosa cells. Concomitant with overall follicle growth is a dynamic interplay at the biochemical level of ovarian and hypophyseal hormones and their specific receptor substrates.

The process of ovulation is not completely understood. The favored hypothesis is a slow oozing process that reflects enzymatic activities (collagenase) at the periphery of the ovary [5]. Isolation of the specific enzyme(s) has not been achieved. It seems clear, however, that rupture of the follicle is not due to increased intrafollicular tension since reduced hydrostatic pressure just prior to ovulation has been well-documented. The discharge of the ovum leaves a tear in the wall of the follicle which closes rapidly via a clotlike formation and a local healing process. The granulosa cells lining the follicle rapidly proliferate and luteinize. The cells transform to become predominantly progesterone synthesizing elements. The thecal layer is similarly affected and the final structure becomes a large mass of cells, the corpus luteum, which is active in a single regard: steroid synthesis. The corpus luteum provides the steroid milieu to sustain other components of the reproductive system in the event of fertilization. This body exists for approximately 13 days provided it receives no additional endocrine information, e.g., placental hormones of a developing conceptus. The demise of the corpus luteum signifies the end of that cycle as described previously and withdrawal of the endocrine support for the endometrium. However, if conception has occurred, this organ is "rescued" and will remain functional in response to the trophic influence of a placental hormone (human chorionic gonadotrophin, HCG) having luteotrophic properties [6]. The ovarian trophic need is subsequently reduced and replaced by placental functions so that by the sixth to eighth week after conception complete maternal gonadectomy and hypophysectomy do not result in abortion.

There are additional activities and changes in the physiology of the female during the normal menstrual cycle. Thus, a behavioral correlate has been described whereby an increase in coitus occurs at midcycle [7]. Progesterone has long been known to have a thermogenic effect and is responsible for the luteal phase rise in basal body temperature. There is increased edema and swelling of the breasts during the luteal phase which often leads to complaints of congestion and is most marked prior to menstruation. Abdominal pain near the middle of the cycle, presumably a reflection of the ovulatory event, has also been reported.

G. The Pituitary and Hypothalamus

The pituitary gland lies at the base of the brain in a bony depression, the sella turcica, and is connected to the hypothalamus by the infundibular stalk. The anterior portion of the gland, the adenohypophysis, is epithelial in origin and derived from Rathke's pouch during early embryologic development. The formation of this structure is thought to be induced by adjacent neural tissue. The adenohypophysis is regionally divided into the pars distalis, the major portion; the pars tuberalis, a cufflike superior region that surrounds the descending stalk; and the pars intermedia, a zone of tissue adjacent to the posterior pituitary. The posterior pituitary, neurohypophysis or pars nervosa, is entirely neural and represents the axonal endings of neurons whose cell bodies originate in the hypothalamic region. The communication between the brain-hypothalamus and adenohypophysis is through a unique blood supply. Endocrine information from the brain is transferred to and transported in a capillary network in the hypothalamic region that unites to form a series of parallel long portal vessels which traverse the stalk, enter the pituitary, and divide into a capillary bed, thereby providing 90% of the organ's blood supply. In addition, evidence has been obtained indicating a return flow of blood in a parallel vascular network [8] which would suggest a possible local means of pituitary regulation of the hypothalamus-brain.

The adenohypophysis is the source of many hormones. Each hormone bears on reproductive cycles in some way but most important are the gonadotropins FSH and LH (follicle-stimulating and luteinizing hormones). Other relevant adenohypophyseal hormones include prolactin, thyroid-stimulating hormone (TSH), growth hormone (GH), and adrenocorticotropin (ACTH). The latter is a small fragment of a much larger molecule, β-lipotropin, which yields other fragments, i.e., endorphins, enkephalins, and β-melanocyte-stimulating hormone (β-MSH). Each such fragment has its characteristic bioactivity, e.g., endorphins are opiates. Endorphins also modify adenohypophyseal hormone secretion (prolactin). This family of newly discovered endocrine factors promises much in the way of understanding pain, mood, etc., and should prove valuable in applied human biology. While these same hormones have also been localized in the brain [9], it remains to be determined if the brain is a native site of synthesis or possesses specific uptake mechanisms for these hormones.

The neurohypophyseal hormones (vasopressin and oxytocin) are produced in brain neurons as part of larger precursor proteins which migrate to their axonal endings and are stored. Their secretion depends upon neural stimulation although endocrine factors may be involved. These hormones have significant actions linked to reproductive processes, e.g., vasopressin is a general pressor and body fluid regulator influencing renal functions while oxytocin affects specific components of the reproductive system. Oxytocin influences the contractility of the uterine myometrium, modulates oviductal irritability, and stimulates mammary myoepithelial cell contraction. In its latter function, oxytocin is the endocrine component of a neural response initiated by breast stimulation that culminates in lactation of the suitably prepared tissue. A behavioral role for breast stimulation during coitus in humans would appear important since this evokes release of oxytocin and provides an endocrine stimulus to the genital tract which favors transit of both ovum and spermatozoa. Visual and auditory cues may be equally significant factors in this particular response mechanism.

Each pituitary hormone is produced by a characteristic cell type. The two gonadotropins appear, however, to be produced by the same cell. These glycoproteins each exist in subunit form (α and β) held together by weak noncovalent bonding. The α subunits are identical for both gonadotropins while each β subunit differs, thereby allowing for their different bioactivities and specific target cell interactions. Interestingly, the placental hormone HCG possesses LH-like bioactivity, is also a glycoprotein comprised of α and β subunits, and has the same α subunit composition as both LH and FSH. Quantitation of these different hormones in biological fluids is now routinely performed by highly specific and sensitive radioimmunoassay systems which take into consideration the unique antigenic determinents of their β subunits [10]. The gonadotropins provide the endocrine support for the ovary: FSH stimulates follicle growth and development which is characterized by ovarian steroidogenesis (estrogens, androgens); LH augments the action of FSH, is critical for the ovulatory event, and causes luteinization of the ovulatory follicle with concomitant progesterone synthesis. The action of both gonadotropins is mediated through initial interaction with specific cell receptors.

The hypothalamic control of hypophyseal function is discussed in greater detail in Chapter 2. Briefly, hypothalamic releasing factors for the gonadotropins and for TSH were obtained in pure form and characterized following heroic isolation procedures from porcine and ovine tissues [11]. The factor responsible for TSH secretion, thyroid-releasing factor thyroid-stimulating hormone releasing factor (TRF), is a tripeptide which also stimulates prolactin release. The factor that controls LH and FSH synthesis and secretion is a decapeptide variously termed luteinizing hormone-releasing hormone (LHRH), luteinizing hormone/follicle-stimulating hormone-releasing factor (LH/FSH-RF), and gonadotropin-releasing hormone (GnRH). The latter term seems more appropriate given the ability of the hormone to regulate both gonadotropins simultaneously. The availability of synthetic GnRH and its analogs provides useful tools in the management of reproductive dysfunctions which have underlying hypothalamic bases as well as providing research tools for the study of peptide hormone action. The synthesis of native GnRH is influenced by the prevailing steroid milieu [12] and its measurement in the periphery is complicated by both systemic dilution and rapid enzymic degradation. The study of GnRH regulation in reproductive biology therefore necessitates analysis at its site of origin (hypothalamus or portal vessels) or its site of action (pituitary). Recent investigations have revealed extrahypophyseal effects of GnRH. As discussed in Chapter 4, GnRH may exert a role in animal behavior thereby suggesting central nervous system sites of action which may relate to the finding of GnRH throughout the brain. Additionally, GnRH alters ovarian and testicular steroidogenesis when administered in pharmacologic doses [13]. This suggests the contraceptive potential of the native peptide.

II. The Menstrual Cycle: Biochemical Aspects

The preceding description of the menstrual cycle has been limited to the obvious repetitive endocrine-related phenomena. The following discussion is meant to develop the underlying cellular bases for these events. It should become apparent that molecular interactions are themselves repetitive and equally characteristic of reproductive cycles. The focus of this section is on the mechanism of hormonal action during a menstrual cycle.

The sequence of events in any hormone's action includes the following: (1) synthesis, (2) secretion into the vascular space, (3) transport to all cells, (4) uptake by all cells, and (5) retention only by specific cells. Specific cellular retention of hormone is the touchstone of modern endocrinology and is the basis for the receptor concept. Our present use of this concept has its origins in the turn of the century (1896) "lock and key" idea of Fischer for understanding enzyme-substrate interactions. During the same period (1908) Ehrlich, in his Nobel address, described how it was that specific toxins affected only specific cell types. He thereupon speculated that these cells contained unique binding entities which he termed "receptors" [14]. In the intervening 60 years, the growing pharmaceutical industry utilized the receptor concept in an operational manner. Further understanding of receptors did not occur until the endocrinologists Jensen and Jacobson [15] succeeded in incorporating an isotope of hydrogen (tritium) into a steroid molecule. This achievement allowed research investigations to proceed on a firm basis with specific target cell receptor entities. The radiolabeled product permitted the physiologic, rather than pharmacologic, study of a hormone and initiated the current era of molecular endocrinology.

It is important to note that most schemes of hormone action are necessarily simplistic. A complete scheme must incorporate diverse but significant physiological variables. Such variations would include endocrine secretions in prohormone form that require modification external to the site of origin (proinsulin), biotransformation of precursor hormones (steroids) in the periphery (androgen → estrogen) that are sex-, weight-, and age-related, and the extent of binding of hormones by transport proteins in the blood, e.g., sex hormone or testosterone binding globulin (SHBG, TeBG) for testosterone and estradiol; corticosteroid binding globulin (CBG) for the corticosteroids and progesterone.

A. Hormone Receptors

The endocrine information in the vascular space is processed at the cellular level through interaction with specific receptors. This appears to be an orderly event that begins as a highly selective recognition process. Thus, the uterus grows and develops in response to estrogens and progestins but not the gonadotropins, while ovarian follicles grow and develop in response to the gonadotropins but not glucocorticoids. The precision of this discrimination is based on the respective tissue content of specific cellular receptors. Hormone and target organ specificities, however, are but two criteria used to define receptors. The property of binding affinity is very important to the receptor concept since the interaction between receptor and hormone (association, K_a, and dissociation, K_d, constants) must be sufficiently "tight" to allow stable complex formation in the presence of the low physiological concentrations of the hormone in the circulation. The hormone-receptor interaction should also be saturable so that a limited number of receptor sites characterize the responsive cell; a nonsaturable binding entity indicates a low affinity relationship. There are examples in normal physiology, however, when excess receptors exist (spare receptors) in a cell concomitant with maximal stimulation by hormone [16]. The latter property also indicates that a correlation of the binding event to a specific physiologic response must exist. As an example, the binding of LH by specific receptors in classic target organs (gonads) can be correlated with increased enzyme production or activity and steroidogenesis (progesterone or testosterone). The absence of receptors correlates with the absence of a classic response as noted for androgen insensitivity in the testicular feminization syndrome.

Hormone receptors are customarily separated into two classes according to their distribution in the cell: membranous and nonmembranous. Receptors that are incorporated into the outer cell membrane are specific for the peptide and protein hormones and the catecholamines. It is postulated that these receptors exist in subunit form: a recognition site which titrates the extravascular-extracellular space for hormone which is coupled to a more interior oriented catalytic subunit (adenylate cyclase). It is believed that the perturbation of the coupled sites increases cyclic AMP production effecting a cascade phenomenon. The cascade involves the activation of enzymes and their subsequent action on specific

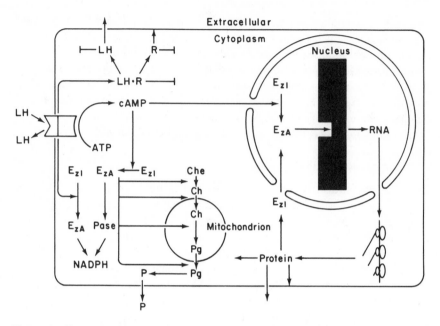

Figure 3 Current concepts of protein hormone action involving the membrane-bound receptor for LH in a luteinized granulosa cell. The end result of this scheme is to promote steroid (progesterone) synthesis. The level of circulating LH is titrated by the recognition subunit of the receptor and coupled to a catalytic (adenylate cyclase) subunit. Two possible modes of action follow: (1) the conversion of endogenous nucleotide (ATP) to the second message (cAMP) with a resultant cascade effect involving a series of enzyme activations ($E_zI \rightarrow E_zA$) at cytoplasmic and nuclear levels or (2) a non-cAMP-dependent action. The latter, as well as one of the former activations, yields increased necessary cofactor (NADPH) for steroid synthesis. The cAMP cascade yields activated enzyme which (1) increases the phosphorylase involved in NADPH production, (2) effects side chain cleavage of cholesterol ester (Che), the precursor for cholesterol (Ch), (3) regulates Ch availability to the mitochondrion where (4) the biotransformation to pregnenolone (Pg) occurs, and (5) influences the transport of Pg out of the organelle and hence its availability to the progesterone (P)-synthesizing apparatus of the cell. At the nuclear level, cAMP also effects activation of enzymes involved in the transcription of DNA to yield characteristic mRNA. The latter is translated by the protein synthesizing apparatus (ᕴ) to yield (1) enzymic proteins or proteins for (2) membrane incorporation, (3) export, or (4) other intracellular processes. The LH bound to receptor may be released after activation of the adenylate cyclase and returned to the extracellular space. Alternatively, the entire LH-receptor complex may be internalized and degraded (⊣), or dissociated into hormone and receptor components which themselves are degraded or returned to the membrane (R) and externalized (LH).

substrates to ultimately yield the characteristic cell response. Figure 3 summarizes current concepts of membrane-bound receptor hormone interactions in an ovarian granulosa cell whose secretory product is progesterone. The fate of the hormone following the binding event is uncertain. Glycoprotein hormones have been dissociated from their receptor and subsequently shown to bind additional receptor [17] which suggests that the bioactivity of the hormone may not be compromised by the binding event. The fate of the membrane associated receptor following binding with hormone is not clear. Some evidence has been obtained indicating the internalization of intact receptor-hormone (LH) complexes by the responsive cell [18]. Receptors (LH) appear to be randomly distributed in patches about the cells surface rather than restricted to one region [19].

The second class of receptors encompasses the presumed intracellular binding entities. These receptors are not bound to membranes and are free and soluble in the extracysternal spaces (nonmembranous) of the cell. The receptors for the steroids (estrogens, progesterone, androgens, gluco-, and mineralocorticoids) represent this class. Current concepts for the mechanism of steroid hormone action involving the nuclear apparatus are shown in Figure 4. The lipid-rich cell membranes do not restrain the lipophilic steroids which appear to enter the cell by simple diffusion. Once inside the target cell it is thought that the steroid is recognized by its specific receptor, an activation (transformation) of the proteinaceous receptor occurs, and the steroid-receptor complex becomes competent to proceed further to the nuclear membrane. The steroid-protein complex must cross this potential barrier and thereupon interact with the genetic apparatus. This interaction is also a highly specific recognition phenomenon, i.e., there is a genomic receptor (acceptor) for steroid receptor. Acceptors for steroid hormone receptors appear to be nonhistone proteins of the nuclear chromatin. The preceding outline is termed the two-step concept of steroid hormone action [20] and is keyed to initial receptor transformation followed by receptor translocation. This concept is based upon cell disruption (broken cell) studies and autoradiographic analyses of the distribution of radioactivity for selected target organs following in vitro incubation with radiolabeled hormone. There are exceptions to this mode of steroid hormone action. The possibility of membrane-mediated events [21], organellar interactions [22], as well as a failure to demonstrate the extranuclear receptor in classic steroid-responsive tissues [23] have been noted. An alternative view has also been posed that does not support the necessity of a two-step phenomenon in estrogen target tissues. Thus, receptor translocation from the operationally defined cytoplasmic to nuclear compartments may occur prior to transformation or be followed by a transformation within the nucleus [24]. The rate at which this event occurs differs according to target tissue and, possibly, age [25]. The described intranuclear receptor processing phenomenon also calls into question the native locus for the steroid receptors, i.e., cytoplasmic or nuclear? Indeed, there is evidence that estrogen receptors may reside within the nuclear compartment [26,27], or interact with microsomes [28], not unlike the

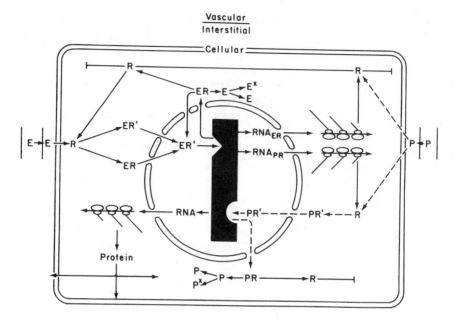

Figure 4 Current concepts of steroid hormone actions. Two hormones, 17β-estradiol (E) and progesterone (P) are considered in this scheme. Cell membranes are not a barrier to the lipophilic steroids; the proteinaceous E and P receptors (R) reside within the cytoplasm. Following entrance to the cell, E is recognized by R yielding a complex (ER) which must then traverse the intracellular and nuclear membranes. This translocation may or may not involve a nonenzymic activation (ER') of the steroid-protein complex. At the nuclear level, where activation may also occur, the ER' is recognized by a population of acceptor molecules, also proteins, which are necessary for the "turning-on" of the appropriate gene sequences. Much controversy exists regarding the nature of this recognition process, the number of specific binding sites, acceptor saturability, etc. The interaction, however, yields ER which can be (1) recycled intact, (2) dissociated to release hormone that can reassociate (E) with receptor or be catabolized (E^x), and (3) receptor available to bind additional hormone (R) or be degraded (→). The interaction of ER with the genome results in characteristic mRNA product(s). Two examples suffice: (1) mRNA for the estrogen receptor and (2) mRNA for the progesterone receptor. The newly synthesized R for E is added to the intracellular pool of receptor. The R for P is available to bind any P that enters the cell. The mode of action of P is similar to E in that characteristic mRNA(s) is transcribed (↷) following PR-acceptor interactions. However, PR is subsequently inactivated and no longer available to bind P. Both R and P are subject to degradation and catabolism at extranuclear sites. In addition, P interferes with the synthesis of the R for E thereby limiting E action to the latter's reutilization of R.

apparent nuclear [29] and mitochondrial [30] loci identified for thyroid hormone (thyroxine). It may be speculated that these metabolically effective hormones do not require a sequence of protein interactions and transit through the complex membranous labyrinth of the target cell. Regardless of the logistics of steroid receptor distribution within the cell, steroid recognition is followed by an amplification of a specific set of genes whose product messenger RNAs increase through activation of DNA-dependent RNA polymerases. Further, the exit of the new mRNA to the extranuclear ribosomal protein synthesizing apparatus yields new proteins. Characteristic cell proteins for secretion, growth, and cell regulation ultimately result from this sequence of events.

B.   Receptor Regulation

The endocrine indices of (1) preovulatory increases in circulating estrogens, (2) periovulatory gonadotropin surges, and (3) postovulatory blood progesterone changes are guides to describing the menstrual cycle and useful in predicting impending ovulation and menstruation and assessing fertility. Specific hormone receptors underlie each tissue response to each hormone. Therefore, it follows that receptor regulation could be important to our understanding of the menstrual cycle. The following discussion of receptor relationships in the developing ovarian follicle and the uterus during a cycle are examples of current concepts in molecular endocrinology as applied to human physiology. An understanding of receptor regulation in reproduction is also useful in understanding general physiology and disease states. Proven receptor relationships have aided in the management of specific pathobiologies of the reproductive system, e.g., breast and endometrial carcinoma. In these examples, steroid receptor quantity, quality, and subcellular distribution were important clues to the patients' predicted response to subsequent endocrine or surgical therapy.

1. The Ovary

The ovary is divided into three functionally and anatomically interrelated compartments: (1) the follicular apparatus, (2) corpora lutea, and (3) the intervening stroma. The follicular apparatus is further divided into the ovum, the inner layer of granulosa cells, and the external layer(s) of theca cells. The process a primary follicle and its ovum undergo in preparation for ovulation requires FSH and LH. Receptor involvement in follicle development occurs as follows. Small follicles specifically bind LH in their thecal layer but the binding of FSH is restricted to the adjacent granulosa cells [31]. This anatomic distribution corresponds to what has long been described for ovarian steroidogenesis: thecal cells produce androgens which can be transformed to estrogens by enzymes (aromatase) present in granulosa cells. The production of estradiol by a follicle in response to gonadotropin stimulation, therefore, is initially via conversion of redistributed precursor androgen. The estrogen synthesized is secreted, transported throughout the body, and selectively taken up and retained by estrogen receptors in the hypothalamus and pituitary where action involves modulation of the hypophysio-tropic GnRH and hypophyseal LH and FSH. A local effect of estradiol at the follicle cell level is also postulated but poorly defined. Thus, exogenously administered estrogen to hypophysectomized animals promotes follicular cAMP production in response to FSH [32] and is correlated with the induction of LH receptors in granulosa cells. This does not occur in small follicles. The appearance of the granulosa LH receptor coincides with the ability of the cell to respond to LH by activation of adenylate cyclase [33] and progesterone synthesis [34]. In an apparent fulminating runaway process, LH-receptor interactions are linked to enhanced responsiveness to both FSH and LH inducing a further increase in LH receptor etc., as can be seen in larger follicles [35]. The follicle soon attains a size suitable for ovulation, is positioned near the surface of the gonad, and awaits both the ovulatory surge of gonadotropins and the local actions of unknown factors (progesterone-mediated collagenase?) that permit rupture of the overlying ovarian surface. An unsettled issue in this scenario, however, is defining the process that selects the follicle most suitable for ovulation. One hypothesis concerns the activity of the aromatase enzyme system in the granulosa cells. The ability to convert precursor androgen produced by the theca to estrogen would provide the appropriate local endocrine signal favoring the induction of the necessary complement of FSH and LH receptors. Coupled with this headstart would be the local enhancement of blood flow promoted by the estrogens and therefore an increased availability of the gonadotropins. The recent documentation of reduced granulosa aromatase activity [36] and excessive antral androgens [37] as biochemical bases for anovulation are most compelling in this regard. However, these observations are limited to a local effect (single ovary) and do not reveal the events occurring in the contralateral ovary. Unlike rodents and other species which ovulate numerous ova at each cycle, the human normally provides one ovum from a single gonad. The existing in vivo control mechanism must therefore be interovarian as well as intraovarian. The sequence of events in follicle maturation and ovulation is depicted in Figure 5.

2. The Uterus

The uterine endometrium and myometrium contain intracellular receptor systems for 17β-estradiol and progesterone, while myometrial cells also possess membrane oxytocin receptors. The interactions between these three hormones through their receptors is not absolutely clear. It would appear that estrogen and oxytocin promote uterine contractility whereas progesterone has a more quiescent effect, however, these need not be receptor-mediated processes. Much more is known about the two steroids, their receptors, their nuclear interactions, and their regulation during the menstrual cycle. The patterns of uterine sex steroid receptor levels and intracellular distributions to be described applies to both endometrium

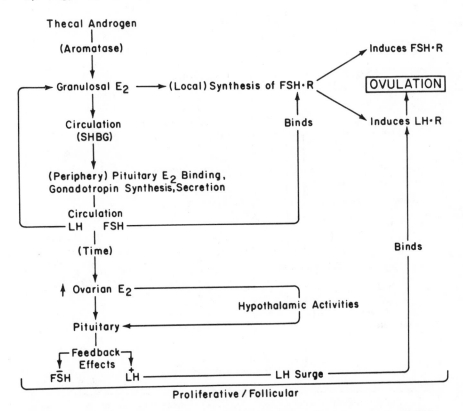

Figure 5 Receptor interactions typifying the development of an ovarian follicle which will culminate in ovulation. Additional details are found in the text. The upper half of the chart considers the first half of the follicular phase. As this progresses (time), the continued low levels of gonadotropins have sufficiently "up-regulated" their own follicular receptors to favor (1) estrogen synthesis and (2) cell responsiveness to the specific gonadotropin. The change in receptor levels and responsiveness primes the follicle for the preovulatory surge of LH.

and myometrium. The sequence of events in receptor interactions during a normal menstrual cycle is shown in Figure 6. While it is clear that the sex steroids exert major effects via genomic interactions and may influence conductive properties of cell membranes, they also are active in altering specific enzymic activities. It is to be noted also that the distribution of estrogen and progesterone receptors in the uterus may [38] or may not [39] be uniform, that endometrial receptor concentrations exceed those of the myometrium, and that their binding properties may vary according to the physiologic state [40].

The levels of both estrogen and progesterone receptors differ according to

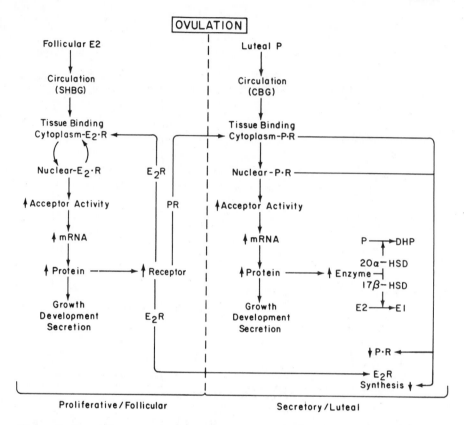

Figure 6 Steroid hormone interactions in endometrial cells during the menstrual cycle. Details are found in the text. The two cycle stages are offset by the ovulatory event. The importance of luteal P can be clearly seen through (1) stimulation of the genome, (2) inactivation of its own R, (3) modulation of the ER population, and (4) activation of enzyme systems which reduce the bioactivity of both E and P.

cycle stages [41-43]. The concentration of estrogen receptor is highest in the follicular phase, lower during the secretory phase, and lowest at menstruation. This pattern obtains whether the available, total, or nuclear levels of receptors are determined. The existing level of estrogen receptor at any one time is a reflection of its synthesis and degradation or inactivation. Estrogen is the driving stimulus for production of its own receptor [44], i.e., up-regulation, and following the nuclear acceptor recognition and action, estrogen receptor may be reutilized. The recycling process returns receptor to the cytoplasmic compartment where it is available to bind additional hormone, hence be recycled. Estrogen also up-regulates the intracellular receptor for progesterone [45]. The profile of increasing endogenous estrogen during the late follicular/proliferative phase of the cycle (Fig. 2) effects an increase in both the tissue estrogen- and progesterone-receptor populations. The greater effectiveness of progesterone treatment following estrogen priming is clearly related to the prior induction of the specific recognition sites for the hormone. The intracellular effect of progesterone, as seen during the secretory/luteal phase, is to cause a reduction (down-regulation) of its own receptor [46] following the characteristic steroid uptake, transfer, nuclear localization, and genomic stimulation scheme [47]. This down-regulation of receptor implies that a maximal response may be achieved and refractoriness will follow, given the diminution of available specific receptor sites. Progesterone also reduces the cellular level of the available estrogen-receptors. The mechanism whereby this dual effect of a single steroid on dissimilar receptors comes about has been determined in studies involving rodents and nonhuman primates. Therefore, progesterone is antiestrogenic by inhibiting the synthesis but not recycling of the estrogen receptor [48]. Estrogen receptor levels are reduced but receptor is nonetheless available during the luteal phase for binding to endogenous hormone.

A coordinated series of enzymic functions that regulate the bioactivity of the steroid hormones exists in addition to the complex interplay of the steroids and receptors in their uterine target cell [49]. 17β-Estradiol is converted to a less potent estrogen, estrone, by a 17β-hydroxysteroid dehydrogenase. This enzymic activity varies during the cycle but is greatest in the secretory/luteal phase. The progesterone secreted during this interval modulates enzyme synthesis and increases the available pool of enzyme in endometrial cells [50]. Progesterone also stimulates 20α-dihydroxysteroid dehydrogenase, an enzyme that transforms progesterone to the less bioactive 20α-dihydroxyprogesterone [51]. Thus, through regulation of enzyme activities as well as target cell receptor densities, luteal phase progesterone serves a pivotal role in total uterine physiology.

III. Summary

Our current understanding of the menstrual cycle of the human female is in many ways similar to that which obtained more than 40 years ago. The descriptive aspects are essentially unchanged but knowledge of the underlying endocrine bases has been significantly expanded. The union of radioisotope and immunologic techniques has allowed an understanding of the interactions between hormones and their specific tissue receptors and brought us to our current era of molecular endocrinology. Further biochemical dissection of the reproductive system will no doubt occur. A more complete understanding of the menstrual cycle, however, will benefit from the additional considerations of related psychologic and behavioral phenomena whose underlying biochemical bases, if existent, are presently unknown.

20   Linkie

References

1. G. W. Corner, *The Hormones in Human Reproduction.* Princeton University Press, New York, 1942.
2. G. T. Ross and R. L. Vande Wiele, in *Textbook of Endocrinology,* 6th Ed. (R. H. Williams, ed.). Saunders, Philadelphia, 1981, pp. 355-399.
3. M. Ferin, F. Halberg, R. M. Richart, and R. L. Vande Wiele, (eds.), *Biorhythms and Human Reproduction.* John Wiley, New York, 1974.
4. T. G. Baker, *Proc. R. Soc. Biol.* 158:417 (1963).
5. P. Rondell, *Biol. Reprod.* 2:64 (1970).
6. R. L. Vande Wiele, R. J. Bogumil, I. Dyrenfurth, M. Ferin, R. Jewelewicz, M. Warren, G. Mikhail, and T. Rizkallah, *Recent Prog. Horm. Res.* 26:63 (1970).
7. J. R. Udry and N. M. Morris, *Nature* 220:593 (1968).
8. R. M. Bergland and R. B. Page, *Science* 204:18 (1979).
9. D. T. Kreiger and A. S. Liotta, *Science* 205:366 (1979).
10. A. R. Midgley, G. D. Niswender, V. L. Gay, and L. E. Reichert, *Recent Prog. Horm. Res.* 27:235 (1971).
11. J. Meites, *Science* 198:594 (1977).
12. H. Kuhl, C. Rosniatowski, and H.-D. Taubert, *Acta Endocrinol. (Copenh.)* 87:476 (1978).
13. A. J. W. Hseuh, C. Wang, and G. F. Erickson, *Endocrinology* 106:1697 (1980).
14. P. Ehrlich, in *The Collected Papers of Paul Ehrlich,* (F. Himmelweit, ed.), *Chemotherapy,* Vol, 3. Pergamon Press, Elmsford, New York, 1960.
15. E. V. Jensen and H. I. Jacobsen, *Recent Prog. Horm. Res.* 18:387 (1962).
16. K. J. Catt and M. L. Dufau, *Nature* 244:219 (1973).
17. P. Cuatrecasas and M. D. Hollenberg, *Adv. Protein Chem.* 30:251 (1976).
18. P. Gorden, J. Carperntier, P. Freychet, and L. Orci, *J. Histochem.* 28:811 (1980).
19. A. J. W. Hseuh, M. L. Dufau, S. I. Katz, and K. J. Catt, *Nature* 261:710 (1976).
20. E. V. Jensen and E. R. DeSombre, *Ann. Rev. Biochem.* 41:203 (1972).
21. E.-E. Baulieu, *Mol. Cell. Endocrinol.* 12:247 (1978).
22. C. M. Szego, in *Structure and Function of the Gonadotropins* (K. W. McKerns, ed.). Plenum, New York, 1978, p. 431.
23. P. J. Sheridan, *Life Sci.* 17:497 (1975).
24. D. M. Linkie and P. K. Siiteri, *J. Steroid Biochem.* 9:1071 (1978).
25. D. M. Linkie, *Endocrinology* 101:1862 (1977).
26. R. A. Carlson and J. Gorski, *Endocrinology* 106:1776 (1980).
27. A. Geier, R. Beery, D. Levran, J. Menczer, and B. Lunenfeld, *J. Clin. Endocrinol. Metab.* 50:541 (1980).

28. M. Little, P. Szendro, C. Teran, A. Hughes, and P. W. Jungblut, *J. Steroid Biochem.* 6:493 (1975).

29. J. H. Oppenheimer, H. L. Schwartz, M. I. Surks, D. Koerner, and W. H. Dillman, *Recent Prog. Horm. Res.* 32:529 (1976).

30. K. Sterling, P. O. Milch, M. A. Brenner, and J. H. Lazerus, *Science* 197:996 (1977).

31. A. J. Zelesnik, A. R. Midgley, and L. E. Reichert, *Endocrinology* 95:818 (1974).

32. J. S. Richards, J. J. Jonassen, A. I. Rolfes, K. Kersey, and L. E. Reichert, *Endocrinology* 104:765 (1979).

33. M. Hunzicker-Dunn and L. Birnbaumer, *Endocrinology* 99:198 (1976).

34. A. J. Zelesnik, P. L. Keyes, K. M. J. Menon, A. R. Midgley, and L. E. Reichert, *Am. J. Physiol.* 233:E299 (1977).

35. J. J. Ireland and J. S. Richards, *Endocrinology* 102:1458 (1978).

36. G. F. Erickson, A. J. W. Hseuh, M. E. Quigley, R. W. Rebar, and S. S. C. Yen, *J. Clin. Endocrinol. Metab.* 49:514 (1979).

37. K. P. McNatty, D. M. Smith, A. Makris, C. DeGrazia, D. Tulchinsky, R. Osathanondh, I. Schiff, and K. J. Ryan, *J. Clin. Endocrinol. Metab.* 50: 755 (1980).

38. D. M. Robertson, J. Mester, J. Beilby, S. J. Steele, and A. E. Kellie, *Acta Endocrinol. (Copenh.)* 68:534 (1971).

39. F. Bayard, S. Damilano, P. Robel, and E.-E. Baulieu, *C.R. Acad. Sci. [D] (Paris),* 281:1341 (1975).

40. M. T. V. Hai and E. Milgrom, *J. Endocrinol.* 76:21 (1978).

41. F. Bayard, S. Damilano, P. Robel, and E.-E. Baulieu, *J. Clin. Endocrinol. Metab.* 46:635 (1978).

42. B. M. Sanborn, H. S. Kuo, and B. Held, *J. Steroid Biochem.* 9:951 (1978).

43. B. Kreitmann, R. Bugat, and F. Bayard, *J. Clin. Endocrinol. Metab.* 49: 926 (1979).

44. J. H. Clark, J. N. Anderson, and E. J. Peck, *Adv. Exp. Med. Biol.* 36:15 (1973).

45. J. H. Clark, A. J. W. Hseuh, and E. J. Peck, *Ann. N.Y. Acad. Sci.* 286:161 (1977).

46. E. Milgrom, M. T. L. Thi, M. Atger, and E.-E. Baulieu, *J. Biol. Chem.* 248: 6366 (1973).

47. B. W. O'Malley and D. O. Toft, *J. Biol. Chem.* 246:117 (1971).

48. A. J. W. Hseuh, E. J. Peck, and J. H. Clark, *Endocrinology* 98:438 (1978).

49. E. Gurpide, *J. Toxicol. Environ. Health* 4:249 (1978).

50. L. Tseng, S. B. Gusberg, and E. Gurpide, *Ann. N.Y. Acad. Sci.* 286:190 (1977).

51. L. Tseng and E. Gurpide, *Endocrinology* 94:419 (1974).

2 The Neuroendocrinologic Control of the Menstrual Cycle

MICHEL FERIN   College of Physicians and Surgeons, Columbia University, New York, New York

The human menstrual cycle is the result of a series of events occurring in several areas of the reproductive system including the hypothalamus, anterior pituitary gland, ovaries, and uterus. In this chapter, we will consider the ways by which these events in organs distant from each other are integrated and review the available information on the endocrine signals which carry the relevant messages. Most of the information will deal with experimental work done in the human or subhuman primate.

As outlined in Chapter 1, the menstrual cycle is divided into two parts, the follicular and luteal phases [1]. During the follicular phase, follicular maturation and secretory activity are initiated under the stimulation of follicle-stimulating hormone (FSH) and luteinizing hormone (LH), 17β-estradiol being the principal secretory product of the follicle. With approaching follicle maturity estradiol secretion increases rapidly, with resulting changes in this hormone's peripheral targets: proliferation of endometrial glands, increased fluidity of the cervical mucus, and cornification of the vaginal smear index. The midcycle estradiol peak is soon followed by a surge in both LH and FSH. This in turn induces the release of the oocyte from the ovarian follicle and its expulsion into the Fallopian tube, a switch in the secretory activity of the follicle from estradiol to progesterone (preovulatory progesterone peak), as well as the invasion of the remaining follicular cells by blood vessels to form the corpus luteum which heralds the luteal phase. In the human, the corpus luteum secretes not only 17β-estradiol but also progesterone, which counteracts estradiol's effects on the reproductive target organs. Progesterone also exerts its effects on the hypothalamic thermo-regulatory center, so that the basal body temperature increases during the luteal phase of the menstrual cycle. The lifetime of the corpus luteum is limited, and within 7 to 9 days of its induction, this structure starts to degenerate, and estra-diol and progesterone levels decline rapidly. This decrease in the secretion of luteal steroids causes sloughing of the uterine lining and menstruation. Normal function of the corpus luteum is dependent on the continuing stimulation by LH but, for reasons still unknown, its lifetime does not exceed 13 to 15 days. Be-yond 14 days, increasing amounts of LH are needed to maintain the corpus lu-teum as it becomes less sensitive to the effect of the hormone. As a rule, there-fore, only the length of the follicular phase varies in menstrual cycles of varying duration.

I. Feedback Loops

As in other endocrine systems, communication between distant compartments of the reproductive system is carried on by hormonal signals. The transfer of information involves feedback loops, whereby hypothalamic-hypophyseal hor-mones affect ovarian growth and secretory patterns, which in turn influence hypothalamic-hypophyseal secretion. In the human, the main ovarian feedback hormone is 17β-estradiol. It affects pituitary LH and FSH secretion both in an inhibitory (negative feedback loop) and stimulatory (positive feedback loop) fashion. Pituitary hormone levels throughout the menstrual cycle are for the most part the result of these two feedback loops.

A. Estradiol Negative Feedback Loop

As gonadotropins stimulate estradiol secretion by the ovaries, estradiol in turn "feeds back" to the hypothalamic-hypophyseal complex to decrease the levels of LH and FSH. In this way, estradiol controls day to day or "tonic" levels of LH and FSH throughout the menstrual cycle. At menopause, after castration, or in patients with gonadal dysgenesis, this negative feedback loop is interrupted or absent as the secretion of estradiol is decreased and both LH and FSH levels increase rapidly. Maximal levels, however, are not obtained until 3 weeks after castration, as the synthesizing capacity of the gland increases slowly to reach its maximum. Reinstitution of the feedback loop in these patients by estradiol ad-ministration produces a decrease in both gonadotropins within minutes of injec-tion [2] (Fig. 1).

B. Estradiol Positive Feedback Loop

Under specific circumstances, 17β-estradiol can also exert a stimulatory effect on both LH and FSH release. This occurs spontaneously at midcycle when high

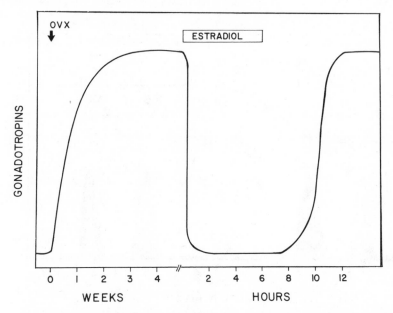

Figure 1 Negative feedback loop of estradiol. After ovariectomy (OVX), there is an increase in gonadotropin levels, as the negative feedback loop is interrupted. Infusion of estradiol at levels mimicking those seen during the early follicular phase of the menstrual cycle rapidly reduce gonadotropin levels. (Adapted from Ref. 2.)

circulating estradiol levels are followed by the gonadotropin surge. That this mid-cycle gonadotropin surge is causally related to increasing estradiol levels has been experimentally demonstrated. In the monkey, antibodies to estradiol, which neutralize circulating estrogens and thereby ovarian signals, prevent midcycle LH and FSH surges with resultant anovulation [3]. In these immunized animals, gonadotropin surges and consequent ovulation could be induced by diethylstilbestrol, a synthetic estrogen not recognized by the antibodies to estradiol (Fig. 2). In normal human subjects, a gonadotropin surge can be induced experimentally, for example by infusing estradiol during the early follicular phase [4]. The control system which responds to the positive feedback action of estradiol by eliciting a LH discharge is activated by increments in circulating estradiol which exceed a threshold (close to circulating estradiol levels at follicle maturity) and which are sustained for 1.5 to 2 days. In contrast to the negative feedback effect, acute exposure, even to massive estradiol levels, is ineffective [5]. Estradiol activates the negative feedback system within minutes; the important difference in the response time of the two estradiol feedback systems clearly ex-

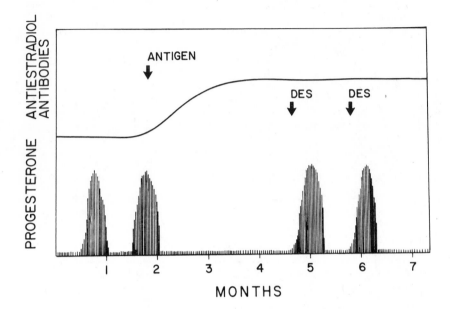

Figure 2 Positive feedback loop of estrogen. An example in a monkey of the causative relationship between estrogen and the gonadotropin surge. During the normal cycle (on the left), the midcycle estradiol rise induces a gonadotropin surge (positive feedback loop) and ovulation (as indicated by a 14 day increase in progesterone secretion). After suppression of the endogenous estradiol signals by antibodies following active immunization to an estradiol-protein antigen, the monkey becomes anovulatory. In this immunized animal, gonadotropin surges and ovulation are induced following diethylstilbestrol (DES) injection (restoration of the positive feedback loop by an estrogen not recognized by the antibodies). (Adapted from Ref. 3.)

plains that administration of estradiol leads first to a decrease in gonadotropins, then only to the gonadotropin surge.

C. Progesterone Feedback Loop

As shown above, 17β-estradiol is the main ovarian feedback hormone during the menstrual cycle. Progesterone has been experimentally shown to modulate or modify the primary estradiol feedback system and may therefore have a physiological role in the control of gonadotropin secretion. The role of progesterone must obviously be minimal during the follicular phase of the cycle, since significant secretion is initiated only at the time of the midcycle LH surge. This steroid has been shown to inhibit, under specific experimental conditions, the estrogen-induced gonadotropin surge and this effect may explain the absence of gonadotropin surges during the luteal phase, even though estradiol concentrations may reach appropriate conditions for a positive feedback [6]. Other experimental data indicate that this hormone may also exert a stimulatory effect on the gonadotropin surge at midcycle. Injections of progesterone at levels seen during the preovulatory period in women pretreated with estrogen were shown to augment the estrogen-induced LH and FSH surges [7]. Progesterone therefore has been postulated to modulate the absolute amounts of LH and FSH released during the midcycle surge.

D. Short Feedback Loop

In addition to the "long" ovarian-hypothalamic-hypophyseal feedback loops described above, some researchers have postulated the existence of a "short" feedback loop through which anterior pituitary hormones may control their own secretion. The physiological role of this feedback loop remains to be determined, but recent experiments in ovariectomized women have demonstrated a decrease in LH (but not FSH) concentrations following the administration of human chorionic gonadotropin (HCG) [8].

II. The Hypothalamus and Endocrine Function

One of the major central regulatory areas of endocrine function is the hypothalamus, the final common pathway between the remainder of the central nervous system and the pituitary gland. It has long been known that hypothalamic lesions or disorders result in disturbances of the secretory function of the pituitary gland.

A. Hypothalamic-Hypophyseal Communications

While the posterior pituitary (neurohypophysis) develops embryologically as a downgrowth from the ventral diencephalon and retains its neural character in adult life, the anterior pituitary (adenohypophysis) lacks a direct nerve supply. The adenohypophysis and the median eminence (a specialized area of the hypothalamus located beneath the inferior portion of the third ventricle and above the pituitary stalk) are connected by portal veins. These originate from the superior hypophyseal arteries, which themselves derive from the internal carotids just prior to their entry into the subarachnoid space. The superior hypophyseal arteries terminate within the median eminence into a dense capillary network, some of which penetrates deeply within the neural tissue and close to the ventricles. These capillaries drain into the "long" portal vessels which then descend along the pituitary stalk and terminate in sinusoids within the adenohypophysis (Fig. 3). A large portion of the blood supply to the adenohypophysis originates from these "long" portal vessels and has therefore been in contact with the hypothalamus. A smaller amount of blood to the anterior pituitary is also supplied by "short" portal vessels

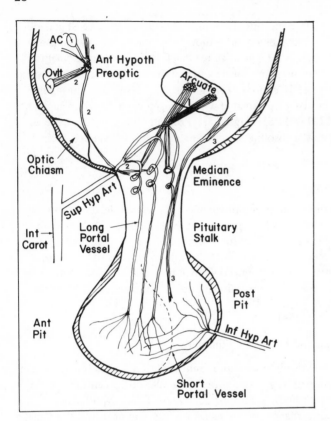

Figure 3 Hypothalamic-hypophyseal portal vasculature and GnRH distribution in the rhesus monkey comprises (1) the tuberoinfundibular tract (arcuate nucleus to median eminence and "long" portal vessels). (2) Tracts from the anterior hypothalamic-preoptic area (Ant Hypoth Preoptic) to the organum vasculosum laminae terminalis (Ovlt) and to the median eminence and "long" portal vessels. (3) Tracts from the posterior hypothalamus to the posterior pituitary (Post Pit). (4) Tracts around the anterior commissure (AC) and into the limbic system. (Adapted from Ref. 12.)

which originate in the neurohypophysis. It is now generally accepted that the main direction of blood flow is from the hypothalamus to the pituitary and therefore the "long" portal system is ideal for the transport of undiluted hypothalamic substances to the pituitary. Interruption of hypothalamic-hypophyseal vascular connections by pituitary stalk section results in a significant decrease or arrest in the secretion of anterior pituitary hormones (except prolactin which is under an inhibitory influence of the hypothalamus), with resultant failure of their target organs [9]. If a barrier is not placed between the cut portions of the stalk, restitution of anterior pituitary function occurs, and this correlates well with a regrowth of long portal vessels and revascularization of the anterior pituitary.

There has recently been discussion of the possibility that blood flows in a retrograde fashion from the pituitary to the hypothalamus. Page et al. [10] have suggested several possible routes for retrograde blood flow, but whether this occurs in physiological situations is not known. The possible significance of this phenomenon is related to the existence of local "short" feedback loops and to the recent discovery of pituitarylike hormones in the brain.

B. Hypothalamic Neurohormonal Networks

The *magnocellular* neural network, carrying oxytocin and vasopressin (and their associated neurophysins), has been recognized as originating from the supraoptic and paraventricular nuclei (oxytocin *and* vasopressin appear to originate in both nuclei). Axons descend into the pituitary stalk to the posterior pituitary from which both hormones are released. Pituitary stalk section also results in disturbances in the secretion of oxytocin and vasopressin. Function is soon restored to a certain degree, however, because the cut neural fibers possess an inherent degree of regeneration and a new neurohemal organ is formed above the level of the cut [11].

Other neurohormonal hypothalamic networks are referred to as *parvicellular.* Tracing of these networks has had to await the identification of the neurohormones they carry and the development of specific antibodies for use in immunocytochemical studies. The structure of three hypothalamic neurohormones has up to now been fully characterized: thyroid-releasing hormone (TRH), a tripeptide; gonadotropin-releasing hormone (GnRH), a decapeptide; and somatostatin, a tetradecapeptide. TRH has been found to release not only thyroid-stimulating hormone (TSH) but also prolactin, while somatostatin inhibits the secretion of growth hormone (GH). In this chapter, we will deal only with GnRH.

In the primate, the GnRH fiber network (Fig. 3) covers quite a large area of the central nervous system [12]. Most important here is the tuberoinfundibular tract which originates from cell bodies in the arcuate nucleus (a structure within the medial basal hypothalamus which contains numerous other small peptides as well), with axons reaching the median eminence and terminating near the long portal vessels into which GnRH is secreted. Lesion of the arcuate nucleus in the monkey results in the arrest of gonadotropin secretion, demonstrating the importance of this tract for normal gonadotropin secretion [13]. Other GnRH fiber networks have also been visualized in the monkey: (1) in the anterior hypothalamic area, which appear to terminate in the organum vasculosum laminae terminalis (OVLT) (a specialized neurovascular structure lying at the rostral end of the third ventricle) as well as in the median eminence; (2) in the posterior hypothalamus, which extend along the pituitary stalk into the neurohypophysis; (3) throughout the limbic system. Although the specific function of the last three groups of GnRH fibers remains to be elucidated, their role in the control of gonadotropin secretion does not appear crucial. Because of the vast area in which GnRH has been found, this factor may also behave like a neurotransmitter or neuromodulator within different circuits of the central nervous system. It has also been suggested that this decapeptide plays a role in sexual behavior, since its injection into the CNS results in the induction of lordosis behavior in the rodent (see Chap. 10).

C. GnRH, the Reproductive Neurohormone

This decapeptide (Pyro glu-his-trp-ser-tyr-gly-leu-arg-pro-glyNH$_2$) originally isolated from ovine and porcine hypothalami releases both LH and FSH within minutes of injection. It does not appear to be species-specific since its biologic activity has been shown in all mammalian species investigated, including the primate. GnRH is essential for normal gonadotropin secretion. Administration of antibodies to GnRH in monkeys rapidly disrupts LH and FSH release. There is good evidence to indicate that this hypothalamic hormone acts at the membrane level of pituitary cells, possibly by modifying the cell's permeability to ions. GnRH is rapidly degraded in the peripheral circulation (with a half-life of less than 5 minutes), but therapeutic use of this factor may be facilitated by the availability of structural analogs which remain in the circulation longer.

The pattern of gonadotropin response to GnRH is known to be influenced by two factors. The first is the endocrine milieu at the time of GnRH administration and, most importantly, prior exposure to estradiol. Ovarian hormonal modulation is best exemplified by the results following administration of identical doses of GnRH at different times of the menstrual cycle [14] (Fig. 4). The amounts of LH and FSH released into the circulation differ greatly depending on the stage of cycle, with greatest release occurring at the end of the follicular phase at the time of maximal estradiol secretion. These differential releases have been postulated to be related to changes in two functionally distinguishable pools of pituitary gonadotropins, one characterized as "readily releasable," the other as "pituitary reserve" (or not so readily releasable) [15]. Both pools increase during the follicular phase but the reserve pool undergoes a preferential increase during the late follicular phase, presumably as a build-up to the midcycle gonadotropin surge. A second factor which influences gonadotropin response is prior exposure to GnRH itself. For example, challenge of the pituitary gland to submaximal pulses of GnRH has indicated that the pituitary can detect small changes in circulatory GnRH concentrations and that these influence the response of the gland to further stimulation.

How a single neurohormone can control the secretion of two separate hypophyseal hormones, LH and FSH, whose secretory patterns during the menstrual

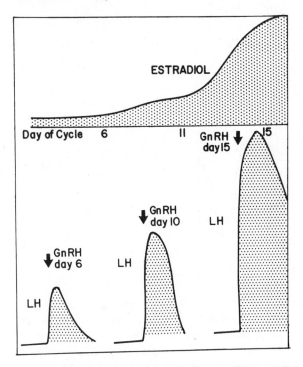

Figure 4 Luteinizing hormone (LH) response to GnRH during the follicular phase. Gonadotropin response to identical doses of GnRH varies with the estrogen milieu. (Adapted from Ref. 14.)

cycle are not exactly parallel, is not entirely known. Several laboratories have searched for a separate hypothalamic hormone which would specifically influence FSH, but with no success to date. One hypothesis is that a nonsteroidal factor ("inhibin") which has been isolated from seminiferous tubules and more recently from ovarian follicular fluid may play a specific role in FSH secretion. Inhibin has indeed been shown to inhibit FSH secretion in the rat, but whether it is present in the circulation in amounts sufficient to influence the pituitary remains to be demonstrated. Another hypothesis is that the response of both gonadotropins is influenced differentially depending on the pattern of GnRH stimulation [13].

D. GnRH Secretion is Pulsatile

In 1972 [6], LH radioimmunoassays on frequent blood samples obtained in ovariectomized monkeys indicated that the secretion of gonadotropins by the anterior pituitary gland is not the result of a continuous process but of an inter-

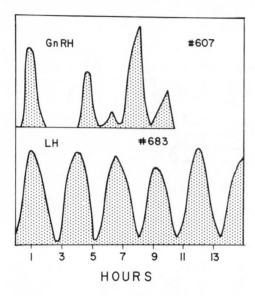

Figure 5 A schematic illustration of the pulsatile release of GnRH and LH in two ovariectomized monkeys (#607 and #683). GnRH release measured in the hypothalamic-hypophyseal portal vessels (it is undetectable in the peripheral circulation) is clearly pulsatile. (The frequency of pulses, however, may be influenced by anesthesia). LH is also released in pulses, occurring at 1-3 h intervals. A simultaneous measurement of GnRH and LH was unfortunately not possible, but it is reasonable to assume that pulsatile pituitary hormone release relates to pulsatile hypothalamic secretory patterns. (Adapted from Refs. 6 and 16.)

mittent one, LH being released in pulses at a frequency of about 1 to 2 h (Fig. 5). This pulsatile pattern of LH secretion has been found to be characteristic of not only the monkey but of most animal species studied. Pulses of FSH are also observed but more difficult to characterize because of the longer half-life of this hormone.

Since it was known that GnRH influences gonadotropin secretion, it had been hypothesized that LH pulses were the result of a pulsatile GnRH pattern of release by the hypothalamus. This hypothesis has been difficult to prove because most radioimmunoassay methods for GnRH are not sensitive enough to monitor the decapeptide's levels in the peripheral circulation. Results in our laboratory, where we were able to measure GnRH directly in hypothalamic-hypophyseal portal blood of rhesus monkeys for prolonged periods of time, clearly demonstrate that GnRH itself is released into the portal circulation in a pulsatile fashion (Fig. 5) [16]. Pulsatile LH release is therefore the consequence of pulsatile hypothalamic activity and not the result of an intrinsic property of the adenohypophysis. Other anterior pituitary hormones are also released in characteristic pulsatile patterns (although of variable frequencies) and it is tempting to speculate that each such pattern is itself the result of pulsatile neurohormonal release activity.

Experiments recently performed in rhesus monkeys lacking GnRH following arcuate nucleus lesion or pituitary stalk section have demonstrated how crucial a pulsatile GnRH release pattern is to "normal" gonadotropin secretion and to the menstrual cycle. When attempts were made in these animals to restore normal gonadotropin secretion by administering GnRH, it was surprising to observe that only temporary elevations in LH and FSH could be obtained with a continuous GnRH infusion, while intermittent, pulsatile GnRH administration produced sustained increases in both hormones [17]. In fact, only with a pulsatile GnRH infusion, mimicking the physiological pattern of hypothalamic release, were the investigators able to restore normal menstrual cyclicity in these amenorrheic monkeys [13]. The reasons for the lack of response of the anterior pituitary to a continuous GnRH stimulation are unknown. Various investigators have postulated a "down regulation" phenomenon, possibly related to a decrease in the number of available GnRH pituitary receptors. Such a phenomenon may explain recent paradoxic results obtained by several investigators following administration of long-acting GnRH analogs. While the authors were attempting to stimulate pituitary response, suppression rather than stimulation of gonadotropin secretion occurred in many patients. A practical consequence of such results involves studies of the use of GnRH analogs as contraceptives.

Initiation of LH pulsatile release patterns occurs during the immediate prepubertal period, when a circadian rhythm emerges with pulsatile release only at night. The number of LH secretory nocturnal episodes correlates well with the number of sleep cycles [18]. In immature female monkeys, it is possible to induce normal menstrual cycles with pulsatile GnRH infusions [19]. However, following disconnection of the infusion, the animals revert to a prepubertal state, until the normal sequence of events is initiated spontaneously. These results indicate that neither the pituitary gland nor the ovaries are limiting factors in the initiation of puberty but that this process depends on the maturation of the hypothalamic system that directs pulsatile secretion of GnRH from the hypothalamus. With completion of puberty, episodic bursts of LH occur throughout the 24 h period and the sleep-associated nocturnal pattern is lost. In the adult, the pattern of pulsatile GnRH and consequently LH release is influenced by ovarian hormones: amplitude as well as frequency of the LH pulses differ with each stage of the menstrual cycle and after ovariectomy [20].

III. Ovarian-Hypothalamic-Hypophyseal Functional Integration

A. Estradiol Feedback Sites

Classic feedback concepts, which evolved from a series of experiments performed in rats 20 years ago, describe a dual organization of the hypothalamus in its response to ovarian feedback and control of hypophyseal gonadotropin secretion. Complete deafferentation of the medial basal hypothalamus or anterior hypothalamic lesions resulted in the abolition of estrus cycles and in anovulation, while estradiol implants within the anterior hypothalamus induced gonadotropin surges. Accordingly, the hypothalamus was divided into two areas: the medial basal hypothalamus as the site concerned with tonic gonadotropin secretion (and responsive to the negative estradiol feedback) and the anterior hypothalamic-preoptic region dealing with "cyclic" gonadotropin secretion (and responsive to the positive estradiol feedback) [21].

   That these concepts of hypothalamic organization may not be applicable in the primate is illustrated by the results of recent experiments in the monkey, in which attempts were made to duplicate the original experiments. Indeed, complete deafferentation, separating the medial basal hypothalamus from the remainder of the neural system, did not interfere with menstrual cyclicity [22] and LH surges could not be induced following estradiol implants in the anterior hypothalamus. Furthermore, estradiol challenges were shown to induce identical LH and FSH surges in monkeys before and immediately following pituitary stalk section [23] and long-term pulsatile GnRH infusions in these animals in whom the pituitary is isolated from the brain also resulted in normal menstrual cycles [13]. The above results convincingly indicate that in the rhesus monkey, in contrast to the rat, estradiol exerts its positive feedback action directly on the anterior pituitary and not on the hypothalamus. A direct estradiol effect is consistent with the high degree of estradiol uptake in cells of the anterior pituitary [24]. That differences in feedback sites exist between the rat and higher species, such as the monkey, may not be surprising. While estradiol is the crucial signal without which the gonadotropin surge cannot occur in both species, in the rat there is a crucial involvement of a neural clock which is superimposed on the estrogen positive feedback signal, as the LH surge is only observed at a time predetermined by the light cycle. In contrast, in the primate, the LH surge is related only to the time, duration and strength of the estradiol stimulus. Figure 6 summarizes the differences between the primate and rodent. The results in the monkey also demonstrate that a GnRH surge, such as occurs in the rodent at proestrus prior to the LH surge [25], is not a prerequisite for normal LH and FSH surges and that GnRH therefore plays only a permissive, albeit essential, role in the midcycle gonadotropin surge.

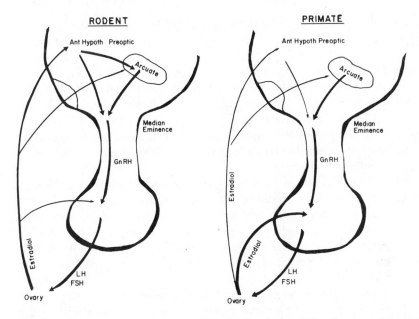

Figure 6 The primary estradiol positive feedback site differs in the rodent and in the primate. In the rat, it is located in the anterior hypothalamic-preoptic area (injection of 17β-estradiol into this site readily induces a gonadotropin surge). In the monkey, it is located in the anterior pituitary (a gonadotropin surge can be readily induced in the stalk sectioned monkey, provided GnRH is infused to maintain the viable gonadotrope). (Adapted from Refs. 13, 21, and 23.)

B. The Role of Neurotransmitters

The factors which control GnRH secretion, and most importantly its pulsatile mode of release, are not precisely known. Among the candidates to be discussed, neurotransmitters occupy an important position. Several neurotransmitters have been identified in the central nervous system. The best known and most frequently implicated in neuroendocrine function are catecholamines, such as dopamine and norepinephrine, and indolamines, such as serotonin. The evidence for their possible involvement in the control of gonadotropin release is voluminous. A clear concept of their mode of action, however, is more difficult to develop, because of the large number of apparently contradictory results which crowd the literature [26]. In the rat, it appears that LH release is regulated by a dual catecholaminergic system, in which norepinephrine exerts a stimulatory effect and dopamine an inhibitory one. Serotonin appears to play a predominantly inhibitory role in gonadotropin secretion. The role of biogenic amines in controlling gonadotropin secretion in the primate is even less clear, as few experiments have been performed. β-Adrenergic blockers have been shown to suppress pulsatile LH secretion in the monkey, but the dose used also had profound effects on the animal's physiology [27]. Dopamine administration in women resulted in a decline in LH levels, but the effects were not profound [28]. Pimozide, a dopamine blocker, was also reported to inhibit the midcycle LH surge. Further experimentation in the primate is clearly needed because the results of different species are difficult to transpose.

Concentration of biogenic amines is greatest in the hypothalamus, and most importantly in the portions of the hypothalamus which contain the cell bodies of the hypophysiotropic neurohormones. A prominent dopaminergic system arises within the medial basal hypothalamus, with axons projecting from the arcuate and periventricular nuclei to the median eminence. A serotonin pathway originating in the medial basal hypothalamus has also been described. However, the majority of neural cell bodies synthesizing biogenic amines are located outside the hypothalamus in the mesencephalon and brain stem. Norepinephrine fibers arise principally in the locus coeruleus, dopamine in the substantia nigra, and serotonin fibers in the mesencephalic and pontine raphé nuclei.

Most investigators postulate a hypothalamic site of action for these neurotransmitters, possibly by modulating the release of GnRH. Anatomic relationships between neurotransmitters and neurohormones suggest several loci at which hypothalamic hormone secretion could be modified by neurotransmitters. Recent observations have shown that catecholamines varicosities and GnRH terminals are located in identical regions within the arcuate nucleus and in the median eminence [29]. GnRH release into the tuberoinfundibular tract could therefore be modulated by a direct effect of the neurotransmitter on the GnRH cell. Alternatively, the neurotransmitter could control GnRH release into the hypophyseal portal circulation by an axo-axonal mechanism (Fig. 7). There have been several reports of significant changes in the activity of biogenic amines in the rat hypothalamus, coincident with the proestrus LH surge. These include decreases in dopamine and increases in norepinephrine turnover. These probably result from an effect of estradiol, which is highest at that time of the cycle and is relatively concentrated in these areas of the brain. The presence of densely labeled estradiol in the same hypothalamic area as GnRH and catecholamines favors a potential interaction among these substances in the regulation of pituitary release of gonadotropins. An intriguing link between estrogens and monoamines is the report of the capability of the hypothalamus to form catecholestrogens such as 2-hydroxyestrone and 2-hydroxyestradiol. Because of their structure, these compounds may act as competitive inhibitors of amine metabolizing enzymes and thereby influence reproductive processes [30].

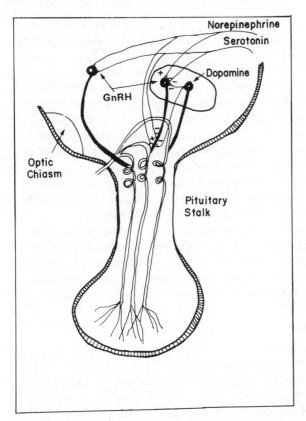

Figure 7 Hypothetical representation of biogenic amine modulation of GnRH release (from results in the rodent). Dopamine and serotonin appear to exert an inhibitory effect while norepinephrine has a stimulatory effect on GnRH release into the hypothalamic-hypophyseal portal circulation. Dopamine is also secreted into the long portal vessels to inhibit prolactin release directly at the pituitary level. (Adapted from Refs. 29 and 31.)

Although most effects of biogenic amines are exerted at central sites, the possibility of a direct pituitary action should also be considered. In this case, the amine could be derived from the peripheral pool of neurotransmitters or reach the pituitary gland via the hypophyseal portal circulation. In support of the latter are the recent demonstrations of high density monoamine boutons in the neurohemal zone of the median eminence, not necessarily in association with neurohormonal terminals and, more importantly, of high levels of dopamine in pituitary stalk portal blood [31]. Hypothalamic control over prolactin secretion is known to be predominantly inhibitory, as isolation of the pituitary from the hypothalamus results in increased prolactin secretion. It is now thought that dopamine is in fact at least one of the prolactin inhibitory factors. Indeed, dopamine itself or its agonists, such as bromoergocryptine, causes an acute lowering of prolactin levels and stops lactation in patients with hyperprolactinemia and galactorrhea [32]. Drugs which block dopaminergic receptor sites, such as phenothiazines, induce a rapid release of prolactin, and their long-term administration may cause hyperprolactinemia, galactorrhea, and amenorrhea. Most probably, dopamine inhibits prolactin by a direct pituitary action following its secretion into the hypophyseal portal circulation. In support of this are experiments which have shown a suppressive effect of dopamine on prolactin release in vitro on pituitaries in culture or in vivo after pituitary stalk section [33]. In this regard, therefore, dopamine behaves more like a neurohormone than a neurotransmitter.

Not only biogenic amines, but also other neurotransmitters, such as acetylcholine, histamine, γ-aminobutyric acid (GABA), and several newly identified peptidergic neurotransmitters, such as substance P, neurotensin, and others, have been in some way or another linked to neuroendocrine functions. Their role in the integration of specific neuroendocrine events remains to be fully appreciated.

C. The Role of Opioid Peptides

Some of the newer central compounds which have been under intense investigation are the opioid peptides. There is good evidence in the primate literature that β-endorphin, which is found in the hypothalamus and pituitary, can induce prolactin release [34]. This effect is reverted by naloxone, an opiate antagonist. Several investigators have suggested that this action is exerted on the hypothalamus, probably by modulating the release of dopamine into the hypophyseal portal circulation [31]. It has also been suggested that β-endorphin plays a role in the control of gonadotropin secretion. Naloxone can increase LH levels in the human, when injected at specific times of the menstrual cycle [35]. In our laboratory, we have observed high levels of β-endorphins (which originate from the arcuate nucleus) in hypophyseal portal blood [36]. No doubt investigations during the next few years will further illuminate the role endorphins have in neuroendocrine function.

III. Dysfunction of the Menstrual Cycle

As shown above, the menstrual cycle is a dynamic system requiring the precise integration of events occurring at the arcuate nucleus of the hypothalamus, pituitary gland, ovaries, and reproductive organs. It is clear, however, that the activity of the arcuate nucleus may be influenced by higher central neural centers and that proper function of the system requires a delicate coordination with the function of other endocrine organs.

Frequent causes of menstrual dysfunction are related to aberrations in CNS-hypothalamic interactions. It is well-known, for example, that serious psychological stress can inhibit ovulation. The most common examples cited in the human are the occurrence of amenorrhea in women in concentration camps during World War II, or in girls entering boarding schools. There are several explanations proposed for the effects of stress on menstrual cyclicity and it is difficult, if not impossible, to relate these to a single cause. In animals, it is known that a wide variety of stimuli not only induce a discharge of catecholamines from the adrenal medulla but also modify the amounts of catecholamines within the arcuate nucleus (but apparently not in other hypothalamic nuclei) [37]. Presumably, humans exposed to stress also undergo changes in catecholamines or their synthesizing enzymes similar to those observed in animals. Psychologic disorders, such as depression, can also produce anovulation and amenorrhea, and again, as in the case of stress, the same neurotransmitters implicated in the clinical pathology of affective disorders are those hypothesized to influence gonadotropin secretion. Drugs, such as phenothiazines which alter CNS catecholamines, are also known to induce dysfunction of the menstrual cycle.

Although adrenal response to stress in the human may not be as dramatic as in the animal, hypercortisolism is usually associated with irregular cycles or anovulation. This effect of cortisol may be related to a decreased response of the gonadotrope to GnRH or of the ovaries to gonadotropins. If hyperandrogenism accompanies elevated cortisol levels, as a result of increased ACTH production, normal estradiol feedback may be altered or interfered with. This is encountered in several pathologic conditions, such as polycystic ovary syndrome, congenital adrenal hyperplasia, Cushing's syndrome, and with androgen-producing tumors. In these cases, estrogen precursor availability is increased and extraglandular production of estrogens may be excessive. Because this rate of estrogen increase is acyclic and not under the control of gonadotropins, the original estradiol feedback may be masked and amenorrhea occurs. Further, estrogen sensitive neurons are seen not only within the pituitary and arcuate nucleus but also in several other regions, including extrahypothalamic areas. There, estrogens may have possible functional roles in the regulation of mood and behavior, and thereby further modulate reproductive cyclicity.

Stress does not involve only hormones of the adrenal axis. Other hormones are also known to increase. For instance, anxiety in the human is a potent stimulus for GH and prolactin release. Hyperprolactinemia has been frequently related to anovulation and the amenorrhea-galactorrhea syndrome has been well documented [38]. Several authors have speculated that prolactin interferes either with gonadotropin response to GnRH stimulation or ovarian response to gonadotropins. However, since this syndrome can be readily reversed by the administration of dopamine agonists such as bromoergocryptine, it has been suggested that the primary defect resides in the dopaminergic system. Similar causes may be found in women who are chronic users of neuroleptics or certain tranquilizers.

Their prolonged use results in decreased gonadotropin release, anovulation, as well as hyperprolactinemia.

Abnormal releases of β-endorphins under stressful or other psychological conditions may also be an important cause of abnormalities in menstrual cyclicity, since endorphins may exert inhibitory effects on gonadotropin release [35].

Finally, it may be of interest to describe briefly here an often-mentioned type of amenorrhea: anorexia nervosa or starvation amenorrhea. Several observers favor psychologic factors as the initiating causes for this symptom. However, in the adolescent population, the incidence of psychiatric disorders appears to be no greater than among the general population of the same age and therefore it is difficult to determine whether the behavioral symptom is primary or secondary to the illness [39]. Endocrine studies reveal low plasma LH and FSH, with presumed low GnRH secretion, as well as low thyroxine and high corticoid levels. Of specific interest in these patients is the correlation between weight loss and regression of the LH secretory pattern from that of an adult one to that seen in early puberty. These patients indeed show the sleep-associated episodic LH bursts characteristic of the early prepubertal period. Following remission and weight gain, a return to the adult LH secretory pattern can be observed. The combination of these abnormalities as well as deficiencies in water and blood regulation suggest a specific hypothalamic disorder.

References

1. R. L. Vande Wiele, R. J. Bogumil, I. Dyrenfurth, M. Ferin, R. Jewelewicz, M. Warren, G. Mikhail, and T. Rizkallah, *Recent Prog. Horm. Res.* 26:63 (1970).

2. S. S. C. Yen, C. C. Tsai, G. Vandenberg, and R. Rebar, *J. Clin. Endocrinol. Metab.* 35:897 (1972).

3. M. Ferin, I. Dyrenfurth, S. Cowchock, M. Warren, and R. L. Vande Wiele, *Endocrinology* 94:765 (1974).

4. S. Monroe, R. Jaffe, and A. R. Midgley, *J. Clin. Endocrinol. Metab.* 34:342 (1972).

5. F. J. Karsch, R. F. Weick, W. R. Butler, D. J. Dierschke, L. C. Krey, G. Weiss, J. Hotchkiss, T. Yamaji, and E. Knobil, *Endocrinology* 92:1740 (1973).

6. E. Knobil, *Recent Prog. Horm. Res.* 30:1 (1974).

7. R. J. Chang and R. B. Jaffe, *J. Clin. Endocrinol. Metab.* 47:119 (1978).

8. A. Miyake, T. Aono, T. Kinugasa, O. Tanizawa, and K. Kurachi, *Acta Endocrinol. (Copenh.)* 88:1 (1978).

9. L. Vaughan, P. W. Carmel, I. Dyrenfurth, A. G. Frantz, J. L. Antunes, and M. Ferin, *Neuroendocrinology* 30:70 (1980).

10. R. B. Page and R. M. Bergland, *Am. J. Anat.* 148:345 (1977).

11. J. L. Antunes, K. M. Louis, S. Huang, E. A. Zimmerman, P. W. Carmel, and M. Ferin, *Ann. Neurol.* 8:308 (1980).
12. A. J. Silverman, J. L. Antunes, M. Ferin, and E. A. Zimmerman, *Endocrinology* 101:134 (1977).
13. E. Knobil, *Recent Prog. Horm. Res.* 36:53 (1980).
14. C. F. Wang, and S. S. C. Yen, *J. Clin. Invest.* 55:201 (1975).
15. C. F. Wang, B. L. Lasley, A. Lein, and S. S. C. Yen, *J. Clin. Endocrinol. Metab.* 42:718 (1976).
16. P. W. Carmel, S. Araki, and M. Ferin, *Endocrinology* 99:243 (1976).
17. P. E. Belchetz, T. M. Plant, Y. Nakai, E. G. Keogh, and E. Knobil, *Science* 202:631 (1978).
18. R. J. Boyar, H. Finkelstein, H. Roffwarg, S. Kapen, E. D. Weitzman, and L. Hellman, *N. Engl. J. Med.* 287:582 (1972).
19. L. Wildt, G. Marshall, and E. Knobil, *Science* 207:1373 (1980).
20. S. S. C. Yen, C. C. Tsai, F. Naftolin, G. Vandeberg, and L. Ajabor, *J. Clin. Endocrinol. Metab.* 34:671 (1972).
21. B. Halasz, *Frontiers in Neuroendocrinology* (W. F. Ganong and L. Martini, eds.). Oxford University Press, England, 1969, p. 307.
22. M. Ferin, J. L. Antunes, E. A. Zimmerman, I. Dyrenfurth, A. G. Frantz, A. Robinson, and P. W. Carmel, *Endocrinology* 101:1611 (1977).
23. M. Ferin, H. Rosenblatt, P. W. Carmel, J. L. Antunes, and R. L. Vande Wiele, *Endocrinology* 104:50 (1979).
24. D. W. Pfaff, L. Gerlach, B. S. McEwen, M. Ferin, P. W. Carmel, and E. A. Zimmerman, *J. Comp. Neurol.* 170:279 (1976).
25. D. K. Sarkar, S. A. Chiappa, G. Fink, and N. M. Sherwood, *Nature* 264:461 (1976).
26. E. E. Müller, G. Nistico, and U. Scapagnini, *Neurotransmitters and Anterior Pituitary Function.* Academic, New York, 1977.
27. T. M. Plant, Y. Nakai, P. Belchetz, E. Keogh, and E. Knobil, *Endocrinology* 102:1015 (1978).
28. H. Leblanc, G. C. L. Lachelin, S. Abu-Fadil, and S. S. C. Yen, *J. Clin. Endocrinol. Metab.* 43:668 (1976).
29. T. H. McNeill and J. R. Sladek, *Science* 200:72 (1978).
30. H. Breuer, G. Kuster, H. T. Schneider, and W. Ladosky, in *Brain-Endocrine Interactions, III Neural Hormones and Reproduction* (D. E. Scott, ed.). Karger, New York, 1978.
31. G. A. Gudelsky and J. C. Porter, *Life Sci.* 25:1697 (1979).
32. G. L. Lachelin, S. Abu-Fadil, and S. S. C. Yen, *J. Clin. Endocrinol. Metab.* 44:1163 (1977).
33. W. P. Diefenbach, P. W. Carmel, A. G. Frantz, and M. Ferin, *J. Clin. Endocrinol. Metab.* 43:638 (1976).
34. C. Rivier, W. Vale, N. Ling, M. Brown, and R. Guillemin, *Endocrinology* 100:238 (1977).

35. M. E. Quigley and S. S. C. Yen, *J. Clin. Endocrinol. Metab.* 51:179 (1980).

36. S. L. Wardlaw, W. B. Wehrenberg, M. Ferin, P. W. Carmel, and A. G. Frantz, *Endocrinology* 106:1323 (1980).

37. M. Palkovits, R. M. Kobayashi, J. S. Kizer, D. M. Jacobowitz, and I. J. Kopen, *Neuroendocrinology* 18:144 (1975).

38. G. Tolis, in *Neuroendocrinology* (D. T. Krieger and J. C. Hughes, eds.). Sinauer Assoc., Sunderland, Mass., 1980.

39. R. L. Vande Wiele, in *Neuroendocrinology* (D. T. Krieger and J. C. Hughes, eds.). Sinauer Assoc., Sunderland, Mass., 1980.

3 Neuroendocrine Regulation of Sexual Behavior

PAULA G. DAVIS* and BRUCE S. McEWEN   The Rockefeller University, New York, New York

The studies of neuroendocrinology and of hormones and behavior have advanced markedly in the last 50 years [6,37,96], but progress has been especially noteworthy in the last two decades. By the mid-1960s, the related concepts that sex steroids regulate behavior and neuroendocrine function, and do so by acting directly upon the central nervous system (CNS), were already well-established [37,97]. The elucidation of many aspects of the mechanisms of hormone action followed rapidly upon the technology of the 1970s which included the advent of new and sensitive assays for steroid hormones and receptors [27,38,48].

At least three important neuroendocrine and behavioral end points of adult animals are regulated by the gonadal steroids (testosterone in males, estradiol and progesterone in females). These include the neural control of gonadotropin secretion by the anterior pituitary gland and the regulation of masculine and feminine sexual behavior by the CNS. The relationships between gonadal steroids and reproductive events in adults are determined in part during "critical periods" of perinatal development as a result of steroid-dependent processes. These events, termed the organizational effects of steroids upon sexual differentiation, have *permanent* consequences for the neuroendocrine and behavioral profiles of the adult. In contrast, the regulation of hormone-dependent reproductive events in adults are a result of the activational effects of the steroids, are relatively *reversible,* and are usually dependent upon the actual presence of the hormones.

Both the organizational and activational effects of sex steroids stem, in large

---

*Present affiliation: M.E.D. Communications, Hopelawn, New Jersey.

43

part, from their actions upon the CNS itself. In adults, gonadal steroids act upon the presumably differentiated CNS substrates to regulate the immediate expression of certain sexually dimorphic characteristics. For both effects of steroids, the major mode of action requires binding to intracellular protein receptors. The steroid-cytosol receptor complexes then translocate to the cell nucleus, bind to DNA, and thereby initiate RNA and protein synthesis [19]. It is thought that sex steroids ultimately influence the neural events underlying behavior and other hormone-dependent measures by regulating genomic expression. Despite the common genomic mechanisms of action proposed for both the developmental and activational effects of gonadal hormones, the consequences of steroid-receptor interaction differ significantly at the two time points. The sequelae are permanent in the first case, but relatively reversible in the second. This implies that the developmental status of the substrate is important in determining the consequences of particular steroid-cellular interactions.

In this chapter, we shall compare and contrast the roles of estrogen-receptor interactions in the processes of sexual differentiation and sexual activation. The primary focus will be on feminine sexual behavior in rats, but the control of masculine sexual behavior and gonadotropin secretion will also be considered.

I. Hormonal Regulation of Reproduction in Rats

A. Mating Behavior and the Role of Sexual Differentiation

A brief review of mating behavior in rats will provide a foundation for evaluating steroid effects on reproduction. As adults, male and female rats exhibit sexually dimorphic patterns of reproduction which include sexual behavior itself, the patterns of gonadotropin secretion, and other social and regulatory behaviors.

A sexual encounter between an estrous female and a gonadally intact male consists of a series of well-coordinated behaviors which depend upon a variety of internal and external stimuli for their integration [see 1, for review]. The estrous female displays solicitation or proceptive behaviors typified by darting and hopping movements and by rapid ear vibrations called ear wiggling. These behaviors appear to attract the male and to stimulate him to mount [9]. Olfactory and auditory stimuli, in addition to visual cues, appear to be of considerable import in male-female interactions [3,17]. The male performs a succession of mounts during which he palpates the female's flanks with his forepaws, thereby facilitating or stimulating her assumption of the receptive posture. The receptive or lordosis reflex is a deep dorsiflexion coupled with head and rump elevation and tail deflection [42]. Maintenance of the lordosis permits the male to achieve intromissions which culminate in the ejaculation. Following a refractory period of about 4 to 6 min, copulation may resume [41].

For each sex, these normal reproductive behaviors are hormone-dependent. Feminine sexual behavior is characterized by its intermittent occurrence during

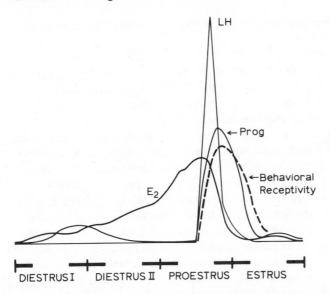

Figure 1 The estrous cycle of the female rat. The rise in estradiol (E$_2$) precedes the surge of luteinizing hormone (LH). Behavioral receptivity is correlated temporally with the secretion of progesterone (Prog).

the 4 to 5 day estrous cycle (Fig. 1). In contrast, masculine copulatory behavior is typified by its relative acyclicity. Castrated animals of either sex show little or no spontaneous sexual behavior; any that does occur is clearly distinguishable from that shown by gonadally intact animals.

For ovariectomized rats, replacement therapy with appropriate doses of the ovarian hormones estradiol and progesterone reinstates the full range of estrous behaviors [14]. Estradiol itself can increase the frequency of the lordosis response [43,98], although progesterone is required to bring about the full complement of estrous behaviors during the estrous cycle [74] and in physiological replacement paradigms [62]. The obligatory role of progesterone is even more clear-cut in other mammals including some rodent species [for review, see 31]. The synergism between progesterone and estrogen depends upon estrogenic priming of target tissue (see below). In rats, the relevant CNS target sites become competent to respond to progesterone at a minimum of 18 to 24 h following onset of estrogen treatment [35]. At that time, behavioral estrus is manifested. Progesterone may play some role in terminating the period of behavioral estrus in rats, an action more clearly documented for other species such as guinea pig and hamsters [see 64, for review]. In rats, the inhibition of subsequent sexual activity by progesterone may depend upon pharmacologic doses of progesterone, but such paradigms have proven useful in unraveling some possible mechanisms of progesterone action [12,13].

The sexual behavior of castrated male rats can be restored by either testosterone or a combination of estradiol and 5α-dihydrotestosterone [5,32,47]. Although testosterone is the major testicular secretion, it is apparent that many of the biologic actions of androgen stimulation are actually the result of metabolic conversions at target tissue sites (see below).

Male and female rats are each most likely to display the *homotypical* mating patterns, but some adults of either sex can be induced to show *heterotypical* mating behavior. Indeed, some individuals show these behaviors quite readily. In particular, females of many species including rats frequently show male-typical mounting [7]. Sometimes they display the intromission motor pattern and, under special conditions, the ejaculatory motor pattern [45,89]. Some gonadally intact males exhibit lordosis behavior when mounted by other males, although this may be a less frequent occurrence than the incidence of male-typical behavior by females. Estimates of heterotypical mating behavior by males may be artificially low because of the difficulties in persuading experienced maters to mount other males. Even when sexually vigorous males mount other males, they may not deliver a constellation of stimuli identical to those that would be received by a receptive female.

The important point about sexual behavior in rats is that the homotypical behaviors have the highest probabilities of occurrence under various hormonal and environmental conditions [70]. One may view the processes of sexual differentiation as events that set these probabilities and provide the physiological substrates for successful reproduction.

B. Sexual Differentiation

Differentiation of the reproductive tract provides a model or analogy for differentiation of the CNS. The relative timing of various developmental events is illustrated in Figure 2. In both genetic males and genetic females, the undifferentiated gonad develops into either testes or ovaries depending upon the type of sex chromosomes present. In XY-bearing mammals (genetic males), the testicular secretions (beginning around day 16 of gestation in rats) regulate the regression of the Müllerian ducts. The factor responsible for Müllerian degenerations is not, however, an androgen, but more likely a peptide of testicular origin [40]. Under androgenic stimulation, the Wolffian ducts develop into epididymis, vas deferens, and seminal vesicles, processes considered to be masculinization. Androgenic secretions also masculinize the remainder of the reproductive tract. In the rat, this process may begin around day 16 of gestation and continue into the beginning of postnatal life. Removal of the testes of the neonate renders the external genitalia relatively insensitive to testosterone administered in later life [10]. In males, the urogenital sinus develops into the prostate, and the genital tubercle

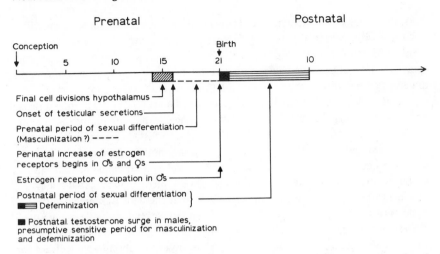

Figure 2 The perinatal period of development in rats, showing events associated with critical periods of sexual differentiation.

gives rise to the penis and scrotum. In the absence of any testicular secretions (i.e., the genetic female or XX individual), the Wolffian ducts degenerate and the Müllerian duct system develops into the feminine phenotype including Fallopian tubes, uterus, and upper vagina. The genital tubercle differentiates into the clitoris and lower vagina. Hormonal intervention while the external genitalia are differentiating can produce varying degrees of masculinization in females and failures to masculinize in males.

As with reproductive tract development, an anhormonal condition during perinatal development results in feminine phenotypic expression [see 74, for review]. In normal females, neonatally castrated males, or males treated neonatally with steroid antagonists, the components of the feminine reproductive phenotype are expressed to a greater or lesser extent. The capacity for cyclic gonadotropin secretion is intact, the potential for feminine sexual behavior is relatively high and that for masculine sexual behavior relatively low. In contrast, normal males and perinatally androgenized females exhibit tonic gonadotropin secretion, suppressed capacity for feminine sexual behavior, and enhanced masculine sexual behavior. Suppression of the capacity for cyclic gonadotropin secretion and for feminine sexual behavior is considered defeminization, whereas potentiation of the capacity for masculine copulatory behavior is considered masculinization [74].

Presumptive sexual differentiation of the brain differs in several important respects from differentiation of the reproductive tract. First, defeminization of gonadotropin secretion and of behavior results from the actions of testicular androgens and their metabolites. But Müllerian duct degeneration, also considered defeminization, appears to result from the action of nonsteroidal factors.

Also, the actions of testicular steroids upon the reproductive tract are primarily inductive with respect to phenotypic expression. In contrast, the most well documented effect of these steroids upon the CNS is the suppression of feminine phenotypic characteristics. It remains to be determined whether the cellular mechanisms underlying these different end points are fundamentally alike or different.

As Beach [8] and others have pointed out, the process of defeminization as it occurs in a normal male results in a relative change in the probability that the individual will show feminine sexual behavior. In contrast, the reproductive tract develops into either a male or female version under normal conditions. The pattern of gonadotropin secretion, however, tends to be either cyclic or tonic and, in that way, is more like reproductive tract development than is sexual behavior. In some cases, such as low-dose androgenization of the neonatal female, a delayed anovulatory syndrome is observed. Such females may initially show normal estrous cycles, but later become anovulatory. At any given time, the capacity for cyclic gonadotropin secretion is either present or absent [see Ref. 33 for review].

Finally, the precise contribution made by peripheral morphologic development and afferent sensory input [2] to the performance of sexual behavior remains unclear. As noted, the capacity of the penis to respond to androgen given in adulthood is related to the age at castration [10]. The closer the surgery is to birth, the greater the later deficit in both penile and behavioral responsiveness to administered hormones. The interactions between the periphery and CNS which might be related to such a covariance require additional investigation.

Despite the foregoing limitations, we now have considerable information about the timing of events related to sexual differentiation, the hormonal conditions mediating these events, and the possible neuroanatomic and biochemical consequences of hormone action. We shall discuss some of these correlations below.

II. Mechanisms of Estrogen Action

A. Topography and Cellular Aspects of Action

1. Adults

Accumulation of labeled steroid hormones by brain tissue has been documented extensively for a variety of vertebrate species [66]. As demonstrated by both biochemical and autoradiographic methods, steroid hormones readily enter the brain from the blood, and are selectively retained in specific brain regions. There are marked similarities in the patterns of hormone uptake from one species to another. In rats, the highest uptake and retention of labeled estradiol and testosterone occur in the hypothalamus and preoptic regions [59-61]. Some steroid-concentrating neurons have also been identified in septum, amygdala, hippocampus, and the midbrain. The neuroanatomic detail afforded by the autoradiographic method provides detailed mappings of steroid-concentrating cells. The distribution of estradiol-concentrating cells in female rat brain [71] is representative of a phylogenetically stable pattern. There are significant numbers of estradiol-concentrating cells in the medial preoptic area, the medial anterior hypothalamus, the arcuate nucleus, and the ventral premammillary nucleus. In addition, there are significant concentrations in the medial and cortical amygdala, the lateral septum, the bed nucleus of the stria terminalis, the olfactory tubercle, the diagonal bands of Broca, the ventral hippocampus, the prepiriform and entorhinal cortices, and the mesencephalic central grey. Many of these regions have been implicated in the control of reproductive function in a number of species (see below).

There are no gross sex differences in the patterns of hormone uptake as shown by autoradiographic and biochemical methods. The existence of similar hormone-concentrating patterns in male and female rats is consistent with the ability of each sex to perform the hetero- as well as homotypical mating behaviors. Such sexual dimorphisms as do exist may be reflected in subtle dimorphisms in brain structure and function (see below). The interesting differences between estradiol and testosterone distributions appear to be related, in large part, to metabolism of testosterone in neural tissue (Fig. 3). Such differences may underlie some aspects of the sex differences in masculine copulatory performance and the control of gonadotropin secretion.

Estradiol accounts for approximately 50% of the radioactivity recovered from brain cell nuclei following injection of tritiated testosterone [48]. The distribution of testosterone-derived estradiol is not identical to that seen when tritiated estradiol is not found in pituitary cell nuclei because the converting enzymes are not present in that tissue [67]. In contrast, the distribution of labeled dihydrotestosterone is the same whether it is injected directly or derived from testosterone (Fig. 4). The distributions of the enzymes responsible for aromatization to estradiol and for 5α-reduction to dihydrotestosterone are coincident with the distribution of the two hormones following tritiated testosterone treatment [26, 67]. Of the two conversions, the functional consequences of aromatization have received the most attention. Testosterone-derived estradiol may have considerable physiological significance as the centrally active steroid for maintaining copulatory behavior and for defeminizing males during sexual differentiation [58,64].

Steroid autoradiographic methods demonstrate the potential hormone-binding of a particular system. The method is limited by the expense of injecting labeled steroids directly into the individual and by the necessity of gonadectomizing the animal. An alternative approach, using an exchange assay, was devised to measure cell nuclear receptor *occupation* by endogenous steroids [81]. Briefly, brain or pituitary cell nuclei, which contain unlabeled estradiol-receptor complexes that have translocated from the cytoplasm, are extracted with 0.4 M KCl to solubilize the receptors. They are then incubated with excess [³H] estra-

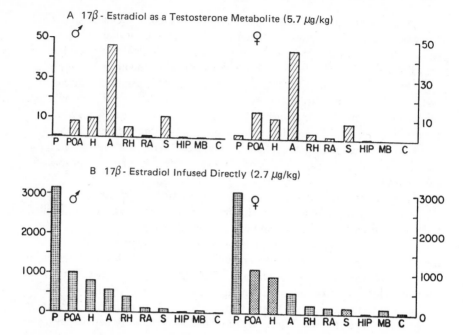

Figure 3   Levels of 17β-estradiol in cell nuclear fractions of gonadectomized-adrenalectomized adult male and female rat brain. Values are expressed as fmol/mg DNA. (A) Levels of radioactivity, identifiable as estradiol, 2 h following injection of tritiated testosterone (5.7 µg/kg). (B) Levels of radioactivity recovered 2 h after injection of tritiated estradiol (2.7 µg/kg). A, corticomedial amygdala; H, basomedial hypothalamus; HIP, hippocampus; C, parietal cerebral cortex; P, whole pituitary; POA, preoptic area; RA, rest of amygdala; RH, rest of hypothalamus; MB, midbrain central grey; S, septum. (From Ref. 48.)

diol to exchange labeled for unlabeled estradiol with an efficiency approaching 100%. The power of this method rests in its ability to provide measurements of estrogen receptor occupation during a variety of hormonal conditions including physiological states. If it were desirable, occupation could then be compared directly with estimates of capacity.

2. Neonates

The distribution of estrogen-concentrating cells in neonates, as measured by exchange or [3H] estradiol uptake, is very similar to that of adults [53,86]. An exception is that estradiol receptors are found in the cortex of neonates and disappear by weaning [52]. As with adults, there are no detectable sex differences in brain estrogen receptors in neonates. These receptors, which are detectable

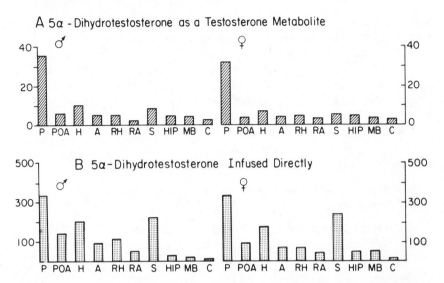

Figure 4 Levels of 5α-dihydrotestosterone in cell nuclear fractions of gonadectomized-adrenalectomized adult male and female rat brain, expressed as fmol/
mg DNA. (A) Levels of radioactivity identifiable as 5α-dihydrotestosterone after
injection of tritiated testosterone (5.7 μg/kg). (B) Levels of radioactivity after
injection of tritiated 5α-dihydrotestosterone (2-4 μg/kg). All determinations
were made 2h following hormone injections. Abbreviations as in Fig. 3. (From
Ref. 48.)

some days before birth [91], increase markedly in concentration starting 1 to 2
days prior to birth, and plateau around day 6 [52]. This may be compared to the
period of sexual differentiation outlined in Figure 2.

In spite of the absence of sex differences in the distribution of estrogen receptors, there are detectable differences in estrogen-receptor occupation in brain
cell nuclei [52]. Testosterone secretion in males begins around day 15 or 16 of
gestation and aromatizing enzyme activity is detectable in brain tissue at that
time (MacLusky et al., unpublished observations). By day 21 of gestation, estrogen-receptor occupation is detectable and coincides with the rapid rise of estrogen
receptors noted above. The brain of the female apparently is protected from
estradiol of maternal origin by the action of α-fetoprotein which binds the estradiol by mass action and prevents it from occupying the receptors and thereby
defeminizing the females [see 54, for review].

Results from autoradiographic studies, cell fractionation, and measurements
of cell nuclear receptor occupation support the view of a genomic mechanism of
action of estradiol in reproduction. Although a complete analysis of this mode
of action is beyond the scope of this chapter, important supporting evidence in-

cludes the following: (1) the time courses of steroid action are measured in hours or days, in contrast to minutes or seconds, which would suggest direct membrane effects [56]; (2) RNA and protein synthesis inhibitors block the biological actions of steroids [76,77]; (3) steroidal and nonsteroidal antagonists of gonadal hormone action compete for nuclear uptake, and such competition is correlated with antagonism of the biological actions of the hormones [29,82]; (4) there is evidence of induction of enzyme activity and of enzyme quantity following treatment with gonadal hormones [49-51].

B. Functional Concomitants of Estrogen Binding in Neural Tissue

1. Neuroanatomic and Biochemical Correlates of Estrogen Action in Mating Behavior

Areas shown by autoradiography and other methods to concentrate estradiol have been linked in several ways to the control of steroid-dependent behaviors. The relationships between steroid concentration and biological activity holds for a number of species and behaviors [66].

Estrogen receptor occupation in preoptic-hypothalamic tissue varies over the estrous cycle, fluctuating with the blood levels of estradiol. Estrogen receptor occupation increases on the second day of the 4-day cycle, whereas peak estrogen receptor occupation occurs on the third day at proestrus. The proestrus peak probably just precedes the time of macimal sexual receptivity [62]. In ovariectomized rats, replacement paradigms designed to provide either subphysiological, physiological, or supraphysiological doses of estradiol indicated that levels that mimicked the proestrous values were sufficient to prime estrous behavior [62].

In rats, as well as in several other species, results of lesion and electrical stimulation studies suggest that the integrity of the preoptic area, a steroid-concentrating region, is crucial to the expression of masculine copulatory behavior [see Ref. 23 for review]. In contrast, similar studies in females point to the ventromedial region of the hypothalamus as critical for feminine sexual behavior [72,73].

One direct means of assessing the functional correlates of steroid uptake in neural tissue entails applying hormones directly to the region of interest in the CNS. In males, implants of either testosterone [39] or estradiol [18,23] in the preoptic area restore copulatory behavior following castration. Similarly, estrogenic implants in the ventromedial hypothalamus facilitate the expression of feminine sexual behavior [4].

Recently, with a technique employing tritiated estradiol diluted with cholesterol, we were able to show that estrogenic stimulation of the ventromedial hypothalamus was sufficient to prime estrous behavior so that the full range of behaviors was exhibited following systemic progesterone treatment [25]. Using a similar approach, Rubin and Barfield [82] demonstrated that such diluted implants were only effective when directly in or immediately adjacent to the ventro-medial nucleus itself. We are now analyzing the spread of radioactivity from our implant sites (Davis et al., unpublished results) to determine precisely which sites within this restricted region are labeled. Our results are consistent with a site of action at the immediate site of implantation. Thus, any biochemical con-sequences of estrogen action critical to the expression of feminine sexual be-havior should occur in the same region, directly around the implant site in the ventromedial hypothalamus. Whether such changes are detectable with the pres-ent technology is problematic. We are able to assess the estrogen-dependent events that occur in less restricted brain regions and at higher doses of the hor-mone. Once these events of interest are identified, it should be possible to ex-amine them under more limiting conditions.

One of the most promising routes for investigation is the analysis of the pro-gestin receptor which has depended for its success upon the use of the synthetic progestin, R 5020. R 5020 has a 10-fold greater affinity for the receptor and it dissociates less rapidly than does the natural hormone [53]. It synergizes with estradiol to promote estrous behavior at a dose one-tenth that required of pro-gesterone itself [13]. Progestin receptor distribution in the brain has been mapped with autoradiography [94] and by cell fractionation studies [11,53].

Progestin receptors are detectable in gonadectomized animals, but estrogen treatment causes an increase in receptor level in some regions of the brain and in the pituitary [53]. Induction of the progestin receptor by estrogen occurs in a subset of the estradiol-concentrating neurons. Specifically, an induction of ap-proximately fourfold occurs in the preoptic area and basomedial hypothalamus. Induction is not detectable in the amygdala or the bed nucleus of the stria ter-minalis. In general, progestin receptor induction tends to occur in midline rather than leteral structures [94]. Table 1 shows a comparison of the properties of estrogen concentrating neurons with respect ot aromatization, 5α-reduction, and progestin receptor induction.

Progestin receptor induction is well-correlated with the appearance of femi-nine sexual behavior in females [68]. Induction of the receptors reaches a maxi-mum approximately 24 to 48 h following the beginning of estrogen treatment. At approximately 18 h after the onset of estrogen treatment, progestin receptors are about 30% of the maximal value and feminine sexual behavior is first ob-served. The peak of the behavioral response coincides with the peak of receptor induction. Moreover, when progesterone is administered intravenously, its ability to facilitate feminine sexual behavior correlates temporally with the translocation of progesterone-receptor complexes to brain cell nuclei [63].

Certain predictions arise relating to estrogenic priming of feminine sexual behavior at the ventromedial hypothalamus with the induction of progestin re-ceptors and the appearance of sexual behavior. First, behaviorally effective doses of estradiol should induce progestin receptors in that subset of the ventromedial hypothalamus containing estrogen-concentrating cells. Then, under controlled

Table 1 A Comparison of the Properties of Estradiol-Concentrating Region of
Brain and Pituitary Tissue of Adult Rats

Region	Aromatization[a]	5'-Reduction[a]	P-Receptor ind.[b]
Anterior pituitary	– –	++	++
Preoptic area	+	+	+
Basomedial hypothalamus	+	+	+
Amygdala	++	+	–

[a] From Ref. 48.
[b] From Ref. 52.

conditions (i.e., minimal doses) of estrogen priming, the effectiveness of locally
applied progesterone in facilitating sexual behavior should be limited to the ventromedial hypothalamus. If induction of the progestin receptor were required
for expression of all components of reminine sexual behavior, doses of estradiol
that do not induce the receptors in the hypothalamus should be incapable of
priming estrous behavior. Thus far, it has been difficult to develop a consistent
assay for measuring progestin receptor induction in discrete hypothalamic nuclei;
but Rubin [83] has shown that implants of progesterone are most effective in
facilitating estrogen primed sexual behavior when they are placed in the ventromedial hypothalamus. The foregoing relationships are suggestive of some of the
possible sufficient conditions for the expression of feminine sexual behavior.
Whether these conditions are also necessary remains to be determined. The interplay between the ventromedial hypothalamus and other portions of the CNS in
the control of reproduction in the gonadally intact animal must also be considered.

Other avenues for investigating estrogen-biochemistry-behavior relationships
include steroid-neurotransmitter interactions. For example, the monoaminergic
neurotransmitters fluctuate over the estrous cycle [46], and also seem to be important in the expression of various components of feminine sexual behavior
[30]. Therefore, it would appear reasonable that estradiol and progesterone
play some role in modulating neurotransmission [see 22, for review]. Indeed,
estradiol regulates hypothalamic monoamines and their enzymes [57] and also
increases muscarinic cholinergic receptors in some estrogen-concentrating cell
groups [78]. It has been suggested that the regulation by steroids of neurotransmitter receptor density may be one way in which steroids could activate particular neural circuits underlying reproductive behavior [55]. Other possibilities in-

clude effects on neurotransmitter metabolism [21], and these mechanisms are not mutually exclusive.

2. Correlates of Estrogen Action During the Perinatal Period of Development

The appearance and occupation of estrogen receptors in the developing rat brain coincide with the period of sexual differentiation (see above and Fig. 2). There is substantial evidence that estrogen receptor occupation reflects the intracellular aromatization of testosterone to a physiologically active metabolite, estradiol. First, estrogens and aromatizable androgens are the most effective agents in defeminizing rats [28,95]. Also agents that antagonize estradiol (antiestrogens such as CI-628) or that block the conversion of testosterone to estradiol (aromatase inhibitors such as ATD) attenuate or prevent defeminization [15,58,92]. When the aromatase inhibitor, ATD (1,4,6-androstatriene-3,17-dione) is administered from days 1 through 10 of life, male rats subsequently show full estrous behavior under estrogen-progesterone treatment [58]. When they remain gonadally intact throughout the course of treatment, they show both estrous and normal masculine copulatory behavior [24]. The capacity for both masculine and feminine patterns of mating behavior supports the view that the substrates for each differentiate independently.

It is possible that the neural substrates for masculine and feminine sexual behavior are either differentially sensitive to hormone treatment or that the processes of masculinization and defeminization occur at different developmental times. Some investigators have suggested that masculinization occurs in large part prior to birth [20,93]. But one major parameter of masculine copulatory behavior, the temporal patterning, is identical in neonatally androgenized females and normal males [85]. The importance of temporal patterning as a measure is that it is relatively independent of external morphologic development which can limit performance (see above).

Females treated with testosterone within 6 h of birth readily show intromission and ejaculatory motor patterns as adults [89]. In comparison, castration of males within 1 h of birth renders them almost identical to normal females when tested for feminine sexual behavior as adults [88]. These data, together with the finding that testosterone surges immediately after birth in male rats [87], suggest that the critical period during the immediate postnatal period may be extremely brief. In this view, the so-called critical period of sexual differentiation which occurs pre- and postnatally in rats would represent the entire interval of the development and waning of sensitivity of neural tissue to gonadal hormones. Hormonal manipulations at any time during the approximately 15 day period might be expected to influence elements of both masculinization and defeminization. But the period immediately around birth may be crucial for setting the complete pattern of adult sexual behavior. It would be of major importance to determine these intervals precisely. Such determinations may be confounded by the possibility that different strains of rats have slightly different gestation lengths [16]. Also, variance in gestation length may account for at least part of the disparate findings on the critical period for sexual differentiation.

An important aspect of sexual differentiation concerns the mechanisms by which estrogen brings about permanent alterations in CNS function. It is clear that sexual dimorphisms in reproductive function are not correlated with either patterns of steroid hormone uptake or progestin receptor induction (see above). The early effects of estrogen may result in morphologic alterations in the CNS and several such sexually dimorphic characteristics of adult brains have been observed. These include: (1) the patterns of dendritic branching in hamster brains [36]; (2) cell nuclear and nucleolar size [69]; (3) the type of synaptic endings [79]; and (4) the size of large nuclear regions. In rats, a region within the preoptic area, termed the sexually dimorphic nucleus (SDN), is larger in males than in females [34].

Steroid hormones exert their permanent, organizational effects upon CNS structure and function during a period of developmental plasticity. One way in which this can occur is through regulation of cell growth and differentiation. Estradiol and testosterone stimulate neurite outgrowth [90] in tissue cultures of preoptic and hypothalamic areas from newborn mouse. The antiestrogen, CI-628, attenuates neurite outgrowth stimulated by testosterone, suggesting that conversion to estradiol is an important step in the process. Such findings are consistent with what is known about the hormonal correlates of sexual differentiation, but it is unknown whether they are the foundation for dimorphisms in reproductive function.

It now appears most likely that sexual dimorphisms in brain structure are related to sex differences in patterns of gonadotropin secretion [80]. As noted previously, it is with respect to that end point that sex differences in the adult are sharpest. It is difficult to imagine that gross, morphologic differences in male and female brains underlie differences in the relative probabilities of particular behavioral responses. Sex differences in mating behavior may result from the interactions of several factors including afferent sensory input, peripheral morphologic structures, individual responsiveness to relevant environmental stimuli, and the state of the CNS substrate, any or all of which may be modulated by hormone-receptor interactions. Relatively subtle alterations in the wiring of relevant portions of the CNS could be important in changing the probability of occurrence of certain behaviors. In addition, some of the biochemical consequences of hormone-receptor interactions that occur in one sex may not occur in the other. These possibilities, alterations of neuronal circuitry and of the biochemical consequences of hormone-receptor interaction as a result of the hormonal milieu of early development, are clearly not mutually exclusive, but offer several prospects for future research.

III. Conclusions

We have examined some of the biochemical and behavioral consequences of estrogen action in rats. Where possible, we have attempted to correlate the uptake and binding of estradiol by neural tissue with the regulation of reproductive function. In rats, and in many other species, these functional relationships are evident during two periods in the life of the individual. As adults, individuals respond to gonadal hormones in a manner determined, in part, by the hormonal milieu of the perinatal period. We have compared the mechanisms of action of steroid hormones during development and in adult life.

The binding of steroids by specific neural regions represents a phylogenetically stable event that has been observed in all classes of vertebrates. Without exception, binding of gonadal hormones is correlated with the regulation of reproductive function. Moreover, the mechanisms of steroid action appear fundamentally similar throughout all species examined. To what extent such relationships hold for humans is presently not well understood. In humans, the expression of reproductive and social behaviors is the result of complex interactions among environment, genetic endowment, and internal physiological events. The precise nature of these interactions remains to be described. While the cellular bases of hormone action in humans are likely to be the same as in other species, it is not now possible to assess the participation of such cellular events in the regulation of behavioral expression in humans.

Acknowledgments

Research from the authors' laboratory, described herein, is supported by USPHS grant NS 07080 and by an institutional grant RF 70095 from the Rockefeller Foundation for research in reproductive biology. Dr. Davis received fellowship support from the USPHS MH 05781. We wish to thank Oksana Wengerchuk for typing the manuscript.

References

1. Adler, N. T. (1978). Social and environmental control of reproductive processes in animals. In *Sexual Behavior, Status and Prospectus* (T. E. McGill, D. A. Dewsbury, and B. D. Sachs, eds.). Plenum, New York, pp. 115-160.
2. Adler, N. T., P. G. Davis, and B. R. Komisaruk (1977). Variation in the size and sensitivity of a genital sensory field in relation to the estrous cycle in rats. *Horm. Behav.* 9:334-344.
3. Barfield, R. J., P. Auerbach, L. A. Geyer, and T. K. McIntosh (1979). Ultrasonic vocalization in rat sexual behavior. *Am. Zool.* 19:469-480.
4. Barfield, R. J., and J. J. Chen (1977). Activation of estrous behavior in

ovariectomized rats by intracerebral implants of estradiol benzoate. *Endocrinology* 101:1716-1725.

5.   Baum, M. J., and J. T. M. Vreeburg (1973). Copulation in castrated male rats following combined treatment with estradiol and dihydrotestosterone. *Science* 182:283-285.

6.   Beach, F. A. (1948). *Hormones and Behavior.* Hoeber, New York.

7.   Beach, F. A. (1967). Factors involved in the control of mounting behavior by female mammals. In *Reproduction and Sexual Behavior* (M. Diamond, ed.). Indiana University Press, Bloomington, pp. 88-131.

8.   Beach, F. A. (1971). Hormonal factors controlling the differentiation, development and display of copulatory behavior in the ramstergig and related species. In *The Biopsychology of Development* (E. Tobach, L. R. Aronson, and E. Shaw eds.). Academic, New York, pp. 249-296.

9.   Beach, F. A. (1976). Sexual attractivity, proceptivity, and receptivity in female mammals. *Horm. Behav.* 7:105-133.

10. Beach, F. A., R. G. Noble, and R. K. Orndoff (1969). Effects of perinatal androgen treatment on responses of male rats to gonadal hormones in adulthood. *J. Comp. Physiol. Psychol.* 68:490-497.

11. Blaustein, J. D., and H. H. Feder (1979). Cytoplasmic progestin receptors in female guinea pig brain and their relationship to refractoriness in expression of female sexual behavior. *Brain Res.* 177:489-498.

12. Blaustein, J. D., and G. N. Wade (1977). Sequential inhibition of sexual behavior by progesterone in female rats: comparison with a synthetic antiestrogen. *J. Comp. Physiol. Psychol.* 91:752-760.

13. Blaustein, J. D., and G. N. Wade (1978). Progestin binding by brain and pituitary cell nuclei and female rat sexual behavior. *Brain Res.* 140:360-372.

14. Boling, J. L., and R. J. Blandau (1939). The estrogen-protesterone induction of mating responses in the spayed female rat. *Endocrinology* 25:359-364.

15. Booth, J. E. (1978). Effects of the aromatization inhibitor Androst-4-ene-3,6,17-trione on sexual differentiation induced by testosterone in the neonatally castrated rat. *J. Endocrinol.* 79:69-76.

16. Butterstein, G. M., and E. S. Freis (1978). Effect of parturition time on the response to neonatal androgen in female rats. *Proc. Soc. Exp. Biol. Med.* 158:179-182.

17. Carr, W. J., L. S. Loeb, and M. L. Dissinger (1965). Responses of rats to sex odors. *J. Comp. Physiol. Psychol.* 59:370-377.

18. Christensen, L. W., and L. G. Clemens (1974). Intrahypothalamic implants of testosterone or estradiol and resumption of masculine sexual behavior in long-term castrated male rats. *Endocrinology* 95:984-990.

19. Clark, J. H., and E. J. Peck, Jr. (1979). *Female Sex Steroids.* Springer-Verlag, Berlin.

20. Clemens, L. G., B. A. Gladue, and L. P. Coniglio (1978). Prenatal endo-
     genous androgenic influences on masculine sexual behavior and genital
     morphology in male and female rats. *Hrom. Behav.* 10:40-53.
21. Crowley, W. R., T. L. O'Donohue, H. Wachslicht, and D. M. Jacobowitz
     (1978). Effects of estrogen and progesterone on plasma gonadotropins
     and on catecholamine levels and turnover in discrete brain regions of ovari-
     ectomized rats. *Brain Res.* 154:345-357.
22. Crowley, W. R., and F. P. Zemlan (1976). The neurochemical basis of
     sexual behavior. In *Neuroendocrinology of Reproduction* (N. T. Adler,
     ed.). Plenum, New York.
23. Davis, P. G., and R. J. Barfield (1979). Activation of masculine sexual
     behavior by intracranial estradiol benzoate implants in male rats. *Neuro-
     endocrinology* 28:217-227.
24. Davis, P. G., C. V. Chaptal, and B. S. McEwen (1979). Independence of
     the differentiation of masculine and feminine sexual behavior in rats. *Horm.
     Behav.* 12:12-19.
25. Davis, P. G., B. S. McEwen, and D. W. Pfaff (1979). Localized behavioral
     effects of tritiated estradiol implants in the ventromedial hypothalamus of
     female rats. *Endocrinology* 104:893-903.
26. Denef, C., C. Magnus, and B. S. McEwen (1973). Sex differences and
     hormonal control of testosterone metabolism in rat pituitary and brain.
     J. Endocrinol. 59:605-621.
27. Diczfalusy, E. (ed.) (1970). Steroid assay by protein binding. *Karolinska
     Symposia: 2nd Symposium* (Geneva), Stockholm, Sweden.
28. Doughty, C., J. E. Booth, P. A. McDonald, and R. F. Parrott (1975). Ef-
     fects of oestradiol-17β, oestradiol benzoate and the synthetic oestrogen
     RU-2858 on sexual differentiation in the neonatal female rat. *J. Endo-
     crinol.* 67:419-424.
29. Etgen, A. M. (1979). Antiestrogens: effects of tamoxifen, Nafoxidine,
     and CI-628 on sexual behavior, cytoplasmic receptors, and nuclear binding
     of receptors. *Horm. Behav.* 2:97-112.
30. Everitt, B. J., K. Fuxe, T. Hökfelt, and G. Jonsson (1975). Role of mono-
     amines in the control by hormones of sexual receptivity in the female rat.
     J. Comp. Physiol. Psychol. 89:556-572.
31. Feder, H. H., and B. L. Marrone (1977). Progesterone: its role in the
     central nervous system as a facilitator and inhibitor of sexual behavior and
     gonadotropin release. *Ann. N.Y. Acad. Sci.* 286:331-354.
32. Feder, H. H., F. Naftolin, and K. J. Ryan (1974). Male and female sexual
     responses in male rats given estradiol benzoate and 5α-androstan-17β-ol-3-
     one propionate. *Endocrinology* 94:136-141.
33. Gorski, R. A. (1978). Sexual differentiation of the brain. *Hosp. Prac.* 13:
     55-62.
34. Gorski, R. A., J. H. Gordon, J. E. Shryne, and A. M. Southam (1978).

Evidence for a morphological sex difference within the medial preoptic area of the rat brain. *Brain Res.* 148:333-346.

35. Green, R., W. G. Luttge, and R. E. Whalen (1970). Induction of receptivity in ovariectomized female rats by a single intravenous injection of estradiol 17β.

36. Greenough, W. T., C. S. Carter, C. Steerman, and T. J. DeVoogd (1977). Sex differences in dendritic patterns in hamster preoptic area. *Brain Res.* 126:63-72.

37. Harris, G. W. (1964). Sex hormones, brain development, and brain function. *Endocrinology* 75:627-648.

38. Jaffe, B. M., and Behrman, H. R. (eds.) (1978). *Methods of Hormone Radioimmunoassay.* Academic, New York.

39. Johnston, P., and J. M. Davidson (1972). Intracerebral androgens and sexual behavior in the male rat. *Horm. Behav.* 3:345-357.

40. Josso, N., M. G. Forest, and J. Y. Picard (1975). Müllerian-inhibiting activity of calf fetal testis: relationship of testosterone and protein synthesis. *Biol. Reprod.* 13:163-167.

41. Karen, L. M., and R. J. Barfield (1975). Differential rates of exhaustion and recovery of several parameters of male rat sexual behavior. *J. Comp. Physiol. Psychol.* 88:693-703.

42. Kow, L. M., M. O. Montgomery, and D. W. Pfaff (1979). Triggering of lordosis reflex in female rats with somatosensory stimulation: quantitative determination of stimulus parameters. *J. Neurophysiol.* 42:195-202.

43. Kow, L. M., and D. W. Pfaff (1975). Induction of lordosis in female rats: two modes of estrogen action and the effect of adrenalectomy. *Horm. Behav.* 6:259-276.

44. Krieger, M. S., and R. J. Barfield (1974). Independence of temporal patterning of male mounting behavior from the influence of androgen during the neonatal period. *Physiol. Behav.* 14:251-254.

45. Krieger, M. S., and R. J. Barfield (1976). Masculine sexual behavior: pacing and ejaculatory patterns in female rats induced by electric shock. *Physiol. Behav.* 16:671-675.

46. Kueng, W., A. Wirz-Justice, R. Menzi, and E. Chappuis-Arndt (1976). Regional brain variations of tryptophan, monoamines, monoamine oxidase activity, plasma free and total tryptophan during the estrous cycle of the rat. *Neuroendocrinology* 21:289-296.

47. Larsson, K., P. Sodersten, and C. Beyer (1973). Induction of male sexual behavior by estradiol benzoate in combination with dihydrotestosterone. *J. Endocrinol.* 57:563-564.

48. Lieberburg, I., and B. S. McEwen (1977). Brain cell nuclear retention of testosterone metabolites, 5α-dihydrotestosterone and estradiol 17β, in adult rats. *Endocrinology* 100:588-597.

49. Luine, V. N., and B. S. McEwen (1977). Effect of oestradiol on turnover of Type A monoamine oxidase in brain. *J. Neurochem.* 28:1221-1227.

50. Luine, V. N., B. S. McEwen, and I. B. Black (1977). Effect of 17β-estradiol on hypothalamic tyrosine hydroxylase activity. *Brain Res.* 120:188-192.

51. Luine, V. M., D. Park, T. Joh, D. Reis, and B. S. McEwen (1980). Immunochemical demonstration of increased choline acetyltransferase concentration in rat preoptic area after estradiol administration. *Brain Res.* 191:273-277.

52. MacLusky, N. J., I. Lieberburg, and B. S. McEwen (1979). The development of estrogen receptors in the rat brain: perinatal development. *Brain Res.* 178:129-142.

53. MacLusky, N. J., and B. S. McEwen (1980). Progestin receptors in rat brain: distribution and properties of cytoplasmic progestin-binding sites. *Endocrinology* 106:192-202.

54. McEwen, B. S. (1980). Gonadal influences on the developing brain. In *Handbook of Biological Psychiatry, Part III, Brain Mechanisms and Abnormal Behavior—Genetics and Neuroendocrinology* (H. M. Van Praag, M. H. Lader, O. J. Rafaelsen, and E. J. Sachar, eds.). Marcel Dekker, New York, pp. 241-278.

55. McEwen, B. S., A. Biegon, T. C. Rainbow, C. Paden, L. Snyder, and V. DeGroff (1981). The interaction of estrogens with intracellular receptors and with putative neurotransmitter receptors: implications for the mechanism of activation of sexual behavior and ovulation. In *Steroid Hormone Regulation of the Brain,* K. Fuxe, J. A. Gustafsson, and L. Wetterberg, eds.). Pergamon Press, London.

56. McEwen, B. S., P. G. Davis, B. Parsons, and D. W. Pfaff (1979). The brain as a target for steroid hormone action. *Ann. Rev. Neurosci.* 2:65-112.

57. McEwen, B. S., L. C. Krey, and V. N. Luine (1978). Steroid hormone action in the neuroendocrine system: When is the genome involved? In *The Hypothalamus* (S. Reichlin, R. J. Baldessarini, and J. B. Martin, eds.). Raven Press, New York, 255-268.

58. McEwen, B. S., I. Lieberburg, C. Chaptal, and L. C. Krey (1977). Aromatization: important for sexual differentiation of the neonatal rat brain. *Horm. Behav.* 9:249-263.

59. McEwen, B. S., and D. W. Pfaff (1970). Factors influencing sex hormone uptake by rat brain regions. I. Effects of neonatal treatment, hypophysectomy, and competing steroid on estradiol uptake. *Brain Res.* 21:1-16.

60. McEwen, B. S., D. W. Pfaff, and R. E. Zigmond (1970). Factors influencing sex hormone uptake. II. Effects of neonatal treatment and hypophysectomy on testosterone uptake. *Brain Res.* 21:17-28.

61. McEwen, B. S., D. W. Pfaff, and R. E. Zigmond (1970). Factors influenc-

ing sex hormone uptake by rat brain regions. III. Effects of competing steroids on testosterone uptake. *Brain Res.* 21:29-38.

62. McGinnis, M. Y., L. C. Krey, N. J. MacLusky, and B. S. McEwen (1981). Steroid receptor levels in intact and castrate estrogen-treated rats: An examination of the quantitative, temporal, and endocrine factors which influence the neuroendocrine efficacy of an estradiol stimulus. *Neuroendocrinology*

63. McGinnis, M. Y., B. Parsons, T. C. Rainbow, L. C. Krey, and B. S. McEwen (1981). Temporal relationship between cell nuclear progestin receptor levels and sexual receptivity following intravenous progesterone administration. *Brain Res.* 218:365-371.

64. Morali, G., K. Larsson, and C. Beyer (1977). Inhibition of testosterone-induced sexual behavior in the castrated male rat by aromatase blockers. *Horm. Behav.* 9:203-213.

65. Morin, L. P. (1977). Progesterone: inhibition of rodent sexual behavior. *Physiol. Behav.* 18:701-715.

66. Morrell, J. I., D. B. Kelley, and D. W. Pfaff (1975). Sex steroid binding in the brains of vertebrates: studies with light-microscope autoradiography. In *Brain Endocrine Interaction II. The Ventricular System* (K. M. Knigge, D. S. Scott, K. Kobayashi, and S. Ishi, eds.). Karger, Basel, pp. 230-256.

67. Naftolin, F., K. J. Ryan, I. J. Davies, V. V. Reddy, F. Flores, Z. Petro, M. Kuhn, R. J. While, Y. Takaoka, and I. Wolin (1975). The formation of estrogens by central neuroendocrine tissues. *Rec. Prog. Horm. Res.* 31: 391-315.

68. B. Parsons, N. J. MacLusky, L. Krey, D. W. Pfaff, and B. S. McEwen (1980). The temporal relationship between estrogen-inducible progestin receptors in the female rat brain and the time course of estrogen activation of mating behavior. *Endocrinology* 107:774-779.

69. Pfaff, D. W. (1966). Morphological changes in the brains of adult male rats after neonatal castration. *J. Endocrinol.* 36:415-416.

70. Pfaff, D. W. (1970). Nature of sex hormone effect on rat sex behavior: specificity of effects and individual patterns of response. *J. Comp. Physiol. Psychol.* 73:349-358.

71. Pfaff, D. W., and M. Keiner (1973). Atlas of estradiol-concentrating neurons in the central nervous system of the female rat. *J. Comp. Neurol.* 151: 121-158.

72. Pfaff, D. W., and Y. Sakuma (1979). Deficit in the lordosis reflex of female rats caused by lesions in the ventromedial nucleus of the hypothalamus. *J. Physiol.* 288:203-210.

73. Pfaff, D. W., and Y. Sakuma (1979). Facilitation of the lordosis reflex of female rats from the ventromedial nucleus of the hypothalamus. *J. Physiol.* 288:189-202.

74. Plapinger, L., and B. S. McEwen (1978). Gonadal steroid-brain interactions

in sexual differentiation. In *Biological Determinants of Sexual Behavior* (J. Hutchison, ed.). John Wiley, New York and London, pp. 193-218.

75. Powers, J. B. (1970). Hormonal control of sexual receptivity during the estrous cycle of the rat. *Physiol. Behav.* 5:831-835.

76. Quadagno, D. M., J. Shryne, and R. A. Gorski (1971). Inhibition of steroid-induced sexual behavior by intrahypothalamic actinomycin-D. *Horm. Behav.* 2:1-10.

77. Rainbow, T. C., P. G. Davis, and B. S. McEwen (1980). Anixomycin inhibits the activation of sexual behavior by estradiol and progesterone. *Brain Res.* 194:548-555.

78. Rainbow, T. C., V. DeGroff, V. N. Luine, and B. S. McEwen (1980). Estradiol 17β increases the number of muscarinic receptors in hypothalamus nuclei. *Brain Res.* 198:239-243.

79. Raisman, G., and P. M. Field (1971). Sexual dimorphism in the preoptic area of the rat. *Science* 173:731-733.

80. Raisman, G., and P. M. Field (1973). Sexual dimorphism in the neuropil of the preoptic area of the rat and its dependence on neonatal androgen. *Brain Res.* 54:1-29.

81. Roy, E. J., and B. S. McEwen (1977). An exchange assay for estrogen receptors in cell nuclei of the adult rat brain. *Steroids* 30:657-669.

82. Roy, E. J., and G. N. Wade (1977). Binding of (^{3}H) estradiol by brain cell nuclei and female rat sexual behavior: inhibition by antiestrogens. *Brain Res.* 126:73-87.

83. Rubin, B. S. (1981). Localization of neural target sites for progesterone action in the regulation of estrous behavior in the female rat. Unpublished doctoral dissertation, Rutgers University, 1981.

84. Rubin, B. S., and R. J. Barfield (1980). Priming of estrous responsiveness by implants of 17β-estradiol in the ventromedial nucleus of female rats. *Endocrinology* 106:504-509.

85. Sachs, B. D., E. I. Pollak, M. S. Krieger, and R. J. Barfield (1973). Sexual behavior: normal male patterning in androgenized female rats. *Science* 181:770-772.

86. Sheridan, P. J., M. Sar, and W. E. Stumpf (1974). Autoradiographic localization of ^{3}H-estradiol or its metabolites in the central nervous system of the developing rat. *Endocrinology* 95:1749-1753.

87. Slob, A. K., M. P. OOms, and J. T. M. Vreeburg (1980). Prenatal and early postnatal sex differences in plasma and gonadal testosterone and plasma luteinizing hormone in female and male rats. *J. Endocrinol.* 87:81-87.

88. Thomas, C. N., and A. A. Gerall (1969). Effect of hour of castration on feminization of neonatally castrated male rats. *Psychon. Sci.* 16:19-20.

89. Thomas, D. A., T. K. McIntosh, and R. J. Barfield (1980). Influence of

androgen in the neonatal period on ejaculatory and postejaculatory behavior in the rat. *Horm. Behav.* 14:153-162.

90. Toran-Allerand, C. D. (1976). Sex steroids and the development of the newborn mouse hypothalamus and preoptic area in vitro: implications for sexual differentiation. *Brain Res.* 106:407-412.

91. Vito, C. C., and T. O. Fox (1979). Embryonic rodent brain contains estrogen receptors. *Science* 204:517-519.

92. Vreeburg, J. T. M., P. D. M. van der Vaart, and P. van der Schoot (1977). Prevention of central defeminization but not masculinization in male rats by inhibition neonatally of oestrogen biosynthesis. *J. Endocrinol.* 74:375-382.

93. Ward, I. L. (1969). Differential effect of pre- and postnatal androgen on the sexual behavior of intact and spayed female rats. *Horm. Behav.* 1:25-36.

94. Warembourg, M. (1978). Uptake of ^{3}H labeled synthetic progestin by rat brain and pituitary. A radioautographic study. *Neurosci. Lett.* 9:329-333.

95. Whalen, R. E., and D. L. Rezek (1974). Inhibition of lordosis in female rats by subcutaneous implants of testosterone, androstenedione or dihydrotestosterone in infancy. *Horm. Behav.* 5:157-162.

96. Young, W. C. (1961). The hormones and mating behavior. In *Sex and Internal Secretion,* Vol. 2 (W. C. Yang, ed.). Williams & Wilkins, Baltimore, pp. 1173-1239.

97. Young, W. C., R. W. Goy, and C. H. Phoenix (1964). Hormones and sexual behavior. *Science* 143:212-217.

98. Zemlan, F. P., and N. T. Adler (1977). Hormonal control of female sexual behavior in the rat. *Horm. Behav.* 9:345-357.

4 Hypothalamic Peptides and Sexual Behavior

ROBERT L. MOSS and CAROL A. DUDLEY   University of Texas Health Science Center, Dallas, Texas

Luteinizing hormone-releasing hormone (LHRH) is a decapeptide originally isolated from hypothalamic tissue and identified on the basis of its ability to release both luteinizing hormone (LH) and follicle-stimulating hormone (FSH) from the anterior pituitary gland in all mammalian species including rat and humans [1,2]. In the pituitary gland, LHRH appears to stimulate LH release preferentially. In the normal human female, LHRH injection has profound effects on the menstrual cycle, which suggests both the possibility of enhancing fertility and preventing conception, while in healthy human males, LHRH administration causes an increase in secretions of gonadotropins and testosterone. In addition to these well-defined actions, other biologic effects associated with LHRH have been discovered; perhpas the most important are the behavioral and neuropharmacologic ones [for current review see 3-5].

The notion that LHRH has extrapituitary or extraendocrine actions was first documented in 1973 by this laboratory [6], and a few months later independently confirmed by another laboratory [7]. In general, the two laboratories demonstrated that subcutaneous LHRH administration facilitated female sexual behavior in estrogen-primed ovariectomized rats and that this extraendocrine action of LHRH occurred independent of the presence of the pituitary and adrenal glands. In further experimentation this potentiation of lordosis behavior was found to be specific to LHRH. Administration of estrogen alone or estrogen in combination with either thyrotropin-releasing hormone (TRH), LH, or FSH was ineffective in enhancing mating behavior [6,8]. Evidence for a role of LHRH in male sexual behavior soon appeared. In 1975, subcutaneous LHRH administration was found to decrease the time necessary to achieve intromission and ejaculation both in the intact and testosterone-primed castrated male rat [9]. Thus LHRH in the presence of low exogenous levels of estrogen in the ovariectomized female and testosterone in the castrated male rat enhances sexual behavior.

By this time, the observation that synthetic LHRH facilitates mating behavior in both male and female rats generated considerable interest in the possibility that LHRH therapy may be useful in the treatment of human sexual dysfunction. A number of experiments have since been published [10-17]. In some cases, LHRH administration has enhanced sexual activities in the normal, hypogonadal and in the psychogenetic, secondary impotent human male, while in other cases no observable changes in behavior were demonstrated with LHRH administration. Thus, the evidence of LHRH's ability to enhance human sexual potency is suggestive at best and requires support by additional experiments. Nonetheless, the action of LHRH on mating behavior appears to be somewhat universal. LHRH has been shown to enhance mating in the rat [6-9,18-22], mouse [23,24], pigeon [25], lizard [26], and frog (Kelley, personal communication). Furthermore, LHRH also has been shown to increase sociability and friendliness in the chimpanzee [27]. Experiments on the rat and mouse have not only shown LHRH to be effective in female but also in the male of the species [9,23,28].

The physiological importance of the aforementioned findings have been questioned, and at this point the question is whether the action of LHRH on reproductive behavior is pharmacologic or physiological in nature. This report will examine the question of physiological importance as well as the current status of LHRH's ability to enhance sexual behavior.

I. Brain LHRH and Mating Behavior

The demonstration that subcutaneous LHRH potentiates mating behavior suggested that the decapeptide may be acting directly on neural tissue to bring about the reported behavioral changes. The microinfusion of either 20 or 50 ng LHRH into the medial preoptic area (MPOA), arcuate nucleus (ARC), or midbrain central gray (MCG) was shown to potentiate mating behavior. The delay between the microinfusion of LHRH into neural tissue and the onset of mating behavior was approximately 20 min; the behavioral activity lasted for approximately 8 h. Similar infusions of LHRH into the lateral hypothalamus (LHA), cerebral cortex (CC), and reticular formation (RF) were shown to have no effect on potentiating mating activities [18,19,29]. Thus, infusion of LHRH into specific sites involved with regulation of gonadotropin surge potentiates mating behavior, whereas infusions into nonreproductive sites have no effect on mating. Infusion of TRH or saline into the MPOA, ARC, LHA, CC, RF, and MCG did not induce increases in sexual behavior.

These data suggest that there are at least three positive neural sites in the

CNS for the action of LHRH: the MPOA, ARC, and MCG. Experiments have shown that infusions of LHRH into these neural sites potentiate mating behavior. It is interesting to note that these three neural sites have a number of overlapping neuroendocrine-related characteristics, (1) LHRH localization, (2) LHRH responsive neurons, (3) estrogen localization (4) regulation of gonadotropin secretion, and (5) regulation of mating behavior [3,19,29-59].

From the recent work of Samson et al. [29] there appear to be at least three immunoreactive LHRH systems in the rat. The first system has cell bodies in the POA, and its fibers extend to and terminate in the median eminence (ME). This system is involved with the release of LHRH into the portal capillary system where it acts on specific target cells in the pituitary gland for the release of LH and FSH. The other two systems may be involved with the mediation of an LHRH-behavioral system. One is a dorsal system which extends through the stria medullaris with projections towards the MCG, and the other, more ventral than the first, extends from the POA through the mamillary bodies and into the interpenduncular nucleus. Recently, LHRH immunoreactive terminals have been localized in the MCG [Hoffman, personal communication]. An LHRH immunoreactive system which involves the POA, medial basal hypothalamus, and MCG appears to be present not only in rat but also in bird, mouse, guinea pig, cat, monkey, and man [see 30-32 for reviews].

Interestingly, microelectrophoresis of the peptide hormone has revealed both the excitatory and inhibitory effects of LHRH on hypothalamic as well as extra-hypothalamic neurons [33-40]. LHRH responsive neurons are more widely distributed in the CNS than the decapeptide itself as determined by radioimmunoassay and immunocytochemistry. Microelectrophoresis of LHRH has revealed peptide-sensitive neurons throughout the hypothalamus POA, septum, MCG, as well as in the CC [see 5, 44-48 for reviews]. The microelectrophoresis of LHRH agonist analog resulted in responses that were similar in direction (excitatory or inhibitory) and magnitude to that of synthetic LHRH, suggesting the presence of LHRH receptors in the brain proper (Table 1). It also should be noted that on occasion the LHRH agonist analog induced greater and longer lasting effects than observed with the synthetic LHRH.

Autoradiography has shown estrogen-concentrating cells in brains of a variety of species ranging from monkey to fish [49-51]. The results are in good agreement with biochemical investigation of steroid hormone binding in similar species. A comparison of the binding sites in vertebrates has revealed accumulation of estrogen by neurons in discrete brain regions that include the POA, the tuberal region of the hypothalamus (which included the ARC), and various components of the limbic forebrain and mesencephalic regions (which included the MCG) deep to the tectum. It is clear from these data that the MPOA, ARC nucleus, and MCG contain LHRH-stained neuronal elements, LHRH sensitive neurons, and estrogen-concentrating neurons. These nuclei have also been implicated in the regulation of gonadotropin secretion and mating behavior [see 52-80 for review of both areas].

Table 1 Summary of Responses Observed in Medial Preoptic Neurons to the Microelectrophoresis of Releasing Hormones

Releasing hormones	No. tested	Response [a]		
		↑	↓	→
LHRH[a]	170	52 (31)[b]	22 (13)	96 (56)
LHRH[+]	135	49 (36)	15 (11)	71 (53)
LHRH[o]	96	30 (31)	14 (15)	52 (54)
LHRH[−]	25	3 (12)	4 (15)	18 (72)

[a]LHRH = Luteinizing hormone-releasing hormone.

[b]Number in parentheses = %;[+] = agonist analog; [o] = inactive analog;[−] = antagonist analog.

Source: From Ref. 3, 3rd International Symposium of Brain—Endocrine Interaction: Neural Hormones and Reproduction. (Karger, Basel, 1978.)

II. Analogs of LHRH and Sexual Behavior

The aforementioned data provide supportive evidence for a LHRH neural system that mediates the secretion of gonadotropins by the anterior pituitary gland as well as mating behavior; thus endogenous LHRH may act as a neurotransmitter and/or neuromodulator in the central nervous system (CNS) regulating mating events. These findings have also raised a question as to the physiological significance of endogenous and exogenous LHRH in facilitating mating activities. It stands to reason that synthetic peptide analogs of LHRH which have a variety of characteristics on the release of the gonadotropins from anterior pituitary gland, including extended duration of action, higher potency, and antagonist activity, may provide a useful tool for investigating the physiological role of brain LHRH as a modulator of extrapituitary function.

To date, a number of experiments have been conducted utilizing (1) superactive analogs (which are known to be more active than the parent LHRH in stimulating gonadotropin secretion), (2) inactive analogs (which are known to have little, if any, stimulatory effects on gonadotropin secretion), and (3) antagonist analogs (which are known to inhibit the release of the gonadotropins) as well as anti-LHRH antibody to study the mechanism of action of LHRH on mating behavior [81-84]. In one of these studies [83], subcutaneous administration of either the superactive, inactive, or antagonist analog was found to increase lordosis behavior in ovariectomized, estrogen-primed (5 μg estradiol benzoate), female rats. The finding that all three analogs, independent of whether they are stimulatory, inactive, or inhibitory in releasing LH and FSH, produced positive mating responses, is extremely interesting, especially in light of the electrophysiological action of these analogs. The microelectrophoretic deposition of an inactive LHRH analog was found to be just as effective as the parent LHRH and the LHRH agonist analog in modulating neural activity of MPO neurons [3,41]. Thus analogs, independent of whether they are stimulatory or inactive in stimulating gonadotropin release, appear to possess similar potency in modulating neural activity (Table 1). This would suggest that a common sequence contained within the parent LHRH, inactive, and agonist analogs may be responsible for mediating neuronal as well as mating activities.

Two recent reports have described the inhibitory effect of an anti-LHRH antibody on mating behavior in ovariectomized female rats [81,82]. In one experiment LHRH antibody was infused into the lateral ventricle of estrogen-progesterone primed, ovariectomized female rats [81], while in the other study antibody was infused into the MCG of estrogen-primed, ovariectomized female rats [82]. In both experiments anti-LHRH antibody suppressed mating behavior. In a recent study from our laboratory [84], a specific and long-acting antagonist analog of LHRH was infused into the ARC-VMH (ventromedial hypothalamus) region of estrogen-progesterone primed, ovariectomized female rats. It was found that the LHRH antagonist analog suppressed sexual receptivity in sexually active, hormone-primed female rats (Fig. 1). This finding suggests that specific binding sites for LHRH exist in this brain region. Further support for the existence of LHRH receptor sites in the ARC-VMH comes from neurophysiologic studies which have shown that LHRH applied in minute quantities to the membrane of these neurons is capable of rapidly producing increases or decreases in firing rate [85]. These changes in neuronal excitability may reflect the existence of LHRH receptors. It must be emphasized that the ARC-VMH has been implicated in mediating female sexual behavior [86]. In cyclic female rats, lesions of the VMH suppressed mating [87] and in the ovariectomized rat, such lesions reduced the ability of estrogen to induce sexual activity [88]. In addition, VMH implants of estrogen induced receptivity [89] while LHRH infusions into ARC-VMH enhanced mating in ovariectomized estrogen-primed female rats [90]. Thus, the observations that (1) the antagonist analog of LHRH when infused into the ARC-VMH will suppress mating, (2) the antagonist analog competes specifically with LHRH for receptor sites, and (3) the infusion of the parent LHRH into the ARC-VMH will enhance mating, support the hypothesis that the decrement in mating behavior following infusion of the antagonist analog is due to the inability of endogenous LHRH to act at specific receptor sites already bound by the antagonist.

III. Interaction of LHRH, Prolactin, and Sexual Behavior

There has been increasing evidence that prolactin (PRL) is involved in a wide variety of reproductive activities ranging from a role in regulating the hypothalamic-pituitary-gonadal axis to a role in parental behavior [91-95]. Recently, experiments in our laboratory have demonstrated that PRL administered centrally,

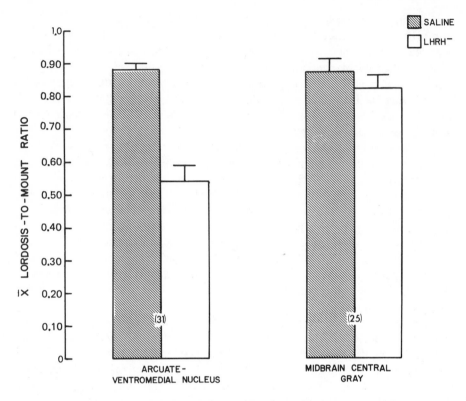

Figure 1 Effect of infusions of an LHRH antagonist analog or saline into the arcuate-ventromedial nucleus or midbrain central gray on the lordosis-to-mount ratio of ovariectomized, estrogen-progesterone primed female rats.

into the third ventricle, can suppress continued female receptivity in estrogen-progesterone primed, ovariectomized rats (Fig. 2). This suggests that centrally acute elevations of PRL can act to inhibit lordosis behavior, whereas the control agents, namely saline and ACTH, were ineffective in inhibiting the high level of sexual receptivity observed in a hormone-primed female rat.

It is proposed that PRL is acting at the level of the hypothalamus via a LHRH system to modulate sexual receptivity. Several lines of evidence support this contention. Firstly, chronic as well as acute hyperprolactinemia as induced by pituitary homografts or by peripheral administration of PRL has been shown to suppress not only male and female copulatory behavior but also levels of plasma LH in male and female rats [96-103]. Secondly, hyper-

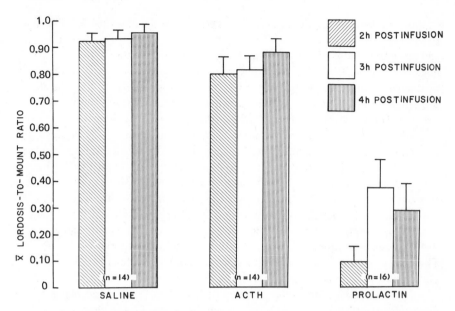

Figure 2 Effect of infusion of prolactin, adrenocorticotropin hormone (ACTH), or saline into the third ventricle on the lordosis-to-mount ratio of ovariectomized, estrogen-progesterone primed female rats. (From Ref. 96.)

prolactinemia has been found to increase hypothalamic LHRH stores [104] and lateral ventricle infusions of PRL have been shown to increase the number of immunofluorescent-positive-stained LHRH cell bodies in the medial basal hypothalamus [105]. These findings suggest that hyperprolactinemia may disrupt LH release and mating behavior, by acting in the CNS to prevent release of LHRH from hypothalamic neurons. Therefore, it is not inconceivable that some PRL-sensitive neurons [106-109] may synthesize and release LHRH or synapse with LHRH-containing neurons, thus modulating the release of the decapeptide for the regulation of gonadotropin secretion and/or mating behavior.

IV. Concluding Remarks

Since the isolation and structural identification of the hypothalamic hypophysiotropic hormones, namely, LHRH, TRH, and somatostatin, many studies have been performed to investigate the biological-endocrine functions of these peptides. In addition to their well-established pituitary gland actions, these peptides have been implicated in a variety of extraendocrine behaviors such as motor activity, pain,

euphoria, stress, epilepsy, thirst, learning, sex, and mental illness [4,5,109-112].
In this chapter, the data presented clearly demonstrate the dissociation of brain
and pituitary actions of LHRH. This decapeptide has been shown to stimulate
release of LH and FSH from the anterior pituitary gland as well as to facilitate
mating behavior in the absence of the pituitary and/or adrenal glands. The ability
of LHRH to enhance sexual behavior also appears to be somewhat universal in
that LHRH modulates mating in a variety of species including humans.

Additional data were also presented addressing the question of whether LHRH
is of physiological importance in mating activities of the rat. Recent electrophysiological as well as behavioral evidence support the hypothesis that LHRH receptor
sites exist in the mediobasal hypothalamus for mediating reproductive function.
It is also suggested that interference with the LHRH receptor sites, as occurs with
the infusion of an LHRH antagonist analog or in hyperprolactinemia, will result
in the suppression of mating behavior. Interestingly, centrally acute elevations
of PRL as well as chronically elevated PRL act to inhibit lordosis behavior.
These data certainly suggest that PRL may be acting through an LHRH neural
system to suppress mating activities.

To date investigation of the influence of LHRH on reproductive behavior in
mammals has offered the most direct evidence of a specific and physiological
CNS-extrapituitary action of the hypothalamic peptide hormones. However, only
continued investigation of a hypothalamic peptide hormone-sensitive brain system,
which mediates sexual activity, will provide the necessary information to critically
evaluate the role of LHRH in mediating reproductive behavior in animals and humans.

Acknowledgments

The authors wish to acknowledge Sue Sauter for the typing of the manuscript,
Drs. Parlow and Raiti of the National Pituitary Agency for prolactin, and Drs.
Vale and Rivier for LHRH. Research from the authors' laboratory referred to in
this chapter was funded by NIH grants NS 10434, HD 11814, and HD 09988.
Dr. Moss is a recipient of a USPHS-NIH Career Development Award, HD 00146.

References

1.   S. S. Yen, *J. Clin. Endocrinol. Metab.* 34:1108 (1972).
2.   W. Vale, J. Rivier, and M. Brown, *Ann. Rev. Physiol.* 39:473 (1977).
3.   R. L. Moss, C. A. Dudley, and W. Vale, in *Brain-Endocrine Interaction III.
     Neural Hormones and Reproduction* (D. E. Scott, G. P. Kozlowski, and A.
     Weindle, eds.). Karger, Munchen, 1978, p. 313.
4.   R. L. Moss, P. Riskind, and C. A. Dudley, in *Central Nervous System Ef-
     fects of Hypothalamic Hormones and Other Peptides* (R. Collu, A. Barveau,

J. R. Durcharme, and J. G. Rochefort, eds.), Raven Press, New York, 1979, p. 345.

5. R. L. Moss, *Ann. Rev. Physiol.* 41:617 (1979).

6. R. L. Moss and S. M. McCann, *Science* 181:177 (1973).

7. D. W. Pfaff, *Science* 182:1148 (1973).

8. R. L. Moss and S. M. McCann, *Neuroendocrinol.* 17:309 (1975).

9. R. L. Moss, C. A. Dudley, M. M. Foreman, and S. M. McCann, in *Hypothalamic Hormones,* (M. Motta, P. G. Crosignani, and L. Martini, eds.). Academic Press, London, 1975, p. 269.

10. R. L. Moss and C. A. Dudley, Presented at the 6th Annual International Symposium on Psychopharmacology, March, 1980, Louisville, Kentucky. Marcel Dekker, New York, in press.

11. C. H. Mortimer, A. S. McNeilly, R. A. Fisher, M. A. F. Murray, and G. M. Besser, *Br. Med. J.* 14:617 (1974).

12. O. Benkert, R. Jordan, H. G. Dahlen, H. P. G. Schneider, and G. Gammel, *Neuropsychobiology* 1:203 (1975).

13. L. Schwarzstein, N. J. Aparicio, D. Turner, J. C. Calamera, J. F. Mancini, and A. V. Schally, *Fertil. Steril.* 25:331 (1975).

14. T. F. Davies, C. Q. Mountjoy, A. Gomes-Pan, M. J. Watson, J. P. Hander, G. M. Besser, and R. Hall, *Clin. Endocrinol.* 5:601 (1976).

15. B. C. McAdoo, C. H. Doering, H. C. Kraemer, N. Dessert, H. K. H. Brodie, and D. A. Hamburg, *Psychosom. Med.* 40:199 (1978).

16. I. M. Evans and L. A. Distiller, *Arch. Sex. Behav.* 8:385 (1979).

17. R. H. Ehrensing and A. J. Kastin, *Pharmacol. Biochem. Behav.* 5:89 (1976).

18. M. M. Foreman and R. L. Moss, *Horm. Behav.* 8:219 (1977).

19. P. Riskind and R. L. Moss, *Brain Res. Bull.* 4:203 (1979).

20. R. L. Moss and M. M. Foreman, *Neuroendocrinology* 20:176 (1976).

21. D. Modianos and D. W. Pfaff, in *Excerpta Medica International Congress Series,* (V. H. T. James, ed.). No. 402. V International Congress of Endocrinology Proceedings, Hamburg, Excerpta Medica, Amsterdam, 1976, p. 67.

22. J. F. Rodriquez-Sierra and B. R. Komisaruk, *Horm. Behav.* 9:281 (1977).

23. W. G. Luttge and C. S. Sheets, *Pharmacol. Biochem. Behav.* 7:563 (1977).

24. H. E. Gray and W. G. Luttge, *Physiol. Behav.* 21:973 (1978).

25. M. F. Cheng, *J. Endocrinol.* 74:37 (1977).

26. M. R. Alderete, R. R. Tokarz, and D. Crews, *Neuroendocrinology* 30:200 (1980).

27. C. H. Doering, P. R. McGinnis, G. W. Kraemer, and D. A. Hamburg, personal communication, 1979.

28. B. M. Myers and M. J. Baum, *Pharmacol. Biochem. Behav.* 12:365 (1980).

29. W. Samson, S. M. McCann, L. Chud, C. A. Dudley, and R. L. Moss, *Neuroendocrinology* 31:66 (1980).

30. R. Elde and T. Hokfelt, in *Frontiers in Neuroendocrinology* (W. F. Ganong and L. Martini, eds.). Raven Press, New York, 1978, p. 1.

31. A. Silverman and E. Zimmerman, in *Brain Endocrine Interaction III. Neural Hormones and Reproduction* (D. E. Scott, G. P. Kozlowski, and A. Weindl, eds.). S. Karger, Munchen, 1978, p. 83.
32. G. Setalo, B. Flerko, A. Arimura, and A. V. Schally, *Int. Rev. Cytol. [Suppl.]* 7:1 (1978).
33. R. G. Dyer and R. E. J. Dyball, *Nature* 252:486 (1974).
34. K. Kawakami and Y. Sakuma, *Neuroendocrinology* 15:290 (1974).
35. R. L. Moss, M. Kelly, and C. A. Dudley, *Fed. Proc.* 34:219 (1975).
36. R. L. Moss, M. Kelly, M. M. Foreman, and C. A. Dudley, *Physiologist* 18: 326 (1975).
37. L. P. Renaud and J. B. Martin, *Brain Res.* 86:150 (1975).
38. L. P. Renaud, J. B. Martin, and P. Brazeau, *Nature* 255:233 (1975).
39. R. L. Moss, M. Kelly, and C. A. Dudley, 6th Annual Meeting, Society of Neuroscience, *Abstracts*, Toronto, Canada, November 7-11, Vol. 2, 1976, p. 652.
40. L. P. Renaud, J. B. Martin, and P. Brazeau, *Pharmacol. Biochem. Behav.* 5:171 (1976).
41. R. L. Moss and C. A. Dudley, *Brain Res.* 149:511 (1978).
42. R. L. Moss, C. A. Dudley, and M. J. Kelly, *Neuropharmacology* 17:87 (1978).
43. P. Poulain and B. Carett, *Brain Res.* 137:154 (1978).
44. R. L. Moss, *Fed. Proc.* 36:1978 (1977).
45. R. L. Moss, in *Psychopharmacology: A Generation of Progress* (M. A. Lipton, A. DiMascio, and K. F. Killam, eds.). Raven Press, New York, 1978, p. 431.
46. R. L. Moss, in *Frontiers in Neuroendocrinology,* Vol. 4 (L. Martini and W. F. Ganong, eds.). Raven Press, New York, 1976, p. 95.
47. R. L. Moss, P. Riskind, and C. A. Dudley, in *Central Nervous System Effects of Hypothalamic Hormones and Other Peptides* (R. Collu, A. Barbeau, J. R. Ducharme, and J. G. Rochefort, eds.). Raven Press, New York, 1979, p. 345.
48. M. S. Krieger, J. I. Morrell, and D. W. Pfaff, in *Brain-Endocrine Interaction III. Neural Hormones and Reproduction* (D. E. Scott, G. P. Kozlowski and A. Weindl, eds.). Karger, Munchen, 1978, p. 197.
49. D. B. Kelley and D. W. Pfaff, in *Biological Determinants of Sexual Behavior* (J. B. Hutchison, ed.). John Wiley, New York, 1978, p. 223.
50. W. E. Stumpf, M. Sar, L. D. Grant, and A. S. Heritage, in *Brain-Endocrine Interaction III. Neural Hormones and Reproduction* (D. E. Scott, G. P. Kozlowski and A. Weindl, eds.). Karger, Munchen, 1978, p. 212.
51. D. W. Pfaff and M. Keiner, *J. Comp. Neurol.* 151:121 (1973).
52. B. V. Critchlow, *Am. J. Physiol.* 195:171 (1958).
53. J. W. Everett and H. M. Radford, *Proc. Soc. Exp. Biol. Med.* 108:604 (1961).

54. J. W. Everett, in *Major Problem in Neuroendocrinology* (E. Bajuxz and G. Jasin, eds.). Karger, New York, 1964, p. 343.
55. H. F. Carrer and S. Taleisnk, *J. Endocrinol.* 48:527 (1970).
56. O. M. Cramer and C. A. Barraclough, *Endocrinology* 88:1175 (1971).
57. J. Turgeon and C. A. Barraclough, *Endocrinology* 92:755 (1973).
58. G. Fink and M. G. Jamieson, *J. Endocrinol.* 93:947 (1973).
59. J. W. Everett, L. C. Krey, and L. Trey, *Endocrinology,* 93:947 (1973).
60. P. S. Kalra and S. M. McCann, *Prog. Brain Res.* 39:185 (1973).
61. G. Fink and M. S. Aijer, *J. Endocrinol.* 62:589 (1974).
62. H. G. Burger, G. Fink, and V. W. K. Less, *J. Endocrinol.* 54:227 (1972).
63. R. L. Eskay, *Endocrinology* 100:263 (1977).
64. S. Taleisnik and S. M. McCann, *Endocrinology* 68:263 (1961).
65. W. Bishop, P. S. Kalra, C. P. Fawcett, L. Krulich, and S. M. McCann, *Endocrinology* 91:1404 (1972).
66. E. M. Bogdanove, *Endocrinology* 73:696 (1963).
67. B. Flerko, *Arch. Anat. Microsc. Morphol. Exp.* 56:446 (1978).
68. B. Halasz and L. Pupp, *Endocrinology* 77:553 (1965).
69. T. Tejasen and J. W. Everett, *Endocrinology* 81:1387 (1967).
70. S. P. Kalra and C. H. Sawyer, *Endocrinology* 87:1124 (1970).
71. C. A. Blake, R. L. Norman, and C. H. Sawyer, *Proc. Soc. Exp. Biol. Med.* 141:1100 (1972).
72. B. Halasz and R. A. Gorski, *Endocrinology* 80:608 (1967).
73. A. Napoli, J. B. Powers, and E. S. Valenstein, *Physiol. Behav.* 9:115 (1972).
74. R. L. Moss, R. F. Paloutzian, and O. T. Law, *Physiol. Behav.* 12:997 (1974).
75. O. T. Law and W. Meagher, *Am. J. Physiol.* 69:738 (1968).
76. J. J. Singer, *J. Comp. Physiol. Psychol.* 69:738 (1968).
77. B. J. Powers and E. S. Valenstein, *Science* 175:1003 (1972).
78. R. A. Gorski, in *Advances in Psychobiology* (G. Newton and A. H. Rieson, eds.). John Wiley, New York, 1974, p. 1.
79. D. M. Nance, J. Shryne, and R. A. Gorski, *Horm. Behav.* 6:59 (1975).
80. D. W. Pfaff, C. Diakow, R. Zigmond, and L.-M. Kow, in *The Neurosciences, Vol. III* (F. O. Schmitt, F. C. Wirden, eds.). MIT Press, Boston, 1973, p. 621.
81. G. P. Kozlowski and G. Hostetter, in *Brain-Endocrine Interaction III. Neural Hormones and Reproduction* (D. E. Scott, G. P. Kozlowski and A. Weindl, eds.). Karger, Basel, 1978, p. 138.
82. Y. Sakuma and D. W. Pfaff, *Nature* 283:566 (1980).
83. A. K. Kastin, D. H. Coy, A. V. Schally, and J. E. Zadina, *Pharmacol. Biochem. Behav.* 13:913 (1980).
84. C. A. Dudley, W. Vale, J. Rivier, and R. L. Moss, *Peptides* 2:393 (1981).
85. R. L. Moss, C. A. Dudley, and M. J. Kelly, *Neuropharmacology* 17:87 (1978).
86. B. R. Komisaruk, in *Biological Determinants of Sexual Behavior* (J. B. Hutchinson, ed.). John Wiley, New York, 1980, p. 349.

87. G. C. Kennedy and J. Mitra, *J. Physiol. (Lond.)* 166:395 (1963).
88. D. Mathews and D. A. Edwards, *Horm. Behav.* 8:40 (1977).
89. R. D. Lisk and M. A. Barfield, *Neuroendocrinology* 19:28 (1975).
90. M. M. Foreman and R. L. Moss, *Physiol. Behav.* 22:283 (1979).
91. A. G. Frantz, in *Endocrinology* (G. F. Cahill, L. Martini, J. T. Potts, D. E. Nelson, E. Steinberger, and Albert Windegrad, eds.). Grune & Straton, New York, 1979, p. 153.
92. O. Riddle, *Nat. Cancer Inst.* 31:1039 (1963).
93. V. Blüm and K. Flieder, *Gen. Comp. Endocrinol.* 5:186 (1965).
94. J. Terkel and S. Rosenblatt, *J. Comp. Physiol. Psychol.* 65:479 (1968).
95. D. F. Horrobin, *Br. J. Psychiatry* 124:456 (1974).
96. C. A. Dudley, T. S. Jamison, and R. L. Moss, *Endocrinology* 110:677 (1982).
97. R. M. Shapre and A. S. McNeilly, *Mol. Cell. Endocrinol.* 16:19 (1979).
98. A. Bartke, M. S. Smith, S. D. Michael, F. G. Peron, and S. Dalterio, *Endocrinology* 100:182 (1977).
99. A. Bartke, A. A. Kafiez, F. J. Bex, and S. Dalterio, *Biol. Reprod.* 18:44 (1978).
100. F. Drago, B. Pellegrini-Quarantotti, U. Scapagnini, and G. L. Gessa, *Physiol. Behav.* 26:277 (1981).
101. P. C. Doherty, A. Bartke, and M. S. Smith, *Neurosci. Abst.* 6:776, 264.3 (1981).
102. B. Svare, A. Bartke, P. Doherty, I. Mason, S. D. Michael, and M. S. Smith, *Biol. Reprod.* 21:529 (1979).
103. P. C. Doherty, S. D. Michael, and B. B. Svare, *Society of the Study of Reproduction.* Abstract No. 134, Carbondale, Ill., (Aug. 1978).
104. Irit Gil-Ad, V. Locatelli, D. Cochi, R. Carminate, C. Arezzini, and E. Müller, *Life Sci.* 23:2245 (1978).
105. J. Barry, D. Croix, and P. Poulain, in *Progress in Prolactin Physiology and Pathology* (C. Robyn and M. Harter, eds.). Biomedical Press, Elsevier/North Holland, 1978, p. 253.
106. P. Poulain and B. Carette, *Brain Res.* 116:172 (1976).
107. T. Hokfelt and K. Fuxe, *Neuroendocrinology* 9:100 (1972).
108. Y. Yamada, *Neuroendocrinology* 18:263 (1975).
109. G. Toubeau, J. Desclin, M. Parmentier, and J. L. Pasteels, Societe Belge et d'Endocrinologie Seance, *Ann. Endocrinol.* 41:147 (1980).
110. A. J. Kastin, C. A. Sandman, A. V. Schally, and R. H. Ehrensing, in *Clinical Neuropharmacology, Vol. 3* (A. L. Klawans, ed.). Raven Press, New York, 1979.
111. G. G. Yarbrough, *Prog. Neurobiol.* 12:291 (1979).
112. R. L. Moss and C. A. Dudley, in *The Role of Peptides in Neuronal Function* (J. L. Barker and T. G. Smith, Jr., eds.). Marcel Dekker, New York, 1980, p. 455.

5 The Psychology of the Menstrual Cycle: Biological and PSYCHOLOGICAL Perspectives

MARY BROWN PARLEE   City University of New York, New York,

Research on the psychology of the menstrual cycle has, until fairly recently, been conducted with a focus on biological changes. That is, the starting point of the inquiry has been the fact of cyclic changes in physiology occurring throughout (defining) the menstrual cycle. The psychological question asked was: what are the psychological consequences of these physiological changes. In recent years the biologically based perspective on the psychology of the menstrual cycle (the focus on physiological changes and their direct psychological consequences) has been supplemented by a more traditionally psychological perspective. In this perspective, the starting point of the inquiry *is* the psychological changes occurring over the course of the menstrual cycle. The research question asked is: What are these changes and what are the processes, biologic and social, that produce them? A psychological perspective also entails, more or less explicitly, a set of questions about systematic variability: what changes occur in what groups of women under what circumstances?

The two perspectives can lead to quite different lines of research, even when they start from the same empirical data. Suppose, for example, that premenstrual increases in anxiety levels were to be found (increases demonstable with more than one operational measure of anxiety). From a biological perspective, the proper interpretation of such increases as manifestations of physiological changes would depend on demonstration of a relationship between physiological and psychological changes within each of the women in the test population. Research establishing such a relationship would reasonably permit the conclusion that the

77

physiological changes cause the psychological ones. From a psychological perspective, however, the range of possible explanatory domains is more diverse. For example, it might be that women who have reason to be concerned about menstrual onset (e.g., fear of pregnancy, or of being caught unprepared for a heavy flow) might become increasingly anxious as the onset of menstruation approaches. These women would show premenstrual increases in anxiety levels, but the increases would be caused by a complex set of indirect processes, in this case primarily social, linking physiological changes and psychological experiences. Further research from a psychological perspective would be directed toward clarifying some of these processes. It should be evident that a psychological perspective does not replace or alter questions framed from a biological point of view. But it does increase the range and complexity of psychological phenomena and causal processes that can be explored.

A biological perspective, therefore, focuses on psychological changes that are the *consequences* of various physiological changes of the menstrual cycle. The task in understanding the psychology of the menstrual cycle from this perspective is to identify which psychological changes have this causal link to physiology, recognizing that all may not. A psychological perspective, on the other hand, focuses on the psychological *concomitants* of the physiological changes, and leaves open the possibility of complex social processes mediating the relationship between physiological and psychological changes. The task here is to determine the ways in which any particular psychological changes are affected by physiological and social processes.

In a review of the literature on the premenstrual tension syndrome published several years ago, this author concluded that while many women spontaneously attest to its reality, the existence of premenstrual tension as a concomitant of the normal menstrual cycle had not been scientifically established (Parlee, 1973). Since then there has been considerable conceptual and empirical progress. Examples of lines of research resulting from this clarification will be discussed in this chapter. The presentation is organized within the same framework as the earlier review, according to methodologic categories. Given the interrelatedness of method, data, and theory (Scheffler, 1967; Kuhn, 1970), it is perhaps not surprising that research in each of these categories has developed along different lines. In one a biological perspective seems to be more fruitful, in another a psychological perspective.*

Particularly for the reader who is a natural scientist, accustomed to dealing with phenomena from within a single, and therefore taken-for-granted, framework, a prefatory note may be in order regarding the discussion of general "perspectives" which recurs as a theme throughout this chapter. In research on the

---

*Other reviews covering some of the same material can be found in Persky, 1974; Parlee, 1978; Smith, 1975; O'Connor et al., 1974; Redgrove, 1971; Friedman et al., 1980.

psychology of the menstrual cycle—on the relationship between psychological and physiological processes—the major problems arise from the conceptualization and measurement of the psychological processes, not from the physiological measurements. The problems are negative results when a particular hypotheses is being tested or critically evaluated, or scattered, statistically significant findings which are not followed up and do not lead to cumulative empirical or theoretical work. These are serious and challenging problems, increasingly recognized by researchers who want to find *something* solid or scientifically sound about the psychology of the menstrual cycle and do not care in advance what it is. The solution to these problems is not simply more research of the same kind (that is, research conducted from the same perspective as before). Nor is it a problem of "more rigorous" measurement. Rigorous measurement can never make up for flabby or inappropriate concepts. Conceptual clarification occurs in part through new empirical work and thought about it and in part through analysis and rethinking of data already in the literature. Much of the progress in recent years is probably attributable to this latter form of activity, hence the recurring discussion of general perspectives as they guide the formulation of issues and questions for research.

I. Correlational Studies

In scientific discussions of the premenstrual tension syndrome, one of the most frequently cited bodies of research is the pioneering work of Katherine Dalton. Her data, and those of others following her paradigm, have clearly demonstrated a significant correlation between certain behavioral acts of women and the phase of the menstrual cycle the woman was in when she performed the act.

Cumulatively, Dalton's research has shown that women who have committed a crime, had an accident at work, been admitted to a mental hospital, or taken a child to the hospital are significantly more likely to have done so in the premenstrual and menstrual phases of the cycle than at other phases (Dalton, 1959, 1960, 1961, 1970; also Tuch, 1975). Similar results have been found for women who have attempted or completed suicide (Tonks et al., 1968; Mandell and Mandell, 1967; MacKinnon and MacKinnon, 1956). These data are among the best evidence in the scientific literature of a significant relationship between menstrual cycle phase and behavior (Parlee, 1978).

The usual interpretation, explicit or implicit, given to these correlational data is that the physiological changes of the menstrual cycle produce a state of psychological tension during the premenstrual and menstrual phases, and that this psychological state predisposes women to perform the actions under study. According to the usual interpretation (as inferred from the contexts in which the research is cited), these studies provide evidence of the existence of a hormonally caused syndrome of premenstrual/menstrual tension (O'Connor et al., 1974; Moos et al., 1969; Janowsky et al., 1966; Coppen and Kessel, 1963). Clearly, such an interpretation arises from a biological perspective.

Given that the correlational data themselves are so unquestionably significant and reliable, and the usual interpretation of them so ubiquitous, could this interpretation, seemingly so in accord with common sense, possibly be mistaken? It could. There is, however, an alternative interpretation, with supporting data, which opens up and is related to an extremely interesting set of empirical and theoretical issues.*

Evidence for the need to rethink the usual interpretation of correlational studies of the menstrual cycle comes from one of Dalton's less frequently cited papers (Dalton, 1968). In that paper, she examined the relationship between the performance of female students on a nationally administered examination in Great Britain and the phase of the menstrual cycle students were in when the test was administered. Although she does not describe them in this way, data Dalton presents in various tables in this paper clearly show the existence of the same relationship between cycle phase and the occurrence of the behavioral act that she had found in her other studies. That is, *students taking the examination were significantly more likely to be in the premenstrual and menstrual phases than in the remainder of the cycle.* Yet unlike crimes, for example, the timing of the occurrence of the behavior in question was not under the woman's control. The examinations were scheduled in advance by an administrative agency at the national level.

It cannot be the case, therefore, that the physiological changes of the menstrual cycle produced a premenstrual or menstrual state of psychological tension which predisposed the woman to take the examination. But if the usual interpretation of the correlations between cycle phase and behavior found in this study is mistaken, can we be certain the usual interpretation is correct for the other correlational studies in which the results take the same form? Evidence from one of these studies suggests that it probably is not.

In her paper on accidents and the menstrual cycle, Dalton reports data for a category of behavior she calls "passive" accidents: those in which there was

---

*This discussion of correlational studies of the menstrual cycle will not focus on some of the obvious methodological problems with the research: estimation of cycle phase from memory of last menstrual onset, exclusion of subjects who have not menstruated within the previous 28 days (see Frazier, 1959; Matsumoto et al., 1962; Presser, 1974). Dalton's results are unlikely to be simply artefacts of these procedures, since use of the same methods has produced the "opposite" results with a different behavioral measure (significantly fewer women who volunteered to participate in a psychological experiment were in the premenstrual and menstrual phases) (Parlee, 1975; see also Doty and Silverthorne, 1975). It should be noted, however, that a logical error is involved in the usual interpretation of the findings. Viz: the data show that *if* a woman has, for example, committed a crime, *then* she is more likely to be in the premenstrual or menstrual phases of the cycle. From the truth of this statement, however, it is the truth of the inverse that is inferred in the usual interpretation: if a woman is in the premenstrual or menstrual phases of the cycle, then she is more likely to commit a crime. Elementary logic tells us this pattern of inference is not valid. (Although it says nothing about the truth of what is inferred.)

nothing the woman could have done to prevent or avoid an accident to her that was wholly caused by actions of others. Yet *the significant correlation with cycle phase was found for the category of passive accidents as well as for those accidents in which the woman played an active role.* Again, a hormonally produced state of psychological tension in the woman cannot account for the correlation between the premenstrual and menstrual phases of the cycle and the occurrence of the behavior act (the passive accident).

If the usual interpretation is incorrect or unproven, how else might the consistently found correlations between cycle phase and certain behaviors be explained? Again, suggestive evidence comes from Dalton's own work. In the 1968 paper on menstruation and examinations (p. 1388, Fig. 3), Dalton presents a graph showing the number of students menstruating each day in the weeks and days preceding, during, and following the examination. From this graph it seems clear that the menstrual days are not randomly distributed but that, perhaps, the stress of the impending examination has affected the timing of menstrual onset. If this were so, the correlation between cycle phase and the act of taking the examination could be the result of the relationship of each to the common factor of stress occurring before and during the examination.

In the paper on examinations, Dalton explicitly considers the role of stress, but not its implication for the interpretation of the correlational data. She analyzed the individual menstrual records of the women and reports that 38 of the 91 students had alterations in the usual length (not defined) of their menstrual cycles during the examination month. For 11, the cycle was shorter by 4 or more days, for 19 it was longer by 4 or more days, and eight students missed their normal menstruation entirely during the month the examinations were given. She concludes that "the stress of the examination caused an alteration in the length of the menstrual cycle in 42% of the girls," and adds that while the effects of emotional stress on menstruation have long been recognized, "this appears to be the first statistical evidence of its occurrence" (p. 1388). Although her conclusion may be somewhat premature (data from a control group of students of similar ages would be necessary to determine normal variability of cycle length), Dalton has provided evidence strongly suggesting an alteration in cycle length due to stress.

Regardless of what the causal processes turn out to be, the logical and empirical critique of correlational studies of the menstrual cycle seems clear. Logically, the existence of a correlation does not itself demonstrate a causal relationship between cycle phase and behavior. A correlation can be the result of a common causal influence. Empirically, a causal relationship between the correlated variables would be impossible in at least some of the studies. Hypothetically, both menstrual onset and behavior are likely to have been affected by a common causal influence, stress being one possibility.

This alternative interpretation of the correlations between cycle phase and behavior can plausibly be applied to most of the correlational studies carried out by Dalton and others, research in which the results are generalized, by implication, to all women. Most of the behaviors examined in these studies seem likely to have been preceeded or influenced by, stressful situations. The usual interpretation of the correlations between cycle phase and behavior (hormones influence behavior) may, of course, remain applicable to particular groups of women (for example, those predisposed to commit a crime) for whom physiological changes of the menstrual and premenstrual phases effectively lower the threshold for the occurrence of the behavior (see also Friedman et al., 1980).

While stress is clearly not itself an explanatory concept, it does point to a set of phenomena and issues that has been the focus of considerable research that, with some exceptions, has until recently been unrelated to the menstrual cycle (e.g., Spielberger and Sarason, 1978; for exceptions see Osofsky and Fisher, 1967; Russell, 1972; Marinari et al. 1976; Abplanalp, 1977). The applicability of the concept of stress to correlational studies of the psychology of the menstrual cycle (Parlee, 1975, 1978) points clearly to the importance of the menstrual cycle as a *dependent* as well as an independent variable. That is, the physiological states and changes of the menstrual cycle are influenced by social and psychological processes as well as the reverse. The importance of thinking about the physiology and psychology of the menstrual cycle as an interactive system is a point that has recently been persuasively made and comprehensively documented in an important paper by Martha McClintock (1981).

In the same volume as the McClintock paper, the proceedings of the Second Interdisciplinary Menstrual Cycle Research Conference, Randi Koeske offers a reanalysis from this interactive perspective of the already classic psychological study by Wilcoxon et al. (Wilcoxon et al., 1976; Koeske, 1981). Wilcoxon et al. collected self-reports of moods over a 35 day interval and found that stressful events in the lives of their female college student subjects were more closely related to variance in moods than was cycle phase. However, Koeske reanalyzed the data and noted that these women were more likely than the other two groups in the study (men randomly assigned to a "cycle phase," and women taking oral contraceptives) to be in the premenstrual phase of their cycle at the beginning and end of the study, which happened to be times of stress (midterm and final examinations). Koeske suggests the stress of the examinations may have affected cycle length in women not taking oral contraceptives, and notes that this casts doubt on the assumed "independence" of stressful events in the environment and menstrual cycle phase. This assumption is required by Wilcoxon et al.'s conclusion as well as by analysis of variance techniques commonly used in such research. (Here and elsewhere Koeske [1980] discusses other important theoretical, methodological, and empirical issues in research on the menstrual cycle.)

In addition to (and stemming from) some of the research topics and questions discussed by McClintock (1981), the reanalysis of correlational studies underlines the relevance of a set of as yet unanswered descriptive questions. For example, what are the social, psychological, and biological factors that affect the frequency of anovulatory cycles in a particular population of women? (For example, how is the frequency of ovulation, in a particular woman or in a particular group, related to cycle length and regularity, diet, exercise, stressful life events, holidays, job stress, climate/season, etc.?) What social and psychological conditions optimize the likelihood of regular ovulatory cycles? What physiological states and statuses do so?

These and other questions are of considerable practical significance in research on the menstrual cycle and in the clinical management of some types of infertility. It is important to note here that they seem also to point to a set of difficult but potentially solvable scientific problems. Related research findings, fruitful methods, and theories already exist. Some of these questions will probably best be answered by adopting a biological perspective in the research; some require an interactional perspective. The promising aspect of the research, however, is that a paradigm seems to be emerging: a shared set of assumptions, problems, and methods offering the possibility of solid, cumulative data collection and theory construction.

II. Retrospective Questionnaires

In earlier research on the premenstrual tension syndrome, investigators almost invariably regarded women's responses on retrospective questionnaires as evidence that they had in fact experienced the symptom and mood changes asked about on the questionnaire (Moos, 1968; Coppen and Kessel, 1963; Sutherland and Stewart, 1965). Over the past several years, however, the interpretation of such questionnaire data for scientific purposes has become more sophisticated. Much of this new work arises from a concern with the validity (in a technical sense) of retrospective self-report questionnaires.

Important as they are, self-reports and self-report questionnaires pose a perennial problem for psychologists. Apart from issues of reliability, questions always arise regarding the validity and the scientific meaning of questionnaire responses. Do they represent accurate accounts of personal experience, the respondent's judgment of a socially desirable response, socially shared beliefs or stereotypes, or the person's response to factors in the test situation itself (such as the respondent's perception of what the experimenter wants)? None of these questions can be clearly answered by the questionnaire data alone, and psychologists have developed a set of procedures for attempting to clarify and establish the validity of self-reports (Anastasi, 1968).

One early effort to explore the validity of responses on questionnaires covering menstrual distress noted the similarity in procedures for eliciting "self-reports" of menstrual distress and procedures in social psychology for exploring stereotypes individuals hold about particular social groups. Further research showed that men, when asked about what women experience, give similar patterns of responses on a menstrual distress questionnaire as women do when asked about themselves individually or about women in general (Parlee, 1974). (All report that women experience premenstrual increases in pain, tension, irritability, depression, and the like.) By themselves, these data from men do not show that women's responses on menstrual distress questionnaires are *not* accurate self-reports. It is entirely possible that the validity of the questionnaire responses is different for women and men. For example, women could be reporting their own experiences, while men are reporting symptom and mood changes they have observed to occur over the menstrual cycle in women they know well.

But the burden of proof has been shifted. Particular patterns of responses on menstrual distress questionnaires cannot be interpreted as accurate reports of personal experience without further research using other measures or responses to establish the validity of the women's responses as self-reports. (This is not to say that investigators will not in practice need to rely upon the validity of menstrual questionnaires in their research: what people say when asked about their experience is both important and easily obtainable. The point here is that interpretations, tests of hypotheses, or conclusions based on questionnaire data cannot be definitive without additional validity data, and should be presented with appropriate caution.) When the questionnaire data are critical for theory construction, and in the absence of additional validity data, questionnaire responses should be conservatively interpreted, perhaps as socially shared beliefs (or stereotypes) about psychological changes occurring over the menstrual cycle.

Socially shared beliefs about the psychology of the menstrual cycle can be true, true in part, or false. Investigations to evaluate these possibilities, however, have thus far yielded little cumulative research and no clear conclusions, for reasons to be considered shortly.* More promising research, conducted entirely from a psychological perspective, has focused on the beliefs *qua* beliefs.

One line of research has been to explore the ways in which beliefs about the psychology of the menstrual cycle function in explanations of another's and one's own behavior. Conducted within an attribution theory framework in social psychology, Koeske and Koeske (1975) found that negatively evaluated actions performed by women tend to be attributed to the menstrual cycle, even where situations or personal factors are adequate to account for the actions under other circumstances. R. Koeske (1980) has further elaborated these findings, and hypothesizes that beliefs about the menstrual cycle are typically invoked to account for negative, out-of-role behavior for women. This is an attributional pattern that, by assigning cause to biological processes, renders less likely an explanation in terms of personal or interpersonal causes. Also applying an attribution theory

---

*As with research on psychological sex differences, it is somewhat difficult to see what the evaluation of the truth of stereotypes yields in a scientific sense. Knowing whether or not a stereotype is accurate says nothing about the processes producing the phenomena described by the stereotype or about the functional significance of the stereotype for the individual who holds it.

analysis, Rodin (1976) has found evidence suggesting that some women may perform better on intellectual tasks if they tend to attribute their states of bodily arousal to the menstrual cycle rather than to the situation.

Working within the framework of cognitive labeling theory, several investigators have explored the possibility that Schacter and Singer's (1962) theory of emotion could be applied to the self-description of premenstrual psychological states. That is, it might be that the physiological changes of the premenstrual phase are nonspecific in their psychological effects and are given cognitive meaning (labeled) largely in accordance with what the social environment of the individual defines as the appropriate response (Koeske, 1977). Socially shared beliefs about the nature of psychological changes in the premenstrual phase, *when they are made salient for the individual,* would be one means of conveying the social definition of the emotional meaning of nonspecific states of premenstrual physiological arousal (or "arousability," Koeske, 1977).

The most direct test of the hypotheses that beliefs about the psychological changes of the menstrual cycle can affect a woman's description of her current bodily state is a study by Diane Ruble (1977). In a social psychological laboratory experiment, Ruble sought to convince one group of subjects that they were "really" premenstrual (as "shown," they were told, by recordings of their autonomic and electroencephalographic responses). Another group (actually in the same phase of the cycle, between the ovulatory and premenstrual phases) were told in a similar way they were in the ovulatory phase. A control group did not receive any information about cycle phase. All the subjects then filled out the Moos Menstrual Distress questionnaire with the instructions to report each of the moods and symptoms "as you feel now." Although there was no difference between the control and experimental groups, the subjects who had been told they were premenstrual reported higher levels of menstrual-related pain than did those who had been told they were in the middle of their cycles. Thus, Ruble concludes, beliefs about the menstrual cycle can influence women's descriptions, and by inference, their experiences, of their own bodily states. This conclusion necessarily presupposes the success of the experimental manipulation: that the women who were told they were premenstrual believed it. Ruble reports that subjects indicated in a debriefing session after the experiment that this was the case. While an expectancy effect could have operated even in the debriefing (Rosenthal and Rosnow, 1975), Ruble's experiment clearly demonstrates an influence of beliefs about the menstrual cycle on subjects' responses to self-report questionnaires. (Similarly, in another study, Brooks et al. (1977) found that simply asking subjects to respond "as if" they were premenstrual resulted in patterns of responses like those usually reported on retrospective questionnaires for the premenstrual phase.) Friedman et al. (1980) discuss some alternate ways in which beliefs and self-descriptions could be related.

In related research, other investigators have used a variety of self-report measures of symptoms and moods to assess the effects of a subject's awareness that she is participating in research on menstruation. One question in this research is whether a subject's awareness of the purpose of a menstrual study makes beliefs about cycle-related psychological changes more salient and thus influences her questionnaire responses. A second question is whether daily self-reports show cycle-related changes similar to those reported on retrospective questionnaires. The results of this research have been contradictory and confusing.

Parlee found no relationship between retrospective and daily reports (on different mood measures), although significant phase differences were reported on the retrospective questionnaires and were found in the daily reports given by women who were unaware of the purpose of the experiment (Parlee, in press). (An increase of positive moods and decrease of negative moods was found in the premenstrual phases during this 90 day study; retrospectively, the women reported premenstrual increases in negative moods. The results are interpreted for the particular population studied as consistent with cognitive labeling theory and as underlining the importance of individual and group differences; Parlee, 1981). May (1976) found no relationship between daily self-reports and retrospective accounts of menstrual experiences gathered in an interview. In a 35 day study, Swandby (1981) found no significant cycle-related changes in daily reports of moods and physical symptoms in subjects unaware of the purpose of the experiment; no retrospective questionnaire was administered. Using one of the same questionnaires Swandby employed, also studying women unaware of the purpose of the study, Englander-Golder et al. (1978) did find significant fluctuations in daily self-reports of pain over the cycle, Schilling (1981) found no significant cycle-related changes in daily self-reports over 35 days, but did find some consistency between daily and retrospective self-reports on the same questionnaire. Testing at the ovulatory and premenstrual phases, Rogers and Harding (1981) found significant premenstrual increases in the pain, negative affect, and water retention scores on the Moos Menstrual Distress Questionnaire Form T (developed for repeated measurement of current mood state). These investigators also found differences in women's performance on the Kinetic Family Drawing test in the ovulatory and premenstrual phases of the cycle. The women in the premenstrual phase showed significantly more compartmentalization (lines or objects in drawings that separated self from other) and drew themselves larger than did the men in the study.

In sum, however, it appears that this plethora of research data on daily and retrospective mood questionnaires has not been matched by a richness of understanding of the processes involved. The lack of clarity, or even empirical consistency, seems likely to persist until scientific psychologists have achieved a broader empirical and theoretical base for conceptualizing and measuring moods and emotions and their relation to cognitive processes (such as believing). It is perhaps not surprising, then, that the clearest demonstrations of global affective changes associated with the menstrual cycle have thus far come from "softer" measures having a clinical base (Paige, 1971; Ivey and Bardwick, 1968; Benedeck and Rubenstein, 1939). Of these, the most recent is the study by Karen Paige, which used the Gottschlak-Glesser Technique for content analysis of speech samples gathered in an unstructured setting (subjects are asked to talk for 5 min about some recent life event). Paige collected data during the ovulatory and premenstrual phases of the cycle in 102 women and found significant premenstrual increases in anxiety and hostility. The women were supposedly unaware that the menstrual cycle was the focus of the investigation.

From the perspective of academic psychology and a concern with "hard" data, perhaps the most interesting line of work to develop out of research on beliefs about the psychology of the menstrual cycle has been that of Ruble and Brooks-Gunn (1979). It focuses on the way beliefs about menstrual symptoms and moods develop and are maintained, even when the content of the beliefs may differ from personal experiences. Marshalling evidence from research on cognitive processes in a variety of domains, Ruble and Brooks-Gunn suggest that generalized beliefs about an association between symptoms and cycle phase may arise through biases in the processing of information about cyclicity. Connotative meaning, salience, and selectivity in processing information related to the beliefs may contribute to their origins, while cognitive mechanisms such as distortion, autonomy, and category accessibility of the evidence contribute to their maintenance once they are formed. Aside from individual studies that lie within the general framework of attribution theory and of cognitive labeling theory, Ruble and Brooks-Gunn's analysis represents one of the most coherent and successful efforts to integrate research on the psychology of the menstrual cycle into a theoretical and empirical framework (social cognition) of mainstream academic psychology. (Arguments that this may not be a wholly unmixed blessing can be found in Parlee, 1979.)

Despite the interest and importance of the research on beliefs about the psychology of the menstrual cycle, one is nevertheless faced with the question of why this strictly psychological research on the psychology of the menstrual cycle has not progressed further. The past decade has seen an influx of new researchers, perspectives, and data, yet research on the topic does not seem to have arrived at a set of hard but potentially solvable and real scientific problems in the same way that research stemming from correlational studies seems to have done. Instead, recent research seems to have thrown into sharp relief certain problems with psychological concepts and methods.

Despite the importance of beliefs about the psychology of menstruation, as well as the importance of individual and group differences in these beliefs, it seems evident that we do not yet know what women *really* believe are the psychological aspects of menstruation. We know what their responses are on questionnaires, and we know what they say in preliminary interviews leading to the development of such questionnaires. But these traditional psychological research methods inevitably impose the investigator's conceptual categories on the phenomena to be described. That is, we ask people (as "subjects") to respond to our categories (selected symptoms, moods, behavior changes), but we do not ask them how well, or even if, such conceptualizations make sense to them. Investigators who have administered menstrual distress questionnaires to "subjects" who felt free to give their reactions will recognize some of the issues involved.

Almost anyone who has conversed with women or men about menstruation knows that it is a topic of great cognitive interest, emotional involvement, and psychodynamic significance. Current methods used in scientific psychological research on beliefs tap only the cognitive tip (and maybe from an oblique angle) of an aspect of experience characterized by great complexity and depth. As in other areas of scientific psychology, the methods strip the phenomena from context (Mishler, 1979) and focus unduly heavily on the cognitive aspects of experience and behavior. Even within a strictly cognitive framework, the methods do not assure, or even attempt to assess, the validity of the conceptual categories used in theory construction.

The inadequacy of the methods to the complexity of the phenomenon probably accounts for the current lack of cumulative theoretical/empirical research. While we might prefer simply to do programmatic research rather than discuss prescientific issues about it, research on the menstrual cycle conducted from a strictly psychological perspective is still at the question-finding rather than the problem-solving stage. This means that investigators will probably have to choose between use of well-developed psychological methods and theoretical perspectives that are in fact inadequate to the phenomenon (and therefore probably will not yield positive or cumulative empirical results) or they will have to adopt "softer" methods which may yield insight into the phenomenon but which will be less likely to be accepted as valid within scientific psychology. These concerns are relevant to research on the psychology of the menstrual cycle conducted from a biological perspective as well as a strictly psychological one. Research exploring the psychological consequences of physiological processes may so frequently have yielded negative results not because the consequences do not exist but because the conceptualization and measurement of the psychological "side" of the correlation is inadequate.

III. Longitudinal Research

In correlational studies and research using retrospective questionnaires, psychological *changes* over the course of the menstrual cycle are inferred; typically increases in negative behaviors and emotional states (tension, depression, irritability, anxiety, and the like) are inferred in the premenstrual phase of the cycle. The focus is usually on premenstrual tension and menstrual distress, and data that might bear upon the presence or absence of positive changes and behaviors are rarely collected. Furthermore, since research in the past was conducted primarily from a biological perspective, physiological causation of the inferred psychological changes is generally assumed without discussion or exploration, through collection of relevant data, of possible additional or alternative causes. This approach reflects and embodies a particular a priori perspective on the nature of the phenomena, one that is directly or indirectly pathology-oriented and biologically based. Such a perspective is essential in clinical research directed toward alleviating suffering and distress through medical treatment. In early research on the psychology of the menstrual cycle, however, this perspective tended to dominate research implicitly directed toward another goal, that of understanding the nature and causes of psychological changes over the menstrual cycle in different groups of women (Parlee, 1973). Although much of the recent research on the psychology of the menstrual cycle is directed toward this latter goal, the review by Friedman et al. (1980) is perhaps the first to draw the distinction between these goals clearly and to organize the literature as it bears on one or the other of them. With the development of this broader aim and perspective, *inferences* about psychological changes over the cycle become less telling than data from longitudinal investigations in which measurements are actually taken on a regular basis over the course of the menstrual cycle.

Even in longitudinal investigations, however, it is worth noting how difficult it sometimes seems to be to step outside a conceptual framework focused on a syndrome of premenstrual tension. For example, June Redgrove's otherwise very useful review (1971) of the psychology of menstruation is diminished by her interpretation of her own longitudinal data showing improvements in typing accuracy in the premenstrual phase of the cycle. Redgrove suggests that the women are exerting special effort during this phase to overcome the disruptive effects of premenstrual tension. Since behavioral effects of premenstrual tension have not been unambiguously demonstrated to occur in normal women, this interpretation of premenstrual improvement in terms of premenstrual tension is not the most parsimonious that could have been made. Improved performance in the premenstrual phase may be just that; as Freud said, a cigar is sometimes simply a cigar. While the most parsimonious explanation is not necessarily the true one, the absence of parsimony as a criterion in evaluating interpretations of these longitudinal data testifies to the strong grip the concept of premenstrual tension can have on the way researchers view their data.

Despite the numerous practical difficulties involved in conducting longitudinal investigations of the normal menstrual cycle, a relatively small but interesting body of such research has accumulated which explores cycle-related changes in a variety of psychological processes.

Some of the recent longitudinal research on self-reported moods and symptom changes over the cycle were discussed above in the context in which it was carried out: in investigations of the relationship between daily and retrospective self-reports. Other longitudinal research on symptom and mood changes has involved concomitant measurement of physiological status (Kopell et al., 1969;

Little and Zahn, 1974; Patkai et al., 1974). While each of these studies contains some interesting and suggestive data, this research, too, fails to yield consistent or coherent conclusions because of the inadequacy of the way the psychological side of the correlation is assessed. This is not a reflection on the investigators' choices of instruments, but a fact about the state of the art in psychological research on moods.

In classic papers investigating possible changes in dream content, Benedeck and Rubenstein (1939) reported a change from an outgoing active orientation to heterosexual relationships in the ovulatory phase to a focus on the inner self, on potential motherhood, during the premenstrual and menstrual phases. Accounts of dreams were collected from analytic patients during analytic sessions, and cycle phase was established by vaginal smear techniques. Dream analyses and vaginal smears were performed by different investigators (Benedek and Rubenstein, respectively), each unaware of the other's data when analyzing their own.

This work was a landmark accomplishment in two respects. It was one of the first investigations of the menstrual cycle to gather regular, concomitant assessments of psychological processes and physiological changes over the course of the menstrual cycle. And secondly, it was based on a subtle and, within its domain, valid theory about human psychology. Interestingly, the main findings of the Benedek and Rubenstein study have recently been replicated in part by Baron (1977) in a study using a self-report questionnaire concerning remembered dreams.

In other recent research on dreams, Hertz and Jensen (1975) used a modified version of the system for scoring manifest dream content developed by Langs and found that remembered dreams occurring during menstruation showed significantly more expressions of emotional conflict than did dreams of a nonmenstruating control group. In an attempt to study the content of dreams closer to the time of their occurrence, Swanson and Foulkes (1968) awakened subjects during periods of rapid eye movement sleep. Although the study had only four subjects, the investigators report finding significantly higher sexuality in the manifest dream content during the menstrual flow, with self-reports of sexual desire being lowest during this time.

Several years ago, Barbara Sommer (1973) published a comprehensive review of the research up to that time on cognitive and perceptual–motor changes over the course of the menstrual cycle. As she noted, her ability to conclude that such changes do not seem to occur when objective measure of performance are used is noteworthy, in view of the traditional practice in psychology of not publishing negative results. If no cycle-related changes in cognition have been found in longitudinal research since then, it is not for want of trying. Eight years and many published and unpublished papers and dissertations later, the picture is substantially the same: basic cognitive processes, measured through means other than self-report, do not seem to vary over the menstrual cycle (see Dan, 1979, for a more recent review). This is true despite the fact that within psychology cognition is a relatively well-developed area, both theoretically and empirically. The investigation by Komnenich and her colleagues (1978), in fact, seems to be the only *published longitudinal study* in which significant changes in cognitive performance have been found over the course of the menstrual cycle. (This statement would have to be qualified if time estimation is considered a cognitive process; Kopell et al. (1969) found fluctuations in time estimation over the cycle.)

A conclusion of "no change" from a review of the literature on the cognition and the menstrual cycle is never entirely satisfactory, however. Fluctuations may occur in modes of cognitive functioning that have not yet been tested or are not compatible with the information-processing paradigm that presently dominates research on basic cognitive processes in psychology. As a heuristic device for identifying whatever modes of cognition might exhibit cycle-related fluctuations, one could look to cognitive and perceptual processes that have been found to vary in relation to biological rhythms other than the menstrual cycle. The literature on rhythms in psychological processes is most substantial in the area of diurnal rhythms (Colquhoun, 1971; Ferin et al., 1974; Luce, 1970), and scattered studies suggest the usefulness of this literature for suggesting psychological measures and tasks that might be fruitful in menstrual cycle research. For example, performance on the Stroop color-word interference test varies over the course of the day (Hartley and Shirley, 1976) and may also vary with the phase of the menstrual cycle. Broverman et al. (1968) would predict, on the basis of their theory, that it would; (see also Parlee, 1972). Klein and Armitage (1979) demonstrated 90 to 100 min oscillations on verbal and spatial matching tasks, fluctuations they suggest may be psychological consequences of the roughly 90 min cycles in rest/activity proposed by Kleitman (1963). Appropriate longitudinal research may show that such tasks also vary with the phase of the menstrual cycle. In considering literature on psychological rhythms, however, it is important to focus carefully on what psychological processes were actually tested in any particular experiment. It would clearly be a mistake, for example, to seek empirical consistency among the widely varied investigations of what are labeled "verbal" and "spatial" tasks and/or abilities, without an analysis of the particular processes involved in any investigation.

Sexual activity at different phases of the menstrual cycle has been the focus of longitudinal investigations using methods other than dream analysis, with results that differ depending on the procedures and methods used. An investigation by Englander-Golden and her colleagues (1980) found that phase of the cycle at which highest self-reported sexual desire occurred was related to whether or not the subjects were aware of being in a study of the menstrual cycle. Udrey and Morris (1968) report finidng a midcycle peak and a premenstrual rise in the frequency of coitus. Adams et al. (1978) also found a significant increased in female-initiated sexual behavior at the time of ovulation, but not in male-initiated behavior. The ovulatory peak of female-initiated sexual activity was not found among women using oral contraceptives. In a related study of rhesus monkeys,

Michael and Herbert (1963) report that the time spent by the female in grooming the male is at a minimum around the time of ovulation, while the male's grooming of the female is at a maximum during this phase. This basic pattern of grooming activity was true of each of the four females observed, but the authors note that the behavior patterns of each pair was highly individual. Persky et al. (1978) investigated husbands' and wives' initiation of and responsivity to sexual activity over the menstrual cycle and found wives' testosterone levels at their ovulatory peak to be related to coital frequency. Taken together, these longitudinal investigations suggest the importance of looking not only at coital frequency but at the frequency of different types of sexual activity, and at behaviors more relevant to interactions between the couple (initiation, responsiveness) which may or may not result in intercourse.

Of all the longitudinal research investigating psychological changes over the menstrual cycle, however, clear evidence of fluctuations can be found most consistently not in dreams, cognition, or sexual activity. It is to be found in research on basic sensory and sensory motor processes. Many of these findings seem to have been serendipitous; the investigators were not primarily interested in menstrual cycle changes, nor did they expect to find them. Sensory changes do not, furthermore, seem to be part of the socially shared beliefs about psychological changes accompanying the menstrual cycle. It seems reasonable that the sensory changes are consequences of the physiological changes of the menstrual cycle, and that they can most productively be studied from a strictly biological perspective. Most importantly for research, the study of sensory processes is one area of psychology where the methods and theories are well-established and, unlike work in personality and social psychology, research based on them has proved to be cumulative.

Because sex differences in basic perceptual and sensory processes have not been a major focus of research, the literature showing such differences has until recently been widely scattered. Baker (1974, 1975) was one of the first to bring it together and to discuss explicitly the potential theoretical significance of the findings. Henkin's (1974) review covers some of the same material; it focuses directly on a possible explanation for the sex differences: the menstrual cycle. Billingsley and Hudgens' 1978 selected bibliography of "Human Performance: Sex Differences and the Influence of the Menstrual Cycle" also covers some of the same literature, although it includes more recent references. Parlee (1978) contains additional references.

The findings of this research are diverse, since the investigations were generally not focused on a common problem or set of questions. Rather than summarize each of the individual studies, selected examples will be very briefly discussed to give the reader a flavor of the work.

In a lengthy study of auditory processes, Wynn (1971) found that a subject with perfect pitch showed systematic variations over the menstrual cycle in selecting the frequency she judged to be the A above middle C (440 Hz). The frequency heard as A peaked around the times of ovulation and menstruation. The presence of migraine headaches, respiratory illness, and the like disrupted the regularity of the auditory cycle. Millodot and Lamont (1974) tested corneal sensitivity to pain over the course of the menstrual cycle and found threshold increases during the premenstrual phase of the cycle compared to the ovulatory phase. Glanville and Kaplan, (1965) report changes in quinine test thresholds over the cycle.

A topic on which there is beginning to be systematic research rather than isolated studies is changes in visual thresholds over the menstrual cycle. Using slightly different procedures, Wong and Tong (1974) and DeMarchi and Tong (1972) explored the visual threshold for the resoltuion of two paired pulses of light. Both used a modified signal detection analysis and found evidence which they interpret as showing shifts in sensitivity (Wong and Tong) and criterion (DeMarchi and Tong) over the course of the cycle. Diamond et al. (1972) also report, using yet another procedure, significant changes in visual threshold. Kopell and his colleagues (1969) found a tendency toward higher two-flash thresholds during the premenstrual phase, but the trend was not significant. In a recent and relatively well designed study, Ward et al. (1978) found changes over the menstrual cycle on what they also call visual detection tasks. (The actual tasks used, however, are quite different from the versions of the two-flash threshold tasks used by the other investigators.)

DeMarchi and Tong, Wong and Tong, and Ward et al. were all interested in roughly the same question: are visual threshold changes over the menstrual cycle the result of fluctuations in sensory sensitivity or criterion shifts, or both? Although the findings are not yet consistent, prospects for answering this and related questions (about underlying mechanisms) seem much more promising than, for example, the prospects of finding consistency in longitudinal studies of moods. Sensory processes, complex as they are, seem to be more amenable to study through established scientific methods than are moods, affects, cognitions, and actions.

In sum, longitudinal investigations of the menstrual cycle have yielded more positive results in some areas of psychological functioning than in others. Most of this research seems at present compatible with a biological perspective, at least in the first stages of the work. For researchers who want to adopt a biological perspective and do programmatic research, sensory processing seems the most productive area at present. For those who want to tap an area of richer psychological significance, dreams would seem to merit further exploration. Investigations of cognitive changes over the menstrual cycle may become more fruitful as researchers seek to link this work to potentially related research on cognitive changes associated with other biological rhythms. Research on mood changes over the menstrual cycle seems at present likely to continue to produce the same picture: negative, nonrepeatable, or contradictory results. What is needed to brighten this empirical picture is some hard thinking, from biological, interactive, and psychological perspectives, about the way an individual's experience and actions are influenced by biological and social contexts. Progress in research on the psychology of the menstrual cycle has been substantial over the past decade, and we still have a long way to go.

References

Adams, D. B., Gold, A. R., and Burt, A. D. (1978). Rise in female-initiated sexual activity at ovulation and its suppression by oral contraceptives. *N. Engl. J. Med.* 299:1145-1150.

Abplanalp, J. M., Livingston, L., Rose, R. M., and Sandwisch, D. (1977). Cortisol and growth hormone responses to stress during the menstrual cycle. *Psychosomatic Medicine* 39:158-177.

Anastasi, H. (1968). *Psychological Testing,* 3rd ed. MacMillan, New York.

Baker, M. A. (1974). Sex bias in perception research. *Sex Differences or Sex Bias?* (R. Unger, chair). Symposium presented at the 82nd Annual Meeting of the American Psychological Association, New Orleans, 1974.

Baker, M. A. (1975). The study of sex differences in sensation and perception: The need, the findings and the value for research in the social sciences. JSAS *Catalog of Selected Documents in Psychology* 5:319.

Baron, J. (1977). Menstrual hormone changes and instinctual tendencies in dreams. *Motiv. Emot.* 1:273-282.

Benedek, T., and Rubenstein, B. B. (1939). Correlations between ovarian activity and psychodynamic processes. Parts I and II. *Psychosom. Med.* 1:245-270; 1:461-485

Billingsley, P. A., and Hudgens, G. A. (1978). *Human Performance: Sex Differences and the Influence of the Menstrual Cycle (A Selected Bibliography).* U.S. Army Human Engineering Laboratory, Aberdeen Proving Ground, Maryland.

Brooks, J., Ruble, D. N., and Clarke, A. E. (1977). College women's attitudes and expectations concerning menstrual-related changes. *Psychosom. Med.* 39:288-298.

Broverman, D. C., Klaiber, E. L., Kobayashi, Y., and Vogel, W. (1968). Roles of activation and inhibition in sex differences in cognitive abilities. *Psychol. Rev.* 75:23-50.

Colquhoun, W. P. (ed.) (1971). *Biological Rhythms and Human Performance.* Academic Press, New York.

Coppen, A., and Kessel, N. (1963). Menstruation and personality. *Br. J. Psychiatry* 109:711-721.

Dalton, K. (1959). Menstruation and acute psychiatric illness. *Br. Med. J.* 1:148-149.

Dalton, K. (1960). Menstruation and accidents. *Br. Med. J.* 2:1425-1426.

Dalton, K. (1961). Menstruation and crime. *Br. Med. J.* 2:1752-1753.

√ Dalton, K. (1968). Menstruation and examinstions. *Lancet* 2:1386-1388.

Dalton, K. (1970). Children's hospital admissions and mother's menstruation. *Brit. Med. J.* 2:27-28.

Dan. A. J. (1979). The menstrual cycle and sex-related differences in cognitive variability. In *Sex-Related Differences in Cognitive Functioning* (M. A. Wittig and A. C. Peterson, eds.). Academic Press, New York.

DeMarchi, G. W., and Tong, J. E. (1972). Menstrual, diurnal, and activation effects on the resolution of temporally paired flashes. *Psychophysiology* 9:362-367.

Diamond, M., Diamond, A. L., and Mast, M. (1972). Visual sensitivity and sexual arousal levels during the menstrual cycle. *J. Nerv. Ment. Dis.* 155:170-176.

Doty, R. L., and Silverthorne, C. (1975). Influence of menstrual cycle on volunteering behavior. *Nature* 254:139-140.

Englander-Golden, P., Chang, H. S., Whitmore, M. R., and Dienstbier, R. A. (1980). Female sexual arousal and the menstrual cycle. *J. Hum. Stress* March, 42-48.

Englander-Golden, P., Whitmore, M. R., and Dienstbier, R. A. (1978). Menstrual cycle as focus of study and self-reports of moods and behaviors. *Motiv. Emot.* 2:75-86.

Ferin, M., Halberg, F., Richart, R. M., and Vande Wiele, R. S. (eds.) (1974). *Biorhythms and Human Reproduction.* John Wiley, New York.

Frazier, T. M. (1959). Error in reported date of last menstrual period. *Am. J. Obstet. Gynecol.* 27:915-918.

Friedman, R. C., Hurt, S. W., Arnoff, M. S., and Clarkin, J. (1980). Behavior and the menstrual cycle. *SIGNS: J. Women Culture Society* 5:719-738.

Glanville, E. V., and Kapland, A. R. (1965). The menstrual cycle and sensitivity of taste perception. *Am. J. Obstet. Gynecol.* 92:189-194.

Hartley, L. R., and Shirley, E. (1976). Color-name interference at different times of day. *J. Appl. Psychol.* 61:119-122.

Henkin, R. I. (1974). Sensory changes during the menstrual cycle. In *Biorhythms and Human Reproduction* (M. Ferin, F. Halberg, R. M. Richart, R. L. Vande Wiele, eds.). John Wiley, New York, pp. 277-285.

Hertz, D. G., and Jensen, M. R. (1975). Menstrual dreams and psychodynamics: Emotional conflict and manifest dream content in menstruating comen. *Br. J. Med. Psychol.* 48:175-183.

Ivey, M. E., and Bardwick, J. M. (1968). Patterns of affective fluctuation in the menstrual cycle. *Psychosom. Med.* 30:336-345.

Janowsky, D., Gorney, R., and Kelley, B. (1966). "The curse"—vicissitudes and variations of the female fertility cycle: Part I. Psychiatric aspects. *Psychosomatics* 7:242-247.

Klein, F., and Armitage, R. (1979). Rhythms in human performance: 1-1/2 hour oscillations in cognitive style. *Science* 204:1326.

Kleitman, N. (1963). Sleep and Wakefulness. Chicago: University of Chicago Press.

Koeske, R. K. D. (1977). The interaction of social, cognitive, and physiological factors in premenstrual emotionality. Unpublished doctoral dissertation, Carnegie-Mellon University.

Koeske, R. D. (1980). Theoretical perspectives for menstrual cycle research. In *The Menstrual Cycle, Vol. 1: A Synthesis of Interdisciplinary Research* (A. J. Dan, E. A. Graham, and C. P. Beecher, eds.). New York: Springer.

Koeske, R. D. (1981). Theoretical and conceptual complexities in the design and analysis of menstrual cycle research. In *The Menstrual Cycle, Vol. 2: Research and Implications for Women's Health* (P. Komnenich, M. McSweeny, J. A. Noack, and S. N. Elder, eds.). Springer-Verlag, New York, pp. 54-70.

Koeske, R. K., and Koeske, G. F. (1975). An attributional approach to moods and the menstrual cycle. *J. Pers. Soc. Psychol.* 31:473-478.

Komnenich, P., Lane, D. M., Dickey, R. P., and Stone, S. C. (1978). Gonadal hormones and cognitive performance. *Physiol. Psychol.* 6:115-120.

Kopell, B. S., Lunde, D. T., Clayton, R. B., and Moos, R. H. (1969). Variations in some measures of arousal during the menstrual cycle. *J. Nerv. Ment. Dis.* 148:180-187.

Kuhn, T. S. (1970). *The Structure of Scientific Revolutions* (2nd ed., enlarged). University of Chicago Press, Chicago.

Little, B. C., and Zahn, T. P. (1974). Changes in mood and autonomic functioning during the menstrual cycle. *Psychophysiology* 11:579-590.

Luce, G. G. (1970). *Biological Rhythms in Psychiatry and Medicine.* Public Health Service Publication No. 2088. U.S. Dept. of HEW, Public Health Service.

MacKinnon, P. C. B., and MacKinnon, I. L. (1956). Hazards of the menstrual cycle. *Br. Med. J.* 1:555.

Mandell, A., and Mandell, M. (1967). Suicide and the menstrual cycle. *JAMA* 200:792-793.

Marinari, K. T., Leshner, A. I., and Doyle, M. P. (1976). Menstrual cycle status and adrenocortical reactivity to psychological stress. *Psychoneuroendocrinology* 1:213-218.

Matsumoto, S., Nogami, Y., and Ohkuri, S. (1962). Statistical studies on menstruation; A criticism on the definition of normal menstruation. *Gunma J. Med. Sci.* 11:294-318.

May, R. R. (1976). Mood shifts and the menstrual cycle. *J. Psychosom. Res.* 20:125-130.

McClintock, M. K. (1981). Major gaps in menstrual cycle research: Behavior and physiological controls in a biological context. In *The Menstrual Cycle, Vol. 2: Research and Implications for Women's Health* (P. Komnenich, M. McSweeney, J. A. Noack, and S. N. Elder, eds.). Springer, New York, pp. 7-23.

Michael, R. P., and Herbert, J. (1963). Menstrual cycle influences grooming behavior and sexual activity in the rhesus monkey. *Science* 140:500-501.

Millodot, M., and Lamont, A. (1974). Influence of menstruation on corneal sensitivity. *Br. J. Ophthalmol.* 58:752-756.

Mishler, E. G. (1979). Meaning in context: Is there any other king? *Harvard Ed. Rev.* 49:1-19.

Moos, R. H. (1968). The development of a menstrual distress questionnaire. *Psychosom. Med.* 30:853-867.

Moos, R. H., Kopell, B. S., Melges, F. T., Yalom, I. L. D., Lunde, D. T., Clayton, R. B., and Hamburg, D. A. (1969). Fluctuations in symptoms and moods during the menstrual cycle. *J. Psychosom. Res.* 13:37-44.

O'Connor, J. F., Shelley, E. M., and Stern, L. O. (1974). Behavioral rhythms related to the menstrual cycle. In *Biorhythms and Human Reproduction* (M. Ferin, F. Halberg, R. M. Richart, and R. VandeWiele, eds.). John Wiley, New York, pp. 309-324.

Osofsky, H. J., and Fisher, S. (1967). Psychological correlates of the development of amenorrhea in a stress situation. *Psychosom. Med.* 29:15-23.

Paige, K. E. (1971). Effects of oral contraceptives on affective fluctuations associated with the menstrual cycle. *Psychosom. Med.* 33:515-537.

Parlee, M. B. (1972). Comments on "Roles of activation and inhibition in sex differences in cognitive abilities" by D. M. Broverman, E. L. Klaiber, Y. Kobayashi, and W. Vogel. *Psychol. Rev.* 79:180-184.

Parlee, M. B. (1973). The premenstrual syndrome. *Psychol. Bull.* 80:454-465.

Parlee, M. B. (1974). Stereotypic beliefs about menstruation: A methodological note on the Moos menstrual distress questionnaire and some new data. *Psychosom. Med.* 36:229-240.

Parlee, M. B. (1975). Menstruation and voluntary participation in a psychological experiment. In *A New Psychology of Menstruation* (W. McKenna, chair). Symposium presented at the 83rd Annual Meeting of the American Psychological Association, Chicago, 1975.

Parlee, M. B. (1978). Psychological aspects of menstruation, childbirth and menopause. In *The Psychology of Women: Future Directions of Research* (J. A. Sherman and F. L. Denmark, eds.). Psychological Dimensions, New York, pp. 179-238.

Parlee, M. B. (1979). Psychology and women. *SIGNS: J. Women Culture Society* 5:121-133.

Parlee, M. B. (1981). Gaps in behavioral research on the menstrual cycle. In *The Menstrual Cycle, Vol. 2: Research and Implications for Women's Health* (P. Komnenich, M. McSweeney, J. A. Noack, and S. N. Elder, eds.). Springer, New York, pp. 45-53.

Parlee, M. B. Changes in moods and activation levels during the menstrual cycle in experimentally naive subjects. *Psychology of Women* Quarterly (in press).

Patkai, P., Johannson, G., and Post, B. (1974). Mood, alertness and sympathetic-adrenal medullary activity during the menstrual cycle. *Psychosom. Med.* 36:503-512.

Persky, H. (1974). Reproductive hormones, moods, and the menstrual cycle. In *Sex Differences in Behavior* (R. C. Friedman, R. M. Richart, R. L. Vande Wiele, and L. O. Stern, eds.). John Wiley, New York, pp. 455-466.

Persky, H., Lief, H. I., Strauss, D., Miller, W. R., and O'Brien, C. P. (1978). Plasma testosterone level and sexual behavior of couples. *Arch. Sex. Behav.* 7:157-173.

Presser, H. B. (1974). Temporal data relating to the human menstrual cycle. In *Biorhythms and Human Reproduction* (M. Ferin, F. Halberg, R. M. Richart, and R. L. Vande Wiele, eds.). John Wiley, New York, pp. 145-160.

Redgrove, J. A. (1971). Menstrual cycles. In *Biological Rhythms and Human Performance* (W. O. Colquhoun, ed.). Academic Press, New York.

Rodin, J. (1976). Menstruation, reattribution and competence. *J. Pers. Soc. Psychol.* 33:345-353.

Rogers, M. L., and Harding, S. S. (1981). Retrospective and daily menstrual distress measures in men and women. In *The Menstrual Cycle, Vol. 2: Research and Implications for Women's Health* (P. Komnenich, M. McSweeny, J. A. Noack, and S. N. Elder, eds.). Springer, New York, pp. 71-81.

Rosenthal, R., and Rosnow, R. L. (1975). *The Volunteer Subject.* John Wiley, New York.

Ruble, D. W. (1977). Premenstrual symptoms: A reinterpretation. *Science* 197:291-292.

Ruble, D. N., and Brooks-Gunn, J. (1979). Menstrual symptoms: A social cognition analysis. *J. Behav. Med.* 2:171-194.

Russell, G. F. M. (1972). Premenstrual tension and "psychogenic" amenorrhea: Psychophysical interactions. *J. Psychosom. Res.* 16:279-287.

Schacter, S., and Singer, J. E. (1962). Cognitive, social and physiological determinants of emotional state. *Psychol. Rev.* 69:379-399.

Scheffler, I. (1967). *Science and Subjectivity,* Bobbs-Merrill, Indianapolis.

Schilling, K. M. (1981). What is a real difference? Content or method in menstrual findings. In *The Menstrual Cycle, Vol. 2: Research and Implications for Women's Health* (P. Komnenich, M. McSweeny, J. A. Noack, and S. N. Elder, eds.). Springer, New York, pp. 82-92.

Smith, S. L. (1975). Mood and the menstrual cycle. In *Topics in Psychoendocrinology* (E. J. Sachar, ed.). Grune & Stratton, New York.

Sommer, B. (1973). The effect of menstruation on cognitive and perceptual-motor behavior: A review. *Psychosom. Med.* 35:515-534.

Spielberger, C. D., and Sarason, I. G. (eds.) (1978). *Stress and Anxiety,* Vol. 5. Halsted, New York.

Sutherland, H., and Stewart, I. (1965). A critical analysis of the premenstrual syndrome. *Lancet,* 1:1180-1193.

Swandby, J. R. (1981). A longitudinal study of daily mood self-reports and their relationship to the menstrual cycle. In *The Menstrual Cycle, Vol. 2: Research and Implications for Women's Health* (P. Komnenich, M. McSweeny, J. A. Noack, and S. N. Elder, eds.). Springer, New York, pp. 93-103.

Swanson, E. M., and Foulkes, D. (1968). Dream content and the menstrual cycle. *J. Nerv. Ment. Dis.* 145:358-363.

Tonks, C. M., Rack, P. H., and Rose, M. J. (1968). Attempted suicide and the menstrual cycle. *J. Psychosom. Res.* 11:319-323.

Tuch, R. H. (1975). The relationship between a woman's menstrual status and her response to illness in her child. *Psychosom. Med.* 37:388-394.

Udry, J. R., and Morris, N. M. (1968). Distribution of coitus in the menstrual cycle. *Nature* 220:593-596.

Ward, M. M., Stone, S. C., and Sandman, C. A. (1978). Visual perception in women during the menstrual cycle. *Physiol. Behav.* 20:239-243.

Wilcoxon, L. A., Schrader, S. L., and Sherif, C. W. (1976). Daily self-reports on activities, life events, moods and somatic changes during the menstrual cycle. *Psychosom. Med.* 38:399-417.

Wong, S., and Tong, J. E. (1974). Menstrual cycle and contraceptive hormonal effects on temporal discrimination. *Percept. Mot. Skills* 39:103-108.

Wynn, V. T. (1971). "Absolute" pitch—a bimensual rhythm. *Nature [Lond.]* 230:337.

6 Cognitive Behavior and the Menstrual Cycle

BARBARA SOMMER   University of California, Davis, California

Do the hormonal changes of the menstrual cycle affect the mental function of women? The preponderance of evidence indicates that cognitive performance or mental ability is not significantly affected by menstrual cycle variables. The weight of the evidence against menstrual cycle phase differences exists despite a publication bias toward positive results. In general, studies showing differences have a greater probability of publication and are more likely to be described in the popular media than those showing no differences. Table 1 shows that out of 81 performance tests carried out in 35 independent studies, only 14 support a hypothesis of either premenstrual or menstrual debilitation. In many of the cases those findings were not replicated by other researchers using similar measures. The better-designed studies were least likely to show menstrual cycle phase effects on behavior; this applies to studies of mood as well as cognition [1].

This is not to deny the possible influence of menstrual cycle variables on behavior. Experimental studies have shown an increased willingness to participate in a psychology experiment during midcycle [2,3]. Activity patterns have also shown a midcycle peak, and the personal space increases in the premenstrual and menstrual phases [4-6].

A small proportion of women, less than 20%, report impairment in concentration or general work performance around the time of menstruation [7,8]. Two studies have found that a disproportionate number of women involved in accidents were either premenstrual or menstruating at the time [9,10]. However, a 3 year study of 94 student nurses failed to find a phase-related increase in acci-

Table 1   Findings Listed by Performance Measures, Outcome, and Evidence for

Measure	Study
Intellectual performance	
Henmon-Nelson Test	Lough, 1937 [20]
Learning of standardized equations	Lough, 1937 [20]
Schoolgirls' weekly work	Dalton, 1960 [24]
Standardized academic examinations	Dalton, 1968 [25]
Watson-Glaser Critical Thinking	Sommer, 1972 [30]
Biweekly Intro. Psych. exams	Sommer, 1972 [30]
Biweekly Intro. Psych. exams	Bernstein, 1977 [31]
Progressive Matrices	Wickham, 1958 [23]
Comprehension of complicated instructions	Wickham, 1958 [23]
Other cognitive functions and perceptual-motor performance	
Ability to reason	Golub, 1976 [35]
Fitting concepts to data	Golub, 1976 [35]
Concept formation	Munchel, 1979 [48]
Rote memory	Golub, 1976 [35]
Ability to think of appropriate wording rapidly	Golub, 1976 [35]
Anagrams	Golub, 1976 [35]
Ideational fluency	Golub, 1976 [35]
Semantic elaboration	Golub, 1976 [35]
Ability to produce words from a restricted area of meaning	Golub, 1976 [35]
Semantic fluency and flexibility	Golub, 1976 [35]
Spelling	Wickham, 1958 [23]
Synonyms and rhymes	Wickham, 1958 [23]
Verbal fluency (speech)	Komnenich, 1974 [39]
Verbal fluency (extemporaneous speech)	Silverman and Zimmer, 1975 [37]
Verbal fluency (oral reading)	Silverman and Zimmer, 1976 [38]
Mechanical comprehension	Wickham, 1958 [23]

Premenstrual or Menstrual Debilitation

Findings	Support for decrement	
	Premenstrual	Menstrual
No phase difference	_[a]	No
No phase difference	No	No
Lower performance in premenstrual and menstrual phase	Yes	Yes
Lower performance in premenstrual and menstrual phase	Yes	Yes
No phase difference	No	No
No phase difference	No	No
No phase difference	No	No
No phase difference	No	No
Better performance in nonperiod phase	Trend	Trend
No phase difference	No	—
No phase difference	No	—
No phase difference	No	—
No phase difference	No	—
No phase difference	No	—
No phase difference	No	—
No phase difference	No	—
No phase difference	No	—
No phase difference	No	—
No phase difference	No	—
No phase difference	No	No
No phase difference	No	No
Premenstrual increase in disfluency	No	Yes
Premenstrual increase in disfluency	Yes	—
No phase difference	No	No
No phase difference	No	No

(continued)

Table 1   (continued)

Measure	Study
Other cognitive functions and perceptual-motor performance (continued)	
Assembly of parts using diagram	Wickham, 1958 [23]
Squares Test—spatial task	Wickham, 1958 [23]
Length estimation	Golub, 1976 [35]
Simple arithmetic calculations	Wuttke et al., 1973 [36]
Arithmetic	Wickham, 1958 [23]
Subtraction	Altenhaus, 1978 [47]
Backward subtraction	Komnenich et al.
Addition	Sommer, 1972 [32]
Speed of closure	Sommer, 1972 [32]
Speed of closure	Golub, 1976 [35]
Letter elimination	Gamberale et al., 1975 [49]
Perceptual speed	Gamberale et al., 1975 [49]
Visualization	Sommer, 1972 [32]
Stroop color reading	Komnenich et al., 1978 [40]
Stroop color naming	Komnenich et al., 1978 [40]
Stroop color-cord without perceptual conflict	Gamberale et al., 1975 [49]
Stroop color-word with perceptual conflict	Gamberale et al., 1975 [49]
Digit symbol, WISC	Komnenich, et al., 1978 [40]
Digit symbol, WISC	Zimmerman and Parlee, 1973 [34]
Human Figure drawing	Dor-Shav, 1976 [45]
Solvable and insolvable puzzles	Althenhaus, 1978 [47]
Insolvable puzzle	Muchel, 1979 [48]
Cognitive battery	Lederman, 1974 [43]
Kinesthetic aftereffect	Baker et al., 1979 [44]
Time estimation	Kopell et al., 1969 [52]
Time estimation	Little and Zahn, 1974 [54]
Time estimation	Gamberale et al., 1975 [49]

Findings	Support for decrement	
	Premenstrual	Menstrual
No phase difference	No	No
No phase difference	No	No
No phase difference	No	—
Increased accuracy in luteal phase; optimum performance premenstrually	No	No
No phase difference	No	No
No phase difference	No	—
Lower performance in preovulatory phase	No	No
No phase difference	No	No
No phase difference	No	No
No phase difference	No	No
No phase difference	No	No
No phase difference	No	No
No phase difference	No	No
No phase difference	No	No
No phase difference	No	No
No phase difference	No	No
No phase difference	No	No
No phase difference	No	No
No phase difference	No	No
Better performance in 3rd week	No	No
No phase difference	No	—
Greater premenstrual persistence in one premenstrual group	No	—
No phase effects	No	No
Increase in aftereffect at beginning and end of cycle	Yes	Yes
Longer intervals produced premenstrually	Yes	—
No phase difference	No	No
No phase difference	No	No

(continued)

Table 1 (continued)

Measure	Study
Other cognitive functions and perceptual-motor performances (continued)	
Time estimation	Schwank, 1971 [53]
Time estimation	Zimmerman and Parlee, 1973 [34]
Cognitive style	
Flexibility of closure	Golub, 1976 [35]
Flexibility of closure	Snyder, 1977 [41]
Flexibility of closure	Sommer, 1972 [32]
Embedded Figures Test	Komnenich et al., 1978 [40]
Embedded Figures Test	Snyder, 1977 [41]
Embedded Figures Test	Dor-Shav, 1976 [45]
Rod and Frame Test	Klaiber et al., 1974 [42]
Rod and Frame Test	Snyder, 1977 [41]
Reflectivity/impulsivity	Snyder, 1977 [41]
Coordination and reaction time	
Aiming	Sommer, 1972 [32]
Arm-hand steadiness	Zimmerman and Parlee, 1973 [34]
Pursuit rotor with arithmetic	Munchel, 1979 [48]
Shock aversion	Tedford et al., 1977 [74]
Reaction time	Pierson and Lockhart, 1963 [51]
Reaction time	Loucks and Thompson, 1968 [55]
Reaction time	Kopell et al., 1969 [52]
Reaction time	Schwank, 1971 [53]
Reaction time	Zimmerman and Parlee, 1973 [34]
Reaction time	Creutzfeldt et al., 1976 [56]
Reaction time	Little and Zahn, 1974 [54]
Reaction time	Landauer, 1974 [50]
Reaction time	Gamerale et al., 1975 [49]
CNS Correlates	
Acquisition of conditioned response measured by heartrate	Vila and Beech, 1978 [65]

Findings	Support for decrement	
	Premenstrual	Menstrual
No phase difference	No	No
No phase difference	No	No
No phase difference	No	—
No phase difference	No	No
No phase difference	No	No
Lower performance in preovulatory phase	No	No
No phase difference	No	No
Better performance in 3rd week	No	No
Change in response from preovulatory to postovulatory phase	?	?
No phase difference	No	No
Shorter latency midcycle	No	No
No phase difference	No	No
Greater steadiness midcycle	Yes	Trend
No phase difference	No	—
Threshold alterations midcycle	No	No
No phase difference	No	No
No phase difference	—	No
No phase difference	No	No
No phase difference	Trend	Trend
No phase difference	No	No
Faster in postovulatory phase and premenstrual decline	Yes	No
No phase difference	No	No
Slowest in perimenstrual period	Yes	Yes
Slower during menstruation	No	Yes
Premenstrual group conditioned more readily	Yes	—

(continued)

Table 1 (continued)

Measure	Study
CNS Correlates (continued)	
Visual pattern discrimination	Ward et al., 1978 [57]
Visual signal detection	Ward et al., 1978 [57]
Visual signal detection	Wong and Tong, 1974 [59]
Visual signal detection	DiMarchi and Tong, 1972 [58]
Visual signal detection	Diamond et al., 1972
GSR amplitude to auditory stimulus	Uno, 1973 [69]
GSR amplitude to auditory stimulus	Zimmerman and Parlee, 1973 [34]
GSR amplitude to auditory stimulus	Little and Zahn, 1974 [54]
Habituation of GSR to auditory stimulus	Friedman and Meares, 1979 [67]
EEG–alpha rhythm	Sugarman, 1970 [70]
EEG–alpha rhythm	Klaiber et al., 1971, 1972 [71,72]
EEG–alpha rhythm	Creutzfeldt et al., 1976 [56]
EEG–alpha rhythm	Leary and Batho, 1979 [73]

[a]– indicates absence of testing for phase.

dents [11]. Two published studies have shown a relationship between menstruation and criminal behavior [7,12]. Two other studies found that premenstrual or menstruating mothers were more likely to bring less seriously ill children to a medical clinic than were mothers in other cycle phases [13,14]. Sommer reviewed other behavioral changes such as absence from work, admission to a psychiatric hospital, and suicide with the general conclusion that their incidence was decreased in the postmenstruation, preovulatory-ovulatory segment of the cycle [15]. These are social behaviors and as such involve motivational factors as well as cognitive variables. One could speculate that the more stable the function, the

| | Support for decrement | |
Findings	Premenstrual	Menstrual
No phase difference	No	No
Greatest sensitivity while menstrual, least in premenstrual phase	Yes	No
No phase difference	No	No
Greatest sensitivity midcycle, least in premenstrual phase	Yes	No
Greatest sensitivity midcycle, lease during menstruation	No	Yes
Greatest response postmenstrual, least premenstrual		
No phase difference		
Increase in ovulatory phase		
Habituation pattern suggested higher CNS arousal in preovulatory and lower arousal postovulatory phase		
Premenstrual decrease in alpha frequency		
Increase in driving response following ovulation		
Some alpha frequency increase in luteal phase with premenstrual decline		
Premenstrual increase in alpha frequency		

less the effect of the normal hormonal fluctuations of the menstrual cycle. Examples of stable characteristics are mental capacity and the performance of well-practiced tasks.

The occasional findings of negative consequences of menstruation, support a prevailing social bias: that the menstrual cycle interferes with a woman's cognitive control. Studies of accidents and criminal behavior have been cited so frequently in secondary sources as to give the impression of a vast body of research supporting their underlying assumptions and assertions. It is important to keep in mind the relative rarity of such events. A 24-year-old woman who has had an accident or committed a crime in the premenstrual phase of her cycle has already surmounted more than 100 such phases without disastrous consequences. An interesting question for future research is why investigators feel compelled to seek evidence of menstrual debilitation.

The effect of menstrual cycle variables on women's behavior and performance has serious and extensive ramifications for the self-perceptions of women as well as for their roles in society. Thus, there are psychological and social, as well as scientific, reasons for taking a very close and critical look at studies of cognition and the menstrual cycle. The first section of this chapter dealing with the relationships between the menstrual cycle and cognitive performance is a review of the studies listed in Table 1. Cognitive performance is broadly construed to cover thinking, reasoning, problem-solving, judgment, learning, and perception. Because boundaries are difficlut to delineate, perceptual-motor behaviors, visual acuity, and some measures of arousal are also included. In the second section of the chapter the direction of the relationship is reversed and consideration is given to the effect of cognitive factors on menstrual events.

I. The Effect of the Menstrual Cycle on Cognitive Performance

Studies which have investigated the relationship between the menstrual cycle and cognitive variables are grouped into three divisions. The first section covers intellectual performance on high-level complex cognitive tasks. The second deals with related although more simple cognitive functions, perceptual-motor skills, and cognitive style. The third section addresses selected sensory-motor functions and CNS correlates.

A. Intellectual Performance

The search for menstrual effects on mental performance has been lengthy, with empirical research reported from the early part of the century. Hollingworth's 1914 dissertation demonstrated the absence of detrimental effects of menstruation on various measures of perceptual-motor and mental ability [16]. Other early studies supported her findings [17-19]. Lough, in 1937, compared scores on two forms of the Henmon-Nelson Test of Mental Ability administered during menstruation and at midcycle. She also studied daily learning on a digit symbol task involving the solution of simple standard nonarithmetic equations. The 96 participants were between the ages of 17 and 24 years, and each served as her own control as scores were obtained throughout the cycle. There were no differences in intellectual performance between the menstruation and midcycle phases, nor were there differences in learning across the cycle. In fact, Lough found a statistically reliable increase in accuracy on the equations on the second day of menstruation. Seward's 1944 review of the psychological effects of the menstrual cycle on women workers once again affirmed the lack of evidence of a direct effect of menstrual cycle fluctuation on performance, as did Smith's 1950 studies of industrial workers [21,22].

Wickham studied two groups of young Englishwomen, Group A (1,525 women with regular menstrual cycles who had been in the service for at least 6 months), and Group B (1,000 new recruits). The groups were given a battery of tests including Progressive Matrices, mechanical comprehension, arithmetic, visual-spatial, and verbal tasks. Group A was tested once and scores were compared between subjects in the Period phase (4 days before and first 4 days of menstruation) and Nonperiod phase (all other days). While slightly lower scores than expected were obtained in the Period phase, the differences were not statistically significant on any of the tests. Group B was retested after 6 weeks. All phase differences were insignificant. Wickham concluded that, for predictive purposes, the menstrual cycle day on which a test is given need not be taken into account [23].

Dalton's two studies of academic performance of English schoolgirls are probably the most often quoted studies of intellectual performance and the menstrual cycle. Both studies support a hypothesis of perimenstrual debilitation, that is, a decline in performance associated with the premenstrual and menstrual phases of the cycle. The first study reported a decline in examination scores of schoolgirls, ages 11 to 17 years, in the premenstrual and menstrual phases (5 days each). Twenty-seven percent of the girls showed the drop. However, 17% improved their performance, and 56% showed no change. There was no statistical assessment of the reliability of the difference between these percentages [24]. In the second study, Dalton examined the scores of teenage English schoolgirls on advanced (A) and ordinary (O) level standardized examinations. On the A level examinations (16- to 19-year-olds) she reported that the average mark was 3% lower for those in the premenstrual and menstrual phases than in the intermenstrual phase, that the pass rate was 13% lower comparing premenstrual with intermenstrual phase, and the distinction rate was 9% lower in the premenstrual phase than in the intermenstrual phase. No statistical tests were reported for these findings. She based her results on the grades assigned to 180 papers obtained from 34 students. This method is inappropriate because it puts disproportionate weight on those individuals submitting more papers in any given cycle phase. Instead, an average performance score by phase should be computed for each person and then comparisons made. This type of confounding continued with the analysis of grades on the O level examinations: 162 scores for 91 individuals. Comparing average score by phase she found a 5% decline in scores for the premenstrual group compared with the intermenstrual one. In addition to the problem of the disproportionate contribution to the average by particular individuals, she claimed, based on differences between groups, that a student suffered an average handicap of 5% when taking the examination in the premenstrual or menstrual phase. Dalton did not compare the performance of the same individuals at different phases of their cycle. Thus, the claim of a 5% decrement is untenable [25]. In the same paper Dalton pointed out that the stress of the exams brought about an alteration in the cycle length in 42% of the young women, and that more of them than expected by chance were menstruating during the examination week. If test anxiety brought about menstruation, it does not make sense to claim that being in the normal premenstrual or menstrual phase was the cause of the diminished performance. It is more tenable to hypothesize that a third factor, anxiety, produced both the menstruation and the poor test performance.

This work merits criticism for its lack of statistical evaluation as well as its methodologic flaws. Despite those limitations, it has, however, been used by others to legitimize, or at lease justify, past and present sex discrimination [26-29]. Further, many who have drawn upon Dalton's conclusions have not only failed to recognize the problems of reliability and external validity, but have also ignored Dalton's own assertion that the alleged handicap was not evenly distributed among the young women studied [25]. A further basis for concern is that no other studies support Dalton's findings on intellectual performance. Sommer studied the performance of college women on two intellectual tasks: the Watson-Glaser Critical Thinking Appraisal and regular class examinations. Equivalent forms of the Watson-Glaser test were given at weekly intervals. Following testing, menstrual cycle data were obtained. Scores from approximately 200 subjects were then categorized on the basis of individual cycle quarter (menstrual, follicular, luteal, and premenstrual) thus permitting comparison of scores of a single test between women in different cycle quarters and also assessment of within-subject variation over time. A similar procedure was used for the classroom examinations. A separate analysis was made for oral contraceptive users. Neither group showed any significant variation associated with the menstrual cycle [30]. Bernstein studied academic performance on biweekly psychology examinations for 126 women who did not use oral contraceptives. Controlling for scholastic ability and motivation, she found no difference in performance between tests taken in the perimenstrual phase (4 days prior to onset and the first 4 days of menstruation) and intermenstrual phase (all other days) [31].

In summary, higher level intellectual function in normal healthy women appears to be stable and independent of menstrual fluctuation.

B. Cognitive Function, Perceptual-Motor Performance, and Cognitive Style

Sommer tested 20 college women at seven intervals over a menstrual cycle using matched forms of the Repetitive Psychometric Measures: aiming, flexibility of closure, number facility, speed of closure, and visualization [32]. None of the subjects used oral contraceptives. While the women retrospectively reported increased negative symptomology in the premenstrual and menstrual phases compared with midcycle, no changes in performance were noted in relation to menstrual cycle phase [33].

Zimmerman and Parlee tested 14 women on a variety of tasks including time estimation and digit-symbol substitution (substituting digits for numerals). There were no phase-related differences in performance except for an increase in arm-hand steadiness during the luteal phase (days 17 to 21) when compared with the premenstrual phase (days 23 to 27) [34].

Golub tested 50 women between the ages of 20 and 45 years on 13 cognitive tasks covering speed and fluency of thought, reasoning, and memory. She also used measures sensitive to depression and anxiety (Depression Adjective Check List and State-Trait Anxiety Inventory). The women were tested twice, first premenstrually (within 4 days of onset of menses) and then while intermenstrual (about 2 weeks after onset). To control for practice effects, the test times were reversed for one-half of the women. There were no statistically significant differences between premenstrual and intermenstrual scores on the cognitive tasks, nor were there reliable correlations between the premenstrual mood and cognitive performance measures [35].

Reporting on 16 normally menstruating women, ages 18 to 25 years, Wuttke et al. found that simple calculations were solved faster in the luteal phase than in the follicular phase, and accuracy increased during the luteal phase with optimum performance 2 to 3 days before menstruation [36].

Silverman and Zimmer tested 12 normally menstruating college students on fluency in extemporaneous speech at ovulation (measured by basal body temperature) and premenstrually (2 to 3 days before expected menstruation) for two consecutive cycles. Nine of the 12 showed an increase in speech disfluencies, particularly revisions or incomplete phrases, in the premenstrual sessions compared with the ovulatory ones [37]. In a later study Silverman and Zimmer evaluated oral reading to determine whether the difficulty was due to motor changes. The first study was duplicated with 20 subjects reading aloud instead of speaking extemporaneously. No differences were found between the phases. The authors concluded that the interference was with language formulation rather than a breakdown in motor-speech production. They suggested anxiety as the causal factor [38]. Komnenich tested four women over a menstrual cycle and their analysis of tape recordings of speech resulted in their report of an increase in disfluencies in the menstrual and luteal phases [39].

Komnenich et al. reported a relationship between estrogen level and task performance. Their work is of particular significance because hormone levels of estrogen, progesterone, testosterone, follicle-stimulating hormone (FSH), and luteinizing hormone (LH) were determined by blood assay. They studied the performance of 14 women not using oral contraceptives, 10 women using oral contraceptives, and 10 men. The dependent variables were performance on color reading and color naming (Stroop test with visual color and written information in conflict). WISC Digit Symbol test, backward subtraction, and the Embedded Figures test (a complex figure is presented and the task is to detect quickly a more simple figure within it). The menstrual cycle for each of the women was divided into four segments with corroboration from the blood sample data: phase 1, low estrogen (days 3 to 5 following menstrual onset); phase 2, prior to ovulation (days 11 to 14); phase 3, progesterone (days 18 to 21); and phase 4, premenstrual days 26 to 28). The men were assigned arbitrary phase designations. Phase differences were found on two of the five tests. The women who were not using oral contraceptives performed less well on the Embedded Figures test and backward subtraction in Phase 2, a time of high estrogen levels. The effect was not found for the oral contraceptive users and the men. While a performance decrement was observed, it occurred during what most researchers have termed the follicular or midcycle phase. They did not find a relationship between woman's average estrogen level and her average performance; subjects with higher overall estrogen levels did not perform more poorly on the two tasks which showed the cycle effect [40].

Snyder investigated similar tasks without the advantage of hormonal assay. There were three studies: a between-group design with testing only once (N=57), a within-subjects repeated measures design with two test sessions (N=75) and another repeated measures design (N=10) with three sessions. She measured field dependence and independence using the Embedded Figures test, Hidden Figures test (similar to embedded figures in that forms are hidden in a larger stimulus array), and the Rod and Frame test. In the Rod and Frame test, subjects are seated in a dark room where only an illuminated square frame surrounding an illuminated rod is visible. Both the frame and rod may be tilted independently either to the left or right. The subject's chair may also be tilted. The test is generally used to measure field dependence/independence, i.e., whether or not the person relies more on external cues (the frame) or internal cues (body position) for determining the position of the rod. Snyder also measured reflectivity/impulsitivity with the Matching Familiar Figures test. No cycle phase differences were found for the field dependence/independence measures. However, during the high estrogen phase (days 17 to 22) subjects exhibited a shorter latency on the Matching Familiar Figures test: they were quicker to respond than during the low phase (days 27, 28, and 1 to 4 of the next cycle). It is not clear whether they were in fact more or less accurate, or simply more quick in the high estrogen phase. The interpretation of the latency change requires more information than was available. However, if a performance decrement was involved (subjects were more impulsive), it did not occur in either the premenstrual or menstrual phases [41].

Klaiber et al. studied two groups of three normally menstruating women using the Rod and Frame test. Measurements were taken daily. When placing the rod in a vertical position, subjects' settings were more affected by the original tilt of the rod, the frame, and their body position in the preovulatory half and less affected by the tilt in the postovulatory half of the cycle. They did not report any phase difference on the dependence/independence dimension, i.e., differential effects of the frame position versus the body position [42].

Lederman tested 32 married mothers on a battery of cognitive tasks: Rod and Frame test, kinesthetic figural aftereffects (recall of size of an object based on touch), size estimation, autokinetic test (perceived movement of a stationary light in a darkened room), and Stroop color-word test. The women were tested in the follicular, ovulatory, luteal, and premenstrual phases, with beginning times varied to control for practice effects. Based on scores on the entire battery, no phase differences were found. On the individual tests, performance on the auto- kinetic measure and the Stroop color-word were best in the ovulatory phase, and performance was lowest premenstrually on the kinesthetic figural aftereffect and size estimation. Presumably better and worse refer on the autokinetic and kinesthetic measures to the degree of perceptual distortion present in the re- sponse [43].

Baker et al. studied kinesthetic aftereffect and the menstrual cycle in three groups of college women (N=47, 14, and 55, respectively). Using one hand only, subjects felt the width of a standard block, rubbed a second and larger block to induce an aftereffect, and then, using a tapered block, recalled by touch the width of the standard. Each subject was tested once. Measured at 3 day intervals over a standardized 29 day cycle, there was a larger kinesthetic aftereffect at the beginning and end of the cycle with a midcycle dip. Based on a chain of logical inferences and empiric connections, the researchers claimed that the aftereffect change was evidence for a reduction of stimulation at the central nervous system level premenstrually and menstrually which in turn was a response to pain and discomfort associated with menstruation. Unfortunately, they did not measure pain and discomfort, thereby failing to test one of their major assumptions [44].

Dor-Shav tested two groups of women, 155 college students, and 116 girls and unmarried women, and reported that their performance on both the Human figure drawing test and Embedded Figures test was better in the third week of their cycle [45].

Rodin manipulated anxiety levels through emphasis on a need for speed and accurate performance and the threat of shock on four tasks: Digit Symbol sub- stitution, Stroop color-word test, anagram solutions, and unsolvable puzzles. Subjects were 60 college students, not using oral contraceptives, who were either in the perimenstrual or midcycle phase. Each phase group was comprised of sub- jects who reported high to moderate levels of menstrual symptoms, or reported no symptoms at all. On the digit symbol and anagrams task, among the anxious subjects, the perimenstrual symptom group performed significantly better than the perimenstrual no symptom group and the midcycle groups. There were no phase differences among the unthreatened subjects [46].

In an effort to create a situation of menstrual debilitation, two researchers deliberately introduced a bias. Altenhaus studied 65 college women performing two perceptual-motor tasks, a subtraction task, and solvable and insolvable puz- zles. Some of the women were told they should perform better in their present menstrual cycle phase and others that they should do worse. She found that while the bogus information affected the women's self-perception of the quality of their performance, it did not affect the performance itself [47]. Munchel, instead of introducing a bias, preselected for it. Using a questionnaire to determine premenstrual attitudes and symptoms, she selected participants who expected performance decrements associated with the premenstrual and menstrual phases. The group was comprised of two types of subjects: those who felt helpless about their menstrual symptoms, and those who reacted against them. Munchel added a group of women who did not consider diminished performance to be a menstrual symptom. She measured performance on three tasks: concept formation, pursuit-rotor combined with arithmetic problems, and tracing. An insolvable task was used to measure motivation (persistence). Contrary to expectation, the subjects who expected to perform poorly premenstrually and felt helpless about it did not show a lower performance, and their persistence premenstrually exceeded that of the other two groups [48].

In a similar instance of preselection, Gamberale et al. studied 12 healthy working women, aged 20 to 34 years, with severe menstrual distress. Phase designations were Premenstrual (6 to 2 days prior to estimated menstruation), Menstrual (first or second day of flow), and Postmenstrual (10 to 18 days from onset). Six psychological tests were used: choice reaction time; time estimation; color-word test, Part 1 (without perceptual conflict) and Part 2 (with perceptual conflict); letter elimination; and perceptual speed. The testing also included physiological measures requiring bicycle exercise. The women also estimated the degree of perceived exertion in the final minute on the bicycle. That estimate varied significantly with menstrual cycle phase. The same exercise intensity (measured objectively by an ergometer) was perceived as more tiring during the menstrual phase than in the pre- and postmenstrual phases, and lower estimates of perceived exertion at the same heart rate were obtained during the pre- and postmenstrual phases than during the menstrual phase. Of the six psychological tests, only choice reaction time showed a phase effect in that it tended to be slower during menstruation [49].

If there is a relationship between the fluctuation of gonadal hormones and performance on cognitive and perceptual-motor tasks, it is not a clear one. As with intellectual performance, the evidence does not favor the hypothesis of menstrual debilitation. Those instances in which phase effects are found might involve more fluid and variable sensory-motor responses than more stable cognitive abilities. Discomfort or other stress associated with the perimenstrual period may also contribute to extra effort. Several studies have shown an improvement in cognitive function either premenstrually or during menstruation [20,36,46,48].

C. Sensory-Motor Function and Central Nervous System Correlates

Landauer compared reaction time among 73 college women using 4 day phase designations with one test session per person. The task was to press a button in response to the appearance of a number on a lighted screen. A distinction was made between *decision* time—the time from the appearance of the signal to the subject's lifting of her finger from its resting position, and *response* time—the time from the beginning of the response movement to the button press. Landauer argued that decision time would be more sensitive to physiological change. Thus, only those times were analyzed. A statistically reliable phase difference was obtained with the slowest performance occurring premenstrually and the second slowest during menstruation [50].

Out of eight other reaction time studies, five showed no phase differences across the menstrual cycle [34,51-54]; one showed no difference but omitted testing in the premenstrual phase [55]; one showed a slowing of choice reaction time during menstruation [49]; and one a postovulatory increase in speed with a premenstrual decline [56].

Ward et al. tested visual detection and visual pattern discrimination in 12 women at four cycle phases. They also assessed mood and collected plasma samples which were radioimmunoassayed for estradiol, progesterone, luteinizing hormone, and follicle-stimulating hormone. None of the participants had used oral contraceptives within the previous 6 months. On the detection task (reported presence or absence of a dot) the group performed best during the menstrual session (days 2 to 4) and worst premenstrually (1 to 3 days before onset). However, on pattern discrimination (distinguishing between patterns of spaced dots and paired dots) there was no reliable difference associated with menstrual cycle phase, with a trend for better performance premenstrually. They did not report a relationship between mood and performance. During the menstrual phase, when visual accuracy was highest, there was a correlation between estradiol level and the percentage of correct detection scores for the 12 subjects; estradiol accounted for 34% of the total variance of perceptual accuracy (detection) [57].

Studying perception of paired flashes, DeMarchi and Tong found low sensitivity premenstrually, an increase in the menstrual phase, and greatest sensitivity in midcycle. However, these results were confounded by potential practice effects [58]. In a replication, Wong and Tong found no phase differences [59]. In contrast, Diamond et al., measuring the ability to detect a test light, found peak sensitivity midcycle remaining high premenstrually and dropping during menstruation [60].

Given the variability of the findings on reaction time and visual acuity it appears that menstrual variables are not sufficiently powerful to override the effects of other factors. Even when carefully assessed in the Ward et al. [57] study using measures of mood and corroboration using hormone samples, there is an odd contradiction of a phase effect for detection but not for pattern discrimination, and the latter results tended to conflict with the former. They did not find the midcycle increase reported in earlier studies.

The menstrual cycle is the target for research because it provides a convenient measure of known hormonal fluctuations and is of interest to researchers concerned with sex differences. However, effects of reproductive hormones on sensory-motor processes may be tangential or indirect through some hypothalamic and/or pituitary interaction with other steroid systems. Henkin and Daly have described the effects of adrenal steroids on auditory detection and perception [61].

A number of researchers have hypothesized differences in arousal as an accompaniment of the menstrual cycle. Some researchers have suggested an increase in CNS arousal and responsiveness premenstrually [62-65]. Others claim support for an increase in arousal in the midcycle phases with a decline in the luteal and premenstrual phases [52,54,66,67].

Asso, attempting to introduce some order to the confused findings, categorized studies of conditioned response acquisition, heart rate, skin potential, skin conductance, and sympathetic autonomic nervous system responsiveness, together as indicators of *autonomic* arousal. She concluded that the evidence supports a premenstrual increase in autonomic arousal. Under the rubric of *cortical* arousal, she grouped studies of electroencephalography (EEG), monoamine oxidase activity, time estimation, and two-flash fusion, and concluded that there is either no change or lowered levels of cortical arousal premenstrually [68]. However, even within these groupings the findings are not consistent.

In support of the increased premenstrual responsiveness view, Marinari et al. found that, in a stressful situation, premenstrual women showed a greater adrenocortical response to psychological stress than midcycle women. A comparison group of oral contraceptive users did not show the increased adrenocortical responsiveness. The group showing the premenstrual increase on the physiological level did not report greater anxiety measured on an adjective checklist [64].

Vila and Beech tested the acquisition of a conditioned response. Learning was defined as a significant change in response measured by heart rate amplitude to the conditioned response (CS) (blue light) following the CS-USC (unconditioned response) association. The UCS was white noise, an aversive stimulus. The intense stimulation of the first presentation of the noise produced a greater acceleration of heart rate for the groups tested in the premenstrual phase, irrespective of oral contraceptive use. With three presentations of the CS and UCS, the premenstrual group showed heart rate *increase,* while the intermenstrual group showed an initial increase followed by a *decrease* (measured over a 10 s period). The authors report other research findings associating a heart rate *increase* with response to noxious stimulation and defensive set against stimulation. The heart rate *decrease* is purportedly associated with responses to novel stimuli and a set to attend to and receive environmental stimulation. They concluded that the premenstrual phobic women showed a defensive response while the intermenstrual phobic women showed an orienting one [65].

However, other studies have failed to show an increased responsiveness of heart rate in the premenstrual phase [49,54,58]. Findings regarding skin conductance are inconsistent, but suggest greater responsiveness in the midcycle phases than around the time of menstruation [54,67,69].

A number of studies have measured cortical changes using EEG frequency over the menstrual cycle. Sugarman et al., studying 15 women twice weekly, found a decrease in EEG frequency in the premenstrual phase [70]. Creutzfeldt et al. measured alpha wave frequency in 16 women with spontaneous menstrual cycles and 16 women using oral contraceptives. No obvious EEG change could be seen with a visual examination of the brain wave patterns but detailed analyses showed a cyclic change in one alpha band with a slight increase during the late luteal phase and a premenstrual decline. The pattern did not occur for the women using oral contraceptives [56].

Massachusetts researchers have studied the relationship between gonadal hormones and autonomic nervous system function. Much of this work has focused on the alpha driving response which they use to assess changes in adrenergic function. The driving response refers to the appearance of alpha waves under specified conditions in response to photic stimulation [71]. The occurrence of the driving response is inversely related to adrenergic function, and they have shown driving response to increase in the postovulatory phase. They did not report specific premenstrual effects. A controlling mechanism involving estrogen and monoamine oxidase is postulated for adrenergic change which is therefore seen as fluctuating systematically with the hormonal changes of the menstrual cycle. Although they have explored measures of cognitive style, relationships between adrenergic function measured by the driving response and cognitive events have yet to be established [66,72].

Leary and Batho recorded EEG for 25 women not using oral contraceptives for two menstrual cycle phases: premenstrual and midcycle. Contrary to the findings of earlier studies, slight premenstrual increases in mean alpha frequency were visually discernable in 20 of the 25 subjects. There were also indications of a premenstrual increase in driving response amplitude [73].

One cannot make any conclusive statements about either an increase or decrease in various forms of arousal in relation to the menstrual cycle. Clearly more studies are needed before drawing conclusions about the effect of gonadal hormones on the brain.

II. The Effect of Cognitive Factors on Menstrual Events

That researchers have repeatedly felt the need to confront the question of menstrual impairment, despite the preponderance of objective evidence to the contrary, underscores the psychological and social power of beliefs about menstruation. For humans, the menstrual cycle must be viewed as a *psychosocial* variable as well as a physiological one. Thus far, the focus of this chapter has been on the menstrual cycle as a physiological variable affecting cognitive behavior. However, a review would be incomplete without considering the psychosocial associations (cognitions, attitudes, etc.) concerning menstruation and their effect on the perception of menstrual function and symptoms.

Cognitive appraisal and its emotional accompaniments may have a direct as well as indirect effect on the hormonal substrate underlying the menstrual cycle. The direct effect lies with the alteration of metabolic factors affecting the pituitary-hypothalamic-gonadal-endocrine axis. A prime example is menstrual irregularity or amenorrhea (absence of menstruation) produced by psychosocial stress. Occasional missed periods have often been attributed to the demands of adaptation to new environments [75]. Amenorrhea has been consistently associated with *anorexia nervosa*, a psychophysiological disorder of life-threatening appetite loss. It is not clear whether amenorrhea accompanying anorexia is caused by the disorder underlying the lack of appetite or whether it is a secondary effect of near-starvation. The latter view is supported by studies of malnutrition and of amenorrhea among strenuous exercisers, whose ratio of fat to lean muscle is altered. However, the association between weight loss and amenorrhea does not eliminate the possibility of emotional factors producing irregularity or other menstrual problems.

Siegel et al. studied 244 college women and failed to find an association between stress (measured by the number of recent life changes) and irregularity of menstruation. However, they found a positive correlation between life change scores, particularly negative events, and the number of symptoms of menstrual discomfort for the women with natural cycles. The correlation was not found for the sample using oral contraceptives [76].

Many people associate the premenstrual and menstrual phases with physical discomfort, debilitating effects on activities, and increased emotionality, especially negative mood. Male and female college students share these stereotypic beliefs about menstruation [77]. Girls who have not yet menstruated already have a clear set of negative expectations, and boys as young as those in junior high school also have a similar set of beliefs about the symptoms experienced by women [78]. For many young women, menarche is viewed as a hygienic crisis rather than a maturational event, and sickness is the implicit metaphor of menstruation. Educational materials emphasize the need to be fastidiously clean and secretive about menses [79,80].

Whether individually accurate or not, a well-defined negative expectation prevails in the culture and can therefore be assumed to affect perception of events and experiences pertaining to menstruation. The experience of pain and discomfort associated with menstruation is sufficiently ubiquitous to reinforce a negative belief system [1]. Expectations, once established, are not readily extinguished and are sustained by occasional confirmation. Proponents of attribution theory have pointed out that both men and women are likely to attribute negative moods occurring in the premenstrual and/or menstrual phases to internal biologic processes. When the negative moods occur at other times, they are attributed to environmental factors [81,82]. Ruble tested the assertion that the perception of menstrual symptoms is influenced by expectation. Volunteer participants were taken into a laboratory and connected to an elaborate EEG machine. They were told by an official-looking person in a white laboratory coat that the brain wave patterns would predict the onset of menstruation. Ruble found an increase in reports of water retention and pain by women who were incorrectly led to believe they were in the premenstrual phase compared with those told they were midcycle and those given no cycle information [83].

While one interpretation of these results is that women's symptoms reports are stereotyped and culturally determined expectations, another is that continued or prolonged association between symptom and cycle phase leads to a conditioned perception, i.e., if I'm premenstrual, I must be bloated. If cultural beliefs alone were responsible for the attribution of negative symptoms to menstruation, there should be an effect on self-reports of mood, as well as the more physical symptoms of water retention and pain. Ruble did not find differences in the reports of negative mood or other behavioral changes between women led to believe they were premenstrual and those led to believe they were midcycle. Nevertheless, the findings do support the hypothesis that expectations plays a part in the perception of menstrual events.

Supporting the argument for the role of stereotypic beliefs is the fact that many women report a greater incidence of menstrual symptoms on retrospective questionnaires than on daily records [32,84]. A 3 year study of student nurses found no significant correlation between ratings of menstrual discomfort on a retrospective questionnaire (Cornell Medical Index) and frequency of calendar reports of menstrual symptoms [11]. Also, while many women expect a decline in ability associated with menstruation, this does not occur even among those with this expectation [15,47,48].

The negative image of menstruation does appear to be changing, perhaps as a result of more research and better education. Schilling found that college women did not attribute their moods to the menstrual cycle to the degree predicted in earlier research [85]. Brooks et al. surveyed 191 undergraduate college women and found that they accepted menstruation as routine and felt fairly positive about it, agreeing, for example, with the statements "Menstruation provides a way for me to keep in touch with my body" or "Menstruation is a recurrent affirmation of womanhood" [86].

III. Conclusion

The results of the studies reviewed in the first part of this chapter may be evaluated in two ways. The first is whether or not they provide support for the hypothesis of premenstrual and menstrual debilitation, and secondly, whether the measures studied fluctuate in accordance with the hormonal changes of the menstrual cycle. The results listed in Table 1 show that problem-solving does not appear to be affected by menstrual variables. When chance findings and the publication bias are taken into account, the evidence does not support a perimenstrual decrement in performance nor changes approximating the cyclic fluctuations of the menstrual cycle. Although there are some hints of alterations in cognitive style, the evidence is not consistent and most of it supports no change. Reaction time, signal detection, and other CNS measures are not sufficiently consistent to support the debilitation hypothesis. However, they do appear to vary in some fashion with the hormonal fluctuations of the cycle. The details of that fluctuation for specific systems remain to be clarified.

A number of researchers have suggested that the failure to find a premenstrual-menstrual decrement in performance or those instances where improved performance occurred were the result of compensatory effort [19,20,31,87]. Redgrove, after an extensive review of the literature on work performance, concluded that the effects of the menstrual cycle on performance would not be observable until a woman was pushed to the limits of her ability [88]. Even if this is the case, and it is a reasonable assertion, it is not at all clear from studies in which limits are reached, such as difficult intellectual tasks and laboratory studies of sensory thresholds, which are the better and worse days of the cycle.

The comparison of several subjects grouped by menstrual cycle phase may obscure individual variation. However, if cyclic variation were consistent or of greater impact than other variables, reliable differences in performance would have been observed. Studies following the same women over time have not yielded greater evidence of systematic change. A given woman may discover a particular effect that her hormonal changes exert upon her behavior. Such knowledge is useful in her personal adaptation. However, there does not appear to be any justification for generalizing such an effect to other women. If anything clear emerges from the lengthy and extensive history of menstrual cycle research, it is the lack of general principles applicable to all women. Individual variability in performance within individuals as well as between them is the most reliable outcome.

The message of this chapter's second section is that cognitive variables may affect the physiological substrate of the menstrual cycle fairly directly with resulting changes in hormonal patterns and symptoms. More pervasively, cognitive variables influence the perception of and response to menstruation. Thus, it is necessary to consider the psychological and social meanings attached to menstruation as well as the hormonal concomitants in those cases where behaviors change relative to the menstrual cycle in reaching conclusions about cause and effect.

References

1. B. Sommer, Menstrual distress, in *The Complete Book of Women's Health* (G. Hongladarom, R. McCorkle and N. F. Woods, eds.), Prentice-Hall, Englewood Cliffs, N.J., 1982.
2. R. L. Doty and C. Silverthorne, Influence of menstrual cycle on volunteering behavior. *Nature* 254:139-140 (1975).

3. M. B. Parlee, Menstruation and voluntary participation in a psychological experiment. Paper presented at the annual meeting of the American Psychological Association, Chicago, Illinois, 1975.

4. A. J. Dan, Behavioral variability and the menstrual cycle. Paper presented at the annual meeting of the American Psychological Association, Washington, D.C., 1976.

5. N. M. Morris and J. R. Udry, Variations in pedometer activity during the menstrual cycle. *Obstet. Gynecol.* 35:199-201 (1970).

6. J. L. Sanders, Relation of personal space to the human menstrual cycle. *J. Psychol.* 100:275-278 (1978).

7. J. H. Morton, H. Addition, R. G. Addison, L. Hunt, and J. J. Sullivan, A clinical study of premenstrual tension. *Am. J. Obstet. Gynecol.* 65:1182-1191 (1953).

8. R. Moos, The development of a menstrual distress questionnaire. *Psychosom. Med.* 30:853-867 (1968).

9. K. Dalton, Menstruation and accidents. *Br. Med. J.* 2:1425-1426 (1960).

10. N. E. Liskey, Accidents: Rhythmic threat to females. *Accident Anal. Prev.* 4:1-11 (1972).

11. E. Friedman, A. H. Katcher, and V. J. Brightman, A prospective study of the distribution of illness within the menstrual cycle. *Motiv. Emot.* 2:355-367 (1978).

12. K. Dalton, Menstruation and crime. *Br. Med. J.* 2:1752-1753 (1961).

13. K. Dalton, The influence of mother's menstruation on her child. *Proc. R. Soc. Med.* 59:1014-1016 (1966).

14. R. Tuch, The relationship between a mother's menstrual status and her response to illness in her child. *Psychosom. Med.* 37:388-394 (1975).

15. B. Sommer, The effect of menstruation on cognitive and perceptual-motor behavior: A review. *Psychosom. Med.* 35:515-534.

16. L. S. Hollingworth, Functional periodicity: An experimental study of the mental and motor abilities of women during menstruation. *Columbia Univ. Centr. Educ., Teach. Coll. Series,* No. 69, 101, 1914.

17. H. E. Eagleson, Periodic changes in blood pressure, muscular coordination and mental efficiency in women. *Comp. Psychol Monogr.* 4:65 (1927).

18. S. C. M. Sowton and C. S. Myers, Two contributions to the experimental study of the menstrual cycle. I. Its influence on mental and muscular efficiency. Industrial Fatigue Research Board, Report No. 45, 72 (1928).

19. G. H. Seward, The female sex rhythm. *Psychol. Bull.* 31:153-192 (1934).

20. O. M. Lough, A psychological study of functional periodicity. *J. Comp. Psychol.* 24:359-368 (1937).

21. G. H. Seward, Psychological effects of the menstrual cycle on women workers. *Psychol. Bull.* 41:90-102 (1944).

22. A. J. Smith, Menstruation and industrial efficiency. II. Quality and quantity of production. *J. Appl. Psychol.* 34:148-152 (1950).

23. M. Wickham, The effects of the menstrual cycle on test performance. *Br. J. Psychol.* 49:34-41 (1958).

24. K. Dalton, Effect of menstruation on schoolgirls' weekly work. *Br. Med. J.* 1:326-328 (1960).

25. K. Dalton, Menstruation and examinations. *Lancet* 2:1386-1388 (1968).

26. D. Barash, Quoted in Womens place is in their genes? (E. Lacitis) Seattle Times, 9/20/79, p. A15, 1979.

27. C. Hutt, *Males and Females.* Penguin, Middlesex, England, 1972.

28. L. Tiger, Male dominance? Yes, alas. A sexist plot: No.   *New York Times Magazine,* 9/25/70, p. 35, 1970.

29. L. Tiger, Quoted in Women's Lib: A second look. *Time Magazine,* 12/14/70, p. 50, 1970.

30. B. Sommer, Menstrual cycle changes and intellectual performance. *Psychosom. Med.* 34:263-269 (1972).

31. B. E. Bernstein, Effect of menstruation on academic performance among college women. *Arch. Sex Behav.* 4:289-296 (1977).

32. B. Sommer, Perceptual-motor performance, mood and the menstrual cycle. Paper presented at the annual of the Western Psychological Assoc., Portland, Oregon (1972).

33. L. J. Moran and R. B. Mefferd, Jr., Repetitive psychometric measures. *Psychol. Rep.* 5:269-275 (1959).

34. E. Zimmerman and M. B. Parlee, Behavioral changes associated with the menstrual cycle: An experimental investigation. *J. Appl. Soc. Psychol.* 3:335-344 (1973).

35. S. Golub, The effect of premenstrual anxiety and depression on cognitive function. *J. Pers. Soc. Psychol.* 34:99-104 (1976).

36. W. Wuttke, P. Arnold, D. Becker, O. Creutzfeldt, S. Langenstein, and W. Tirsch, Hormonal profiles and variations of the EEG and of performance in psychological tests in women with spontaneous menstrual cycles and under oral contraceptives. In *Psychotropic Action of Hormones* (T. M. Itil, ed.). Spectrum Publ., Jamaica, New York, 1976.

37. E-M. Silverman and C. Zimmer, Speech fluency fluctuations during the menstrual cycle. *J. Speech Hear. Res.* 18:202-206 (1975).

38. E. M. Silverman and C. H. Zimmer, Replication of "speech fluency fluctuations during the menstrual cycle." *Percept. Mot Skills* 42:1004-1006 (1976).

39. P. Komnenich, Hormonal influences on verbal behavior in women. *Diss. Abst. Int.* 34:3065B (1974).

40. P. Komnenich, D. M. Lane, R. P. Dickey, and S. C. Stone, Gonadal hormones and cognitive performance. *Physiol. Psychol.* 6:115-120 (1978).

41. D. B. Snyder, The relationship of the menstrual cycle to certain aspects of perceptual cognitive functioning. Diss. Abst. Int. 39(2-B):962-963 (1978).

42. E. Klaiber, D. Broverman, W. Vogel, and Y. Kobayashi, Rhythms in plasma MAO activity, EEG, and behavior during the menstrual cycle. In *Biorhythms and Human Reproduction* (M. Ferin, F. Halberg, R. M. Richart, and R. L. Van de Wiele, eds.). John Wiley, New York, 1974.

43. M. Lederman, Menstrual cycle and fluctuation in cognitive-perceptual performance. *Diss. Abst. Int.* 35:1388-1389B (1974).

44. A. H. Baker, I. W. Kostin, B. L. Mishara, and L. Parker, Menstrual cycle affects kinesthetic aftereffect, an index of personality and perceptual style. *J. Pers. Soc. Psychol.* 37:234-246 (1979).

45. N. K. Dor-Shav, In search of pre-menstrual tension: Note on sex differences in psychological differentiations as a function of cyclical physiological changes. *Percept. Mot. Skills* 42:1138-1142 (1976).

46. J. Rodin, Menstruation, reattribution and competence. *J. Pers. Soc. Psychol.* 33:345-353 (1976).

47. A. L. Altenhaus, The effect of expectancy for change on performance during the menstrual cycle. *Diss. Abst. Int.* 39(2-B):968 (1978).

48. M. E. Munchel, The effects of symptom expectation and response styles on cognitive and perceptual-motor performance during the menstrual phase. *Diss. Abst. Int.* 39(7-B):3531-3532 (1979).

49. F. Gamberale, L. Strindberg, and I. Wahlberg, Female work capacity during the menstrual cycle: Physiological and psychological reactions. *Scand. J. Work Environ. Health* 1:120-127 (1975).

50. A. A. Landauer, Choice decision time and the menstrual cycle. *Practitioner* 213:703-706 (1974).

51. W. R. Pierson and A. Lockhart, Effect of menstruation on simple reaction and movement time. *Br. Med. J.* 1:796-797 (1963).

52. B. Kopell, D. Lunde, R. Clayton, R. Moos, and D. Hamburg, Variations in some measures of arousal during the menstrual cycle. *J. Nerv. Ment. Dis.* 148:180-187 (1969).

53. J. Schwank, The menstrual cycle and performance on various laboratory tasks. Unpublished manuscript, 1971.

54. B. C. Little and T. P. Zahn, Changes in mood and autonomic functioning during the menstrual cycle. *Psychophysiology* 11:579-590 (1974).

55. J. Loucks and H. Thompson, Effect of menstruation on reaction time. *Res. Q.* 39:407-408 (1968).

56. O. D. Creutzfeldt, P. M. Arnold, D. Becker, S. Langenstein, W. Tirsch, H. Wilhelm, and W. Wuttke, EEG changes during spontaneous and controlled menstrual cycles and their correlation with psychological performance. *Electroencephalogr. Clin. Neurophysiol.* 40:113-131 (1976).

57. M. M. Ward, S. C. Stone, and C. A. Sandman, Visual perception in women during the menstrual cycle. *Physiol. Behav.* 20:239-243 (1978).

58. G. W. DeMarchi and J. E. Tong, Menstrual, diurnal, and activation effects on

the resolution of temporally paired flashes. *Psychophysiology* 9:362-367 (1972).

59. S. Wong and T. E. Tong, Menstrual cycle and contraceptive hormone effects on temporal discrimination. *Percept. Mot. Skills* 39:103-108 (1974).

60. M. Diamond, A. Diamond, and M. Mast, Visual sensitivity and sexual arousal levels during the menstrual cycle. *J. Nerv. Ment. Dis.* 155:170-176 (1972).

61. R. I. Henkin and R. L. Daly, Auditory detection and perception in normal man and in patients with adrenal cortical insufficiency: Effect of adrenal cortical steroids. *J. Clin. Invest.* 47:1269-1280 (1968).

62. E. W. Wineman, Autonomic balance changes during the human menstrual cycle. *Psychophysiology* 8:1-6 (1971).

63. D. Asso and H. R. Beech, Susceptibility to the acquisition of a conditioned response in relation to the menstrual cycle. *J. Psychosom. Res.* 19:337-344 (1975).

64. K. T. Marinari, A. I. Leshner, and M. P. Doyle, Menstrual cycle status and adrenocortical reactivity to psychological stress. *Psychoneuroendocrinology* 2:213-218 (1976).

65. J. Vila and H. R. Beech, Vulnerability and defensive reactions in relation to the human menstrual cycle. *Br. J. Soc. Clin. Psychol.* 17:93-100 (1978).

66. W. Vogel, D. M. Broverman, and E. L. Klaiber, EEG responses in regularly menstruating women and in amenorrheic women treated with ovarian hormones. *Science* 172:388-391 (1971).

67. J. Friedman and R. A. Meares, The menstrual cycle and habituation. *Psychosom. Med.* 41:369-381 (1979).

68. D. Asso, Levels of arousal in the premenstrual phase. *Br. J. Soc. Clin. Psychol.* 17:47-55 (1978).

69. T. Uno, GSR activity and the human menstrual cycle. *Psychophysiology* 10:213-214 (1973).

70. A. A. Sugarman and A. T. deBruin, Quantitative EEG changes in the human menstrual cycle. *Res. Commun. Chem. Pathol. Pharmacol.* 1:526-534 (1970).

71. E. L. Klaiber, Y. Kobayashi, D. M. Broverman, and F. Hall, Plasma monoamine oxidase activity in regularly menstruating women and in amenorrheic women receiving cyclic treatment with estrogens and a progestin. *J. Clin. Endocrinol. Metab.* 33:630-638 (1971).

72. E. L. Klaiber, D. M. Broverman, W. Vogel, Y. Kobayashi, and D. Moriarty, Effects of estrogen therapy on plasma MAO activity and EEG driving responses of depressed women. *Am. J. Psychiatry* 128:1492-1498 (1972).

73. P. M. Leary and K. Batho, Changes in electro-encephalogram related to the menstrual cycle. *S. Afr. Med. J.* 55:666-668 (1979).

74. W. H. Tedford, D. E. Warren, and W. E. Flynn, Alteration of shock aver-

sion thresholds during the menstrual cycle. *Percept. Psychophysics* 21: 193-196 (1977).

75. G. F. Russell, Psychological and nutritional factors in disturbances of menstrual function and ovulation. *Postgrad. Med. J.* 48:10-13 (1972).

76. J. M. Siegel, J. H. Johnson, and I. G. Sarason, Life changes and menstrual discomfort. *J. Hum. Stress* 5:41-46 (1979).

77. M. B. Parlee, Sterotypic beliefs about menstruation: A methodological note on the Moos Menstrual Distress Questionnaire and some new data. *Psychosom. Med.* 36:229-240 (1974).

78. A. E. Clarke and D. N. Ruble, Young adolescents' beliefs concerning menstruation. *Child Dev.* 29:231-234 (1978).

79. L. Whisnant and L. Zegans, A study of attitudes toward menarche in white middle-class American adolescent firls. *Am. J. Psychiatry* 132:809-814 (1975).

80. L. Whisnant, E. Brett, and L. Zegans, Implicit messages concerning menstruation in commercial educational materials prepared for young adolescent girls. *Am. J. Psychiatry* 132:815-820 (1975).

81. R. K. Koeske and G. F. Koeske, An attributional approach to moods and the menstrual cycle. *J. Pers. Soc. Psychol.* 31:473-478 (1975).

82. M. Brooks-Gunn and D. Ruble, Menstrual-related symptomatology in adolescents: The effect of attitudes, first menstrual experience, and parental factors. Presented at the Menstrual Cycle: Second Annual Interdisciplinary Research Conference, St. Louis University, May 25-26, 1978.

83. D. Ruble, Premenstrual symptoms: A reinterpretation. *Science* 197:291-292 (1977).

84. J. M. Abplanalp, A. F. Donnelly, and R. M. Rose, Psychoendocrinology of the menstrual cycle: I. Enjoyment of daily activities and moods. *Psychosom. Med.*, 41:587-604 (1979).

85. K. M. Schilling, What is a real difference? Content or method in menstrual findings, in *The Menstrual Cycle, Volume 2* (P. Komnenich, M. McSweeney, J. A. Noack, and N. Elder, eds.), Springer Publishing Co., New York, 1981.

86. J. Brooks-Gunn, D. Ruble, and A. Clarke, College women's attitudes and expectations concerning menstrual-related changes. *Psychosom. Med.* 39: 288-298 (1977).

87. K. Lewin and A. Freund, Untersuchungen sur Handlungsund Affectpsychologie. *Psychol. Forsch.* 13:198-217 (1930); described in G. H. Seward, The female sex rhythm. *Psychol. Bull.* 31:153-192 (1934).

88. J. A. Redgrove, Menstrual cycles, in *Biological Rhythms and Human Performance* (W. P. Colquhoun, ed.). Academic Press, London, 1971.

7 Epidemiological Patterns of Sexual Behavior in the Menstrual Cycle

NAOMI M. MORRIS*   University of Health Sciences/The Chicago Medical School, Chicago, Illinois

J. RICHARD UDRY   University of North Carolina at Chapel Hill, Chapel Hill, North Carolina

I. Our First Finding

In connection with other research we had collected daily sexual data from 40 premenopausal married working women, approximately 60% of whom had not graduated from high school. Most of the women were nonwhite. We graphed their reports of intercourse and orgasm by reverse menstrual cycle day (reverse cycle day 1 being the day before the onset of a menstrual period, reverse cycle day 2 being the day before that, etc.), and saw to our surprise that the percentage of positive reports at midcycle was approximately twice as high as the percentage 1 week before or 1 week after that time. On reverse day 4 an extremely low point was reached, followed by a recovery in the level of positive reports right before the onset of the next menstruation [1]. (Fig. 1.)

II. Mammalian/Nonhuman Primate Patterns

The pattern thus obtained looked very much like one derived from research with rhesus monkeys [2]. Breeding habits of laboratory monkeys have long been studied. The rhesus monkey has been observed to copulate throughout the menstrual cycle, but females living in groups exhibiting physical evidence of being in

---

*Present affiliation: Community Health Sciences Program, School of Public Health, University of Illinois at the Medical Center, Chicago, Illinois.

129

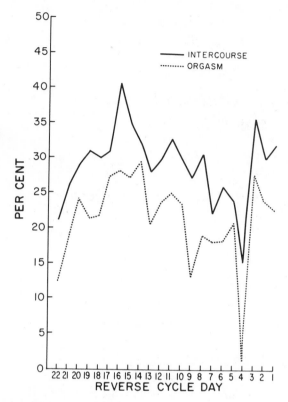

Figure 1 Percentage of women in the original sample reporting intercourse and orgasm by reverse day of menstrual cycle. There were 40 women, and 73-115 cycles represented at each point. (From Ref. 1, reprinted by permission from *Nature,* Vol. 220, No. 5167, pp. 593-596. Copyright (©) 1968 Macmillan Journals Limited.)

the periovulatory period seem to be preferred partners. Males having access to only one female will approach her sexually and ejaculate more often at midcycle [2,3]. This pattern characterizes nonhuman primates, all of which have menstrual cycles rather than estrous periods.

Estrous periods characteristic of lower mammals involve coincident periodic vaginal discharge, receptivity, fertility, and attractivity in the females; at other times the females do not mate and are not fertile. Estrus also involves a period of heightened activity, which in female laboratory rodents is often evidenced by peaks of running on exercise wheels.

Both estrous and menstrual cycles reflect shifting gonadal hormone levels physiologically. With regard to ovulation and hormone status, estrus (the fertile period) is most comparable to midcycle in animals with menstrual cycles. The direction of evolution suggests a weakening of the influence of hormonal factors on behavior as intellectual and psychic factors become more important [4].

Our finding a pattern at all similar to that of a lower species in humans was therefore surprising.

III. Implications of Nonsocial Influences on Human Behavior

If one entertains the possibility of nonsocial influences on the pattern of human sexual intercourse, one can consider some very basic questions, among them (1) what explains the attraction of males to females (and females to males)? and (2) can an inoperative biologic attraction mechanism explain homosexuality?

These questions arise from the following reasoning: for differences in the probability of sexual intercourse to exist from day to day within the menstrual cycle, one particularly has to explain what stimulates the male's motivation, since most students of human behavior agree that coitus usually follows male, rather than female, "demand" [5-7].

IV. Questions We Have Pursued

A. Does the Pattern Really Exist?

1. Findings of Other Investigators

Our first task was to assure ourselves that the pattern created on our graph really exists. A literature search showed that there were data bearing on the question from three sources. The first was retrospective reports. Davis [8] and Terman [9] found increased levels of sexual desire just before and just after menstruation in the histories given by their study subjects. There is no reason to assume, however, that desire is equivalent to consummation. Furthermore, the value of retrospective reports is limited. McCance et al. compared similar retrospective reports with daily recordings of feelings and found no relationship between the two [10]. A new study reinforces this [11].

A second source of data was the psychoanalytic interpretation of dreams. Benedek studied 15 women in therapy and found that the "highest integration of the sexual drive" occurs around the time of ovulation. From her analysis one can predict a midcycle peak in desire, but since she did not collect information on overt sexual behavior no inference can be made about the actual occurrence of coitus [12].

The third source of data is daily reports of sexual activity. McCance et al. collected menstrual cycle records with daily notations of a number of different feelings and behaviors from a sample of white, mostly college-educated women. They reported a peak sexual frequency at day 8 and another elevated period from day 11 to day 17, based on a mathematically standardized 28 day menstrual cycle counted forward from the first day of menstrual bleeding [10].

More recent reports from other investigators using methodology incorporating daily notations have also generally found peaks of sexual desire or intercourse shortly after the end of menstruation or in the follicular phase, and not usually at midcycle [13,14]. There have been exceptions [11,15]. Most such studies have been of students or college-educated women, whose educational level may have a bearing, as we will discuss later. Graphs of the daily probability of intercourse tend to show a depression in the luteal phase.

It should be noted that other investigators have questioned single or married women under a variety of assumptions, about a variety of not well-defined feeling states, fantasies, dreams, and other measures that are difficult to standardize. Although the results may be interesting, replication is problematic. We have tried to confine our studies to women who had equal access to sexual interaction on a daily basis (usually married), and to record definite behaviors. In this way we hoped to minimize subjective interpretation and reinterpretation of feelings in the light of events, and to maximize information on the types of behavior which could be objectively observed as in animal studies (although the participants themselves have been the only observers of their own behaviors).

2. Pattern Variation in Various Groups

The Institute for Sex Research (ISR) Group. The first group in which we actively sought confirmation of our pattern was a sample of 48 middle-class, mostly college-educated women who had contributed sexual calendars to the files of the Institute for Sex Research, Indiana University. The women were asked to record daily on the calendars, which were actually collected only yearly or less often. The data we reported from these calendars represented 818 to 882 menstrual cycles. For years during which some of the women were single, we saw a sharp rise in the rate of intercourse towards the middle of the cycle, followed by a decline in the latter half of the cycle, and a brief recovery before the next menstrual period, much as we had seen in our original group. A parallel in the rates of orgasm was even more striking. For married women, the graph derived from reports of their intercourse did not show a midcycle peak, but suggested some depression in the luteal phase. The graph of orgasm, however, was more like our first pattern. Perhaps the ability to climax more accurately reflects biologic status than does participation in coitus.

Since many of the women in the ISR sample had provided data for years, it was possible to look at patterns characterizing individuals. A wide range of variation in the patterns of intercourse and orgasm was seen within the menstrual cycle. Some women had clear periodicity and others did not. Neither the woman's age, frequency of intercourse, nor the proportion of time they had an orgasm predicted whether or not there would be a pattern to their sexual behavior [1].

We did not consider the ISR women to be necessarily typical of all women, since it is quite unusual for individuals to keep and share such detailed records of their personal lives over long periods of time. We have therefore reexamined periodicity in other groups of women whom we have recruited to participate in studies which we subsequently organized to answer various specific questions.

The Double-Blind Pill Study Group. Fifty-one women recruited from a public family planning clinic, graduate school, and a religious congregation participated in a study designed to measure the effects of the hormones in contraceptive pills on sexual behavior, utilizing a double-blind format. About 25% of the sample were black, the rest white. Their education level ranged from high school to graduate school; wives of graduate students predominated. Data derived from daily reports obtained during nonpill exposure showed a midcycle rise in the probability of intercourse and orgasm, and a luteal phase depression. The graphs were produced by plotting data according to standardized menstrual cycle days. (Standardization converts data from cycles of different lengths to a 28 day cycle, by use of a mathematical formula, as suggested earlier.) This replicated our original finding, although the contrasts produced by the peak at midcycle and trough in the luteal phase were not quite as great [16].

The Pheromone Study Group. Sixty-two couples participated through 3 menstrual months in a study designed to seek pheromonal influences on human sexual behavior. Graphs of their behavior by reverse or standardized menstrual cycle day did not show a midcycle peak. The graph did indicate a higher overall level during the follicular phase of the cycle than during the second half of the cycle [17].

This group of participants differed from previous groups we had studied in that we had purposely recruited high education-level people because we anticipated difficulties in following a relatively elaborate protocol. Only one nonwhite couple volunteered for the study, and most of the women were wives of graduate students or were graduate students themselves.

For the first time, we asked the women in the pheromone study to measure their basal body temperature each morning. We also obtained blood from a subsample of the group and determined luteinizing hormone (LH) levels. We graphed the occurrence of intercourse and orgasm against cycle days lined up either by the basal body temperature nadir or by the day of the luteinizing hormone surge. For only 42% of the cycles reported by women measuring basal body temperature (BBT) could we determine the day of the nadir. Of 43 women contributing blood samples, we detected the LH peak for 35. (We collected 10 to 14 serial midcycle samples and probably missed the LH peak when an unusually long cycle occurred.) Graphing sexual behavior against the BBT nadir, we observed a marked decrease in sexual activity the day before and a sharp rise on the day of the nadir (Fig. 2). Using the LH surge, no midcycle pattern was seen [18].

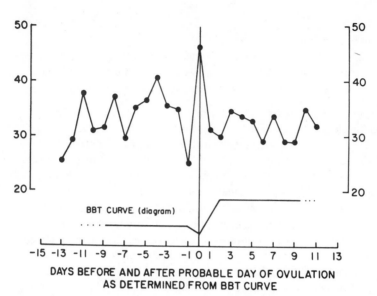

Figure 2 Percentage of husbands reporting intercourse by temperature cycle day as determined from wife's basal body temperature (BBT) curve (includes intercourse at all times of day; excludes cycles where BBT curve did not permit reading of probable ovulation day). Average number of observations per point = 104. (From Ref. 17.)

3. The Effect of Different Methods of Analysis and Measurement

To put into perspective the new patterns obtained from the use of BBT and LH biologic benchmarks, we have compared the effects of different methods of measurement and analysis to the pattern of sexual activity in the menstrual cycle. It is clear that the effects are profound, and that, depending on what portion of the cycle one is interested in, different methods of study are appropriate. For example, forward or reverse menstrual cycle days are not really helpful for studies focused on midcycle. No calculation can substitute for closer measures of the internal events of interest. Reverse cycle days and forward days starting from the beginning or end of menstrual bleeding (providing one carefully defines how much bleeding counts) can bracket the period of menstrual flow, for studies within that segment of the cycle. The further one gets away from the flow, the less certain one can be of the cycle day measure as an indicator of presumably correlated events and hormone levels.

Pulling together daily reports from 85 married couples from whom we had the necessary data (which includes the 62 couples of the pheromone study), we organized menstrual events using six techniques of aggregation [19] (Figs. 3 to 5).

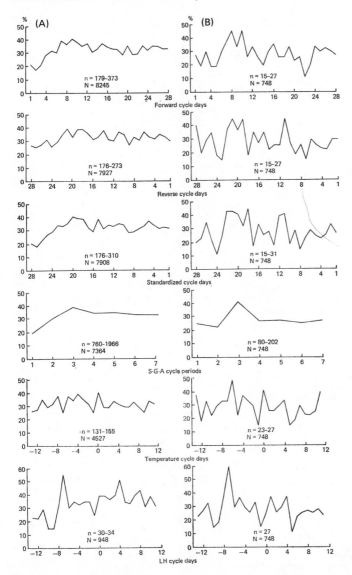

Figure 3 The percentages of women reporting intercourse for each day of the menstrual cycle plotted according to different methods of standardizing data (see text) from (A) all available data for each method and (B) cycles for which data were available for all six aggregation techniques. N = the number of events for each panel; n = the number of events at each point. (From Ref. 19.) Note: The "S-G-A" method of standardizing utilizes a grid that identifies which days of which cycle length are to be assigned to each of seven cycle phases [20].

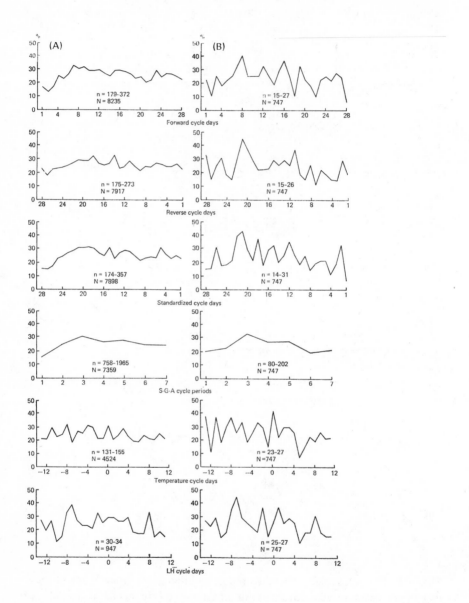

Figure 4 The percentages of women reporting orgasm for each day of the menstrual cycle plotted according to different methods of standardizing data from (A) all available data for each method and (B) cycles for which data were available for all six aggregation techniques. N = the number of events for each panel; n = the number of events at each point. (From Ref. 19.)

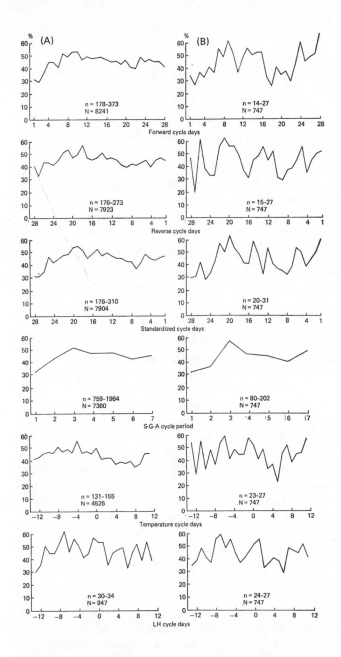

Figure 5 The percentages of women reporting the desire for intercourse for each day of the menstrual cycle plotted according to different methods of standardizing data from **(A)** all available data for each method and **(B)** cycles for which data were available for all six aggregation techniques. N = the number of events for each panel; n = the number of events at each point. (From Ref. 19.)

The luteal phase depression was a consistent finding, especially in a woman's probability of orgasm and her desire for intercourse; and there is an apparent peak about six days before midcycle in many of the graphs. The latter is consistent with the pioneering observations of McCance et al.

We have concluded that different samples of women show different patterns, particularly in the first half of the cycle. We believe the differences among groups are attributable to sociologic phenomena related to differences in the initiation and control of coitus, affected by education, marital status, and unexplored social-psychological processes.

B. How is the Pattern Produced?

If we assume that there *is* an underlying biologic process influencing the pattern of human sexual intercourse within the menstrual cycle, the next question is, what produces the pattern and through what mechanism does this come about?

1. Gonadal Hormone Effects in Mammals/Nonhuman Primates

Investigation of reproductive biology has been extensive in laboratory rodents and to a somewhat less degree in nonhuman primates. We know that the entire neuroendocrine system is involved in the normal mammalian reproductive process, including behavior. Gonadal hormones, estrogens and progesterone in the female and testosterone in the male, may be considered the end products of a neurohormonal system characterized by multiple levels of facilitation and inhibition of hormone release with feedback at every level. Although everything observed in rodents does not apply to primates, and there are differences among primate species, the laboratory findings are useful for seeking explanations of human behavior because of some similarities.

Considering primate behavioral effects of the gonadal hormones, the ovariectomized rhesus female is not attractive to the rhesus male and is not usually approached sexually. Injections of estrogen cause her to be approached again, and sexual interaction, including intromission and ejaculation by male partners, returns to approximate midcycle levels. Adding progesterone to the female's therapy reduces male interest and performance.

Sexual approaches made by the female to the male may be stimulated by giving her testosterone, but unless she is in an estrogenized state, without progesterone having been added, the male will not be responsive to her invitations.

It is believed that estrogen increases and progesterone decreases the probability of heterosexual activity, accounting for periodicity within the menstrual cycle. The usual role testosterone plays in rhesus females is not clear [21,22]. It seems reasonable to us to hypothesize that this holds true for human sexual behavior.

2. Proceptivity, Receptivity, and Attractivity in Mammals/Nonhuman Primates

Heterosexual behavior, however, involves two individuals. A female hormone mechanism implies that variations in hormone concentrations affect the rate of initiation or invitation from the female; affect the receptivity of the female or her willingness to cooperate when invited; or affect her stimulus value for males, thereby affecting the timing of the sexual approaches she receives from males. Frank Beach has referred to these conditions as sexual proceptivity, receptivity, and attractivity, respectively [22].

Attractivity refers to the female stimulus value in evoking sexual responses by the male. Proceptivity connotes various reactions by the female toward the male which constitute her assumption of initiative in establishing or maintaining sexual interaction. Receptivity is defined in terms of female responses necessary and sufficient for the male's success in achieving intravaginal ejaculation.

Beach cites literature showing that estrogen increases female attractivity through both behavioral and nonbehavioral means. Undefined nonhormonal factors also influence attractivity, since males will exhibit preference for one partner over another, all other things apparently being equal; and the substitution of a fresh female in place of a familiar one will in addition attract even a sex-satiated male who has not recently copulated with the new female. This latter phenomenon is fairly common among mammals, and has been called the "Coolidge effect." Attractivity is therefore not a simple condition eliciting totally automatic responses even in lower animals.

Several proceptive behaviors may be observed among mammalian species. The most common is the establishment and maintenance of proximity to the male. Another manifested in virtually all mammals consists of various forms of physical contact initiated by the female. Proceptive behaviors may be stimulated by exogenous gonadal hormones, primarily estrogens in laboratory primates. Beach reserves judgment on the additional effect of androgen because of the possibility that exogenous androgen may be converted to estrogen before it produces its effects on the behavior of the female monkey [22].

Female monkeys express individual preferences, ignoring some males and addressing sexual invitations to others. The bases for selective proceptivity in nonhuman primates or other mammals are unknown, although such selectivity clearly exists. Selectivity is not characteristic only of humans. Beach notes certain recurring differences in male stimulus value for females. Receptive primate females prefer mature and socially dominant males to juveniles or low-ranking adults [22]. Castrated animals of various laboratory species have also been observed to elicit fewer approach responses by females than do normal males.

In most mammals, female sexual receptivity depends upon estrogenic stimulation. In some rodents, progesterone may exhibit a biphasic effect with rising levels facilitating receptivity. In general, after ovulation, progesterone has the opposite effect. Nonhormonal determinants of receptivity include olfactory stimuli and tactile sensations for many laboratory animals. However, individual preferences play a role particularly among primates, as noted for proceptive behaviors.

Baum et al. [23] also discuss the hormonal basis of proceptivity and receptivity in female primates, and conclude that most hormone-dependent changes in sexual interaction associated with the menstrual cycle seem to result from fluctuations in nonbehavioral attributes of female sexual *attractivity*. Thus at midcycle, estrogen levels are high, associated with the female being maximally attractive. During the luteal phase, when sexual interaction is at a low point, the female is secreting less estrogen and more progesterone. The data show that either of these hormonal changes causes a reduction in attractivity, independent of behavior.

3. Pheromones (External Chemical Messengers) in Mammals/Nonhuman Primates

Although many studies on laboratory rodents have demonstrated the clear significance of olfactory stimuli for reproductive development and behavior, only a few investigations of what the nonbehavioral cue might be have been carried out in primates. Michael and colleagues, after experimental olfaction-blocking in rhesus males and hormonal manipulation of ovariectomized females, have concluded that the menstrual cycle pattern of sexual activity in monkeys is in part due to the male's recognition of the female's endocrine status through the olfactory sense. Short chain aliphatic acids isolated from estrogenized female monkeys' vaginal secretions have been shown in Michael's laboratory to be a stimulus for immediate male sexual behavior. These short chain aliphatic acids are also found in the vaginal secretions of other female primates, including humans [21], and are produced by bacteria in the vagina under the influence of estrogen [24]. Attempts to replicate Michael's findings concerning this olfactory stimulus to male copulatory behavior have not been successful [25]. Since not all male monkeys in Michael's labs were capable of responding in this experiment, it is not clear to what extent the findings may be generalized [26].

4. General Activity Patterns in Human Females

The series of studies we began after our original study was designed to test hypotheses derived from the above-mentioned research which seemed to have some promise for explaining human behavior. One of our first simple efforts was to test whether female activity in general varies with gonadal hormone status as it does in lower vertebrates with estrous cycles [27]. We put pedometers on 34 women, 25 of whom participated through three or more complete menstrual cycles. The typical subject was white, married, college-educated, 30-years-old, the mother of two or three children, and not employed outside the home. The women wore the pedometers all day between arising and retiring. We plotted the recorded daily activity, utilizing a standardized 28 day menstrual cycle. A clear midcycle peak and briefer peaks near the beginning and end of the cycle appeared. We concluded that human female activity *is* increased around the time of ovulation, and therefore entertained the idea that a higher probability of sexual intercourse at this time might reflect a higher general activity level. We attempted to replicate this result in our next study but were unsuccessful. The age and parity of the participants in the two studies were different. Few of the women in the second study were employed only in the home. Aside from the possibility that the younger women in the new study had a more regimented lifestyle, we cannot really explain the different results. Previous reports in the literature on cyclic variations in motor activity in relation to the human female menstrual cycle are similarly inconsistent. The issue therefore remains uncertain.

5. Gonadal Hormone Effects in Human Females

The Double-Blind Pill Study. The study after the original pedometer study was the double-blind pill study mentioned above [16]. It was designed primarily for us to learn more about the effects of exogenous gonadal hormones on the pattern of human sexual intercourse. We hypothesized on the basis of animal studies, and anecdotes concerning "loss of libido" in women receiving highly progestogenic contraceptive pills, that the progesterone in contraceptive pills might cause depression of sexual activity. However we found that average sexual frequency was not directly affected by the contraceptive agents subjects used during the first 2 months of use. But there was an immediate change in the periodicity of behavior.

The married women who participated in the double-blind pill study were regularly using some method of contraception other than the pill. As mentioned earlier, there were 51 women, approximately 25% of whom were nonwhite. Their educational levels ranged from high school to graduate school, with wives of graduate students predominating. The women were randomly divided into three groups. For the first cycle, everyone sent in data daily, but no pills were ingested. After the first cycle, one group took 0.1 mg of mestranol combined with 2.0 mg of norethindrone; the second group took 0.08 mg of mestranol, and in the last six pills of each cycle they received 0.08 mg of mestranol, combined with 2 mg of norethindrone. The third group took lactose placebos. Neither the participants nor the investigators knew what any individual was taking. The lactose and the active pills were each stuffed into capsules and looked identical; they did not resemble commercial contraceptive pills. The participants were given the capsules in numbered strands of 60, with instructions to take them continu-

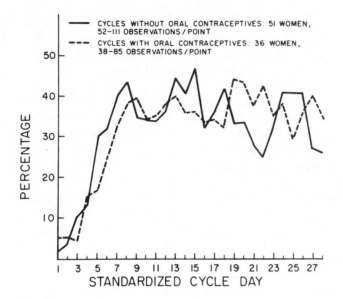

Figure 6 Percentage of women who reported intercourse per standardized menstrual cycle day. (From Ref. 16, reprinted by permission from *Nature,* Vol. 227, No. 5257, pp. 502-503. Copyright (©) 1970 Macmillan Journals Limited.)

ously in consecutive order until they were all used. Women taking capsules containing active ingredients were actually taking them in a cycle of 20 days on and 8 days off, the intervening capsules being lactose.

Intercourse and orgasm data were graphed on a standardized 28 day cycle. Low group rates at the beginning of the cycle coincided with days of menstrual bleeding. Rates of intercourse when *no* pills were taken have a peak halfway through the cycle and are depressed during the luteal phase. Rates of intercourse when pills *were* being taken reach a peak during what would have been the luteal phase had ovulation occurred; no depression can be seen (Fig. 6). The pattern for orgasm rates was similar, with the same change in the luteal phase.

We were very surprised to see that the pills erased the luteal depression. Because we had previously concluded that estrogen increases and progesterone decreases the probability of sexual activity during the menstrual cycle, we expected exogenous progesterone to have an immediate depressant effect. We thought the women might show decreased activity all the time they were taking progesterone; for women receiving combined medication, this would amount to almost the whole cycle; but instead we found that the characteristic luteal depression disappeared and that activity was greatest during that interval. We attributed the disappearance of the characteristic luteal depression of sexual activity to the wiping out of the usual luteal peak of endogenous progesterone, since the oral contraceptives used in this experiment work by inhibiting ovulation. Without ovulation, no corpus luteum is formed, and there is no luteal surge of endogenous progesterone. (The progestogen level provided by the pills is relatively low.) Both types of contraceptive pills work through the same mechanism, and we saw no difference according to type of contraceptive pill taken. The amount of hormones ingested by our participants was proportionately much less than that given to female laboratory primates in whom contraceptive pills over 6 months were seen to be associated with a loss of ejaculatory performance in male partners [21].

Additional analysis of the data from our double-blind pill study interested us even further in the possibility that nonbehavioral cues might help determine patterning within the menstrual cycle. We rejected the notion that, during the luteal phase, the difference in pattern was due to a direct effect of the contraceptive pills on the woman's feeling state or overall activity level, since direct questions and the measurement of activity did not show any difference during contraceptive pill use. We considered the possibility that sex drive in females is affected by androgenic hormones, and that the production of these androgens would be altered by the use of oral contraceptives in a pattern similar to the changes in sexual behavior. Comparing our data with available reports of androgen measurement in females did not seem to support such a relationship but left this question unanswered.

We did observe a difference in the woman's questionnaire responses with regard to the previous 24 hours that her husband had wanted intercourse. During the luteal phase she said "yes" more during pill cycles than nonpill cycles. In other words, the probability of a positive report that he wanted intercourse during those days was higher during the nonpill cycles. We were left looking for an explanation of why he would want intercourse more during this period, therefore stimulating our interest in a nonbehavioral cue [28].

A Pilot Study. The next study was conducted to find out in a nonstructured way about the sequence of events in the heterosexual encounter and possible effects of contraceptive pills. We enlisted approximately 50 participants who were divided into discussion groups according to whether they were male or female, black or white, middle- or working-class. Discussions focused on the role of the various contraceptives which they had used in their reproductive lives. The discussions were stimulated by printed questions which were distributed, but the conversation was relatively free-flowing. Among the results which were very clear was the fact that the men initiated most heterosexual encounters and that the women who were uninterested in having intercourse at any given time had well-developed avoidance techniques which they used, such as staying up to watch a late movie on television, during which time the man often went to bed before the woman.

Comments about contraceptive pills were also valuable. Some women and men observed that contraceptive pill usage reduced the amount of vaginal secretion and therefore made intercourse less easy or less pleasant. Women's psychological depression, nausea, weight gain, and water retention were also prominent symptoms mentioned in the group discussions.

No group made any spontaneous reference to the role of olfaction in their sexual lives. There was no question on the printed sheets relating to odors or smells as turn-ons or turn-offs in sexual life. Our interest in olfactory stimuli only became serious later, reflecting developments in the literature on nonhuman primates.

6. Olfactory Effects in Humans

The "Smeller-Smellee" Pilot Study. To pursue the possibility of an olfactory cue influencing the frequency and timing of coitus by influencing male demand, we designed a preliminary study to determine whether humans could identify another's sex by smell. For the time being, we left open the question of which sex influences which through its odor.

Fourteen male and fourteen female participants were recruited from an undergraduate sociology class. To standardize the format, participants and researchers were instructed to prepare themselves for experimental sessions as follows: they were to bathe with Ivory soap on the day of the session; use no perfumed cosmetics, hair spray, etc., or deodorants; and wear clean clothes. For 2 hours preceding the experiment, they were to refrain from smoking or eating. During the experiment, participants wore freshly aired hospital gowns and surgical caps. Researchers covered their street clothes with surgical gowns and also wore surgical caps. Female participants were requested not to attend sessions during their menstrual periods.

A hospital suite with fairly consistent temperature and humidity was utilized. Participants registered in a waiting area, were oriented to the procedure, received gowns and numbered caps, and retired to dressing areas segregated by sex. Here, researchers applied cotton wads and eye patches for blindfolds. From this point on, efforts were made to conceal the sex of the individuals from one another. Half the group, mixed as to sex, was taken to a row of cots in an adjacent room. The cots were covered with clean sheets, were about 6 feet apart, and were each surrounded by hanging drapes in the manner of a hospital ward. The subjects to be smelled, the "smellees," lay supine on the cots. The other participants, the "smellers," were then paired with researchers and led from cot to cot. As participants stood individually at the side of a cot, they were requested to bend forward. The researcher stopped participants' forward inclination as their heads reached approximately 12 inches from the subjects' upper chest. After they had an opportunity to concentrate on odor, the guessing participants were asked to indicate with a previously agreed-upon hand signal whether the subject was male or female. The guess was forced into one category or the other, even when the cot was empty (two cots in variable locations were left empty). The guessing participants then lowered their head to approximately 4 inches from the subject's chest. Finally they were repositioned approximately 4 inches from the subjects' axillae. In each location, they was asked to guess as before, making a total of three guesses over each subject or empty cot. Only the third guess counted for data analysis below. After each series of three guesses, participants were led away from the cot and asked whether they did indeed smell anything, whether it seemed pleasant or unpleasant, whether they could identify what it was, and whether they noticed anything else which contributed to their guess. Answers were whispered.

The nostrils of the guessing participants were plugged with wet cotton after they had had one or two opportunities to stand next to every subject, and they were taken through the procedure again. After they had made the circuit, they and the subjects were led around in a confusing manner designed to obscure the reshuffling. The two groups at this point were trading roles. The new subjects were placed on fresh sheets on the cots, and the guessing sequence was then repeated as before.

Guesses made at random should have approximated 50% male, 50% female. Over the empty cots, this was the case. When the male participants were exposed to men, they guessed "male" 57% of the time. This does not differ from 50% at the P=0.05 level. However when the male participants were exposed to females, they guessed "female" 63% of the time. This differs from 50% at the P=<0.01 level. With their noses plugged, men's guesses over empty cots and males or females did not differ from random. It therefore appeared that olfaction contributes to the male perception of a female.

Over the empty cots, women's guesses did not differ from a random distribution at the P=0.05 level. The distribution was about 50-50 when female participants were exposed to female subjects. However when the female participants were exposed to male subjects, they guessed "male" 65% of the time. This differs from 50% at the P=<0.01 level. It appears from these data that olfaction contributes to the female perception of a male. Interpretation of the female data, however, was clouded by the performance of the women with their noses plugged. In this condition, regardless of the situation, women guessed "male" more often than they guessed "female" (156 guesses male, 108 guesses female).

Individuals did not improve their performance with experience. Repeated observations in the same pair-encounters suggested that the reliability of the guesses was low.

We did not publish the results of this study, because we considered it preliminary and had many questions about the methodology. However, since this experiment, others have reported that men and women can correctly match the owners of tee shirts which had been worn for a prolonged period, and can distinguish sex via olfaction [29]. An elegant in vitro study by Doty et al. provides a possible explanation for the findings, namely that more intense, less pleasant odors are interpreted as male [30]. That the conclusions agree is reinforcing, but one must question all these experiments because of methodologic weaknesses.

The Synthetic Hyopthetic Human Female Pheromone Study. In our next study, the "pheromone study," we decided to expose couples to the aliphatic acid mixture which had been found in human vaginal secretions and determine whether this influenced the timing of their sexual behavior [17]. We hypothesized that male-reported desire for sexual intercourse, sex play, intercourse, and/or orgasm during the nights following exposure to the mixture would be greater than during nights following placebo or no exposure. We did not expect the mixture to have any effects on the women, because in the literature on nonhuman primates all the testing had been done on male behavior and no changes in female behavior were described. We created four treatments packaged in one-dose containers, numbered consecutively, and randomized so that each of the four treatments appeared twice in 8 days. Only one treatment of the four contained the six short-chain aliphatic acids, the olfactory stimulus of interest. Sixty-two couples completed three cycles of participation. Mean age of the men was 25.5 years. Seventy-six percent of the men were attending the university, all but six at the graduate level. The mean age of the women was 24.8 years. Twenty-four percent were university students, six at the graduate level.

The couples were not told how many different treatments there were. Each woman was asked to apply the contents of one container (0.5 cc total volume) to the skin of her chest each night at bedtime. Wives also measured their basal body temperatures each morning. Both husbands and wives each morning individually recorded on separate forms answers to questions concerning sexual desire and behavior in the previous 24 h. The forms were mailed to the investigators daily. Couples were carefully oriented as to what was expected. Respondents were asked to indicate nights on which they did not go to bed at the same time. Periods of menstruation, illness, and separation were to be reported. To account for intercourse occurring during the day or before the application of the experimental substance, wives recorded on a 24 h scale the time of application of the treatment and the time(s) of coitus. Husbands also recorded intercourse on a time-scale providing a methodologic check.

As mentioned earlier, this group turned out not to show periodicity when the data were organized by reverse or standardized menstrual cycle days. The group therefore did not show the behavior the experiment was designed to explain. No effect of the treatment was found with the following possible exception: a subsample of the couples (12) did exhibit periodic sexual intercourse within the menstrual cycle. We defined periodicity as reporting at least two more episodes of intercourse during reverse days 13 to 15 than during reverse days 6 to 8. Within this subsample there was an elevated sexual response following exposure to the acid mixture (Table 1). The significance test utilized considered the total number of observations. More conservative methods of analysis utilizing the number

Table 1 Percentage of Husbands Reporting[a] Intercourse after Treatment, by Type of Treatment, for Cyclic (N=12) and Noncyclic (N=50) Couples

	Intercourse after treatment	
Treatment	Cyclic (%)	Noncyclic (%)
Alcohol	25.6 (172)	26.8 (735)
Pheromone in alcohol	31.5 (184)[b]	24.2 (765)
Water	26.4 (174)	28.9 (766)
Perfume in alcohol	21.9 (178)	25.8 (749)

[a]Excluding menstrual days and days when couple was not together at bedtime.

[b]$t=1.83$, P is 0.03 for pheromone versus all other treatments, one-tailed test. Numbers of observations in parentheses.

Source: Ref. 17.

of couples as the "N" showed that the amount of difference seen in the behavior was not statistically significant. Analyzing the problems in this experiment, we concluded that the issue was not settled. We could neither reject nor accept the idea that a nonbehavioral cue sometimes operates through the sense of olfaction to influence male sexual demand.

V. Our Present Research

A. Daily Testosterone Measure

The blood samples from which luteinizing hormone was measured are still available for further hormonal analysis. We have planned to correlate other steroid measures including testosterone with the information we have concerning the woman's daily sexual activity. Although information available to us earlier did not suggest that testosterone might be influencing female behavior, all inferences concerning behavior and hormone levels are questionable until the actual measurements are done within individuals for whom behavioral data has been collected.

B. Female-Initiated Behavior

From the couples participating in the pheromone study, we have, as noted above, data from the men as well as the women. Included are answers to a series of questions concerning the process of heterosexual behavior if intercourse occurred, and the reasons why it did not occur if it did not. It has been reported by other investigators that if one focuses on female-initiated sexual behavior, including female fantasies, dreams, and masturbation as well as overt proceptivity, one sees a cyclic pattern within the menstrual cycle with a peak at midcycle [31]. We are analyzing our data to determine whether we can support this finding. Our data do not exactly match the questions used by the other investigators, but we should be able to address the same questions. We have the advantage of the male's explanation for the same event when heterosexual interaction was involved. Preliminary attempts do not appear supportive. Although our data do not include dream and fantasy information, we do have data on masturbation and female-initiated heterosexual intercourse. The latter is a very infrequent event in our samples.

C. Development of Adolescent Heterosexual Behavior

We currently are studying, through field interviews, the development of heterosexual behavior in young adolescents. By observing pubertal development, we have a reflection of the growing levels of gonadal hormones. We are attempting to relate these rising hormone levels to the increasing frequency of sexual fantasies, masturbation, and overt heterosexual behavior. The strength of the biologic correlations as compared with various social correlations may help us assess the importance of nonsocial influences on human sexual behavior.

VI. Future Research

A. Cycle Effects

1. Hypotheses for Study

In reflecting on needed future research, we must now reformulate the fundamental research question. When our research on menstrual cyclicity of sexual behavior began, measures of hormones were primitive, and hypotheses concerning hormone-behavior mechanisms were much less developed than today. Our initial interest in menstrual cycle patterns of sexual behavior reflected the amorphous state of knowledge at that time. Today, global questions concerning the existence and pattern of cyclic sexual behavior need to be dissolved into much more definite questions. Once these questions are asked, the cyclicity questions have served their purpose. Once these questions are answered, the cyclicity questions will have been resolved. The right questions are those about the effects of male and female hormones on human sexual behavior. The research techniques are the measurement of hormones, the manipulation of hormones, and the measurement of sexual behavior, not the arrangement of sexual behavior according to its position with respect to menstrual markers.

The existence of possible effects of one sex's hormones on the sexual behavior of the other sex complicates the research problem. But a focus of these questions on menstrual cycle patterns rather than on specific hormone-behavior relationships is likely to obscure rather than clarify the answers.

Even in cross-sex effects, the preferred research strategy is a direct attack on the hormone-behavior relationship. The existence of a male behavior patterned on the menstrual cycle of his partner is only a sign that there may be an effect of a female hormone on male behavior, and the pattern may suggest the effective hormone. The important questions will still remain: what is the hormone, and what is the behavioral mechanism through which it works?

Five recent findings make plausible a hypothesis relating endogenous testosterone in females to sexual cyclicity with a midcycle peak. First, baseline levels of plasma testosterone are correlated with self-reports of female sexual gratification. Second, testosterone levels peak at midcycle, presumably as a consequence of ovarian function. Third, the height of the midcycle peak in female testosterone is correlated with frequency of marital intercourse. Fourth, frequency of intercourse is not related to male testosterone levels [32]. Fifth, treatment with testosterone is helpful for sexually unresponsive women [33]. These facts make the female testosterone hypothesis rather than a pheromone hypothesis the more parsimonious explanation of a midcycle peak (if any) in sexual intercourse rates. And the testosterone hypothesis depends on cyclic changes in the *behavior* of females, suggesting greater proceptivity on the part of females at midcycle.

In the simplest terms, we now consider the leading hypotheses relating to cyclicity of sexual behavior to be as follows: (1) testosterone increases female proceptivity; (2) estrogen increases female receptivity; (3) progesterone reduces female receptivity; (4) couples whose sexual encounters are sensitive to female sexual states will show midcycle peaks and luteal depressions in sexual behavior.

2. Behavior in Groups Differing by Demographic Measures

Cyclic behaviors and concomitant hormone levels need further study in different social and ethnic groups. A review of our findings showed that the pattern differences by educational level and possibly by race appear to suggest that differences among groups are sociologic phenomena related to differences in the control and initiation of coitus. This needs documentation. Hormone measures are needed to show that the differences are not related to biologic parameters.

3. Behavior by Nutritional Status

Another possibly fruitful area for study is the effect of nutritional status on the proportion of ovulatory cycles, hormone levels, and sexual behavior. In the Second World War, reproductive problems were attributed to disruption of food supplies in both Holland and Russia [34,35]. The assumption seems to have been made that sexual behavior remained the same. This assumption is probably unwarranted, since war disrupts all aspects of life. At any rate, it would be worthwhile to obtain hormone *and* daily sexual behavior information from individuals whose nutritional status has brought them under medical supervision. This would be at the least a fruitful type of research which has not previously been attempted, to our knowledge.

B. Other Hormonal Effects

1. Luteinizing Hormone-Releasing Hormone: Direct Effect?

It is of interest that anecdotal evidence in humans exists for a directly sexual stimulus resulting from a bolus of intravenous luteinizing hormone-releasing hormone (LHRH) [36]. Laboratory rodents given LHRH have been observed to assume copulatory postures [37]. This suggests that, in addition to a possible effect resulting from the release of luteinizing hormone which in turn stimulates the production of gonadal hormones, LHRH might have an immediate effect on sexual behavior. Considering the sharp peak of sexual activity correlating with basal body temperature, one might ask what the relationship is between the LHRH level at midcycle and basal body temperature. There has been at least one study in which basal body temperature was measured in nonhuman primates and correlated with gonadal hormone levels. However a study which included basal body temperature, LHRH, LH, gonadal hormones, and sexual behavior would be very helpful in clarifying further temporal relationships among the spectrum of midcycle events.

2. Puberty, Hormone Analysis, and Behavior

Apter and others have studied children through puberty and adolescence with frequent hormone sampling [38,39]. It would be valuable to add behavioral measures to these precise multiple steroid hormone analyses.

C. Olfactory Stimuli Effects

Much more information is needed on the effects of olfactory stimuli and hormones on reproductive behavior before these factors can satisfactorily be put together to explain nonhuman primate behavior, let alone human behavior.

1. Male-Female Effects

The report by Cowley et al. that androstenol and the aliphatic acid mixture found in primate vaginal secretions modify judgments, acting differently on males and females, suggests an area deserving further study [40]. The notion that *female* sexual behavior might be influenced through olfactory cues has hardly been touched upon in *experiments* on any mammals, with the exception of the ubiquitous finding that most female mammals are more interested in urine from intact males than from males whose testosterone levels are low and that, given a choice, they will approach a normal male rather than a castrated one [22]. Greater human female olfactory acuity for selected musklike odors at midcycle than during menstruation is an old finding responsible for much teleologic speculation [41].

2. Attraction Effects

Patterning aside, the studies which have questioned the pleasant or nonpleasant nature of various sexually related volatile substances via smell experiments might profitably be repeated in homosexuals [42]. It would be interesting to know whether their definition of a pleasant odor is the same or different, and whether the range of substances they are able to detect is different from that of the heterosexual in quality and quantity.

VII. Conclusions

After 16 years of research, we do not have a clear-cut answer to the question of the existence or cause of a pattern of intercourse related to the female menstrual cycle. Our own studies produce inconsistent results, as do those of other investigators. If some couples exhibit cyclic patterns, we now believe that the most likely explanation is not female pheromones influencing male sexual initiation, but hormones of the female influencing her own behavior. The inconsistency of results seeking cyclic patterns, together with the improved knowledge of hormone effects and the improved ability to measure hormone levels, makes further studies using menstrual markers as data organizers unpromising for future research. Hormones must be measured for direct correlations with behavior. The leading hypotheses today are that female testosterone increases and progesterone decreases the readiness of women to seek or engage in coitus. If there is an estrogen-dependent female pheromone affecting male behavior, its timing would correspond to the testosterone peak in women. Under naturally occurring conditions, it is unlikely that the pheromone will produce an effect which could be identified. If women today are more sexually assertive than in the past, and/or if men today are more sensitive to female sexual desires than in the past, as is often stated, then we should expect the pattern of occurrence of coitus in contemporary couples to be more closely associated with female hormone patterns than in the past.

Acknowledgments

For the previously unpublished research mentioned in this chapter, the authors gratefully acknowledge the assistance of Dr. Newton D. Fischer, Otolaryngology; Dr. Charles E. Morris, Neurology; Sue E. Flowers, Physical Therapy; and Alexa Aycock, Maternal and Child Health, University of North Carolina at Chapel Hill, in the olfaction study; and support from Faculty Grant #324-ALU-1(530), University of North Carolina, for the group discussions.

References

1. J. R. Udry and N. M. Morris, *Nature* 220:593 (1968).
2. R. P. Michael and D. Zumpe, *J. Reprod. Fertil.* 21:199 (1970).
3. R. P. Michael, *Proc. R. Soc. Med.* 48:595 (1965).
4. A. H. Maslow, in *Sex Research, New Developments* (J. Money, ed.). Holt, Rinehart, and Winston, New York, 1965.
5. C. Leuba, *The Sexual Nature of Man.* Doubleday, Garden City, New York, 1954, p. 29.
6. P. Wallin and A. Clark, *Sociometry* 21:247 (1958).
7. W. M. Kephart, in *The Family, Society, and the Individual,* 2nd ed. Houghton Mifflin, Boston, 1966, p. 433.
8. K. B. Davis, in *Factors in the Sex Life of 2200 Women.* Harper and Row Pub., New York, and London, 1929.
9. L. M. Terman, in *Psychological Factors in Marital Happiness.* McGraw-Hill, New York, 1938.
10. R. A. McCance, M. C. Luff, and E. E. Widdowson, *J. Hyg.* 37:571 (1937).
11. P. Englander-Golden, H-S Chang, M. R. Whitmore, and R. A. Dienstbier, *J. Human Stress* 6:42 (1980).
12. T. Benedek, in *Psychosexual Functions in Women: Studies in Psychosomatic Medicine.* Ronald Press, New York, 1952.
13. C. J. Spitz, A. R. Gold, and D. B. Adams, *Arch. Sex. Behav.* 4:249 (1975).
14. W. H. James, *J. Biosoc. Sci.* 3:159 (1971).
15. J. R. Cavanagh, *Med. Aspects Hum. Sexuality* 3:29 (1969).
16. J. R. Udry and N. M. Morris, *Nature* 227:502 (1970).
17. N. M. Morris and J. R. Udry, *J. Biosoc. Sci.* 10:147 (1978).
18. N. M. Morris, J. R. Udry and L. E. Underwood, *Fertil. Steril.* 28:440 (1977).
19. J. R. Udry and N. M. Morris, *J. Reprod. Fertil.* 51:419 (1977).
20. C. J. Spitz, A. R. Gold, and D. B. Adams, *Arch. Sex. Behav.* 4:249 (1975).
21. R. P. Michael, in *The Use of Non-Human Primates in Research on Human Reproduction* (E. Diczfalusy and C. C. Standley, eds.). WHO Research and Training Centre on Human Reproduction, Karolinska Institutet, Stockholm, 1972, p. 322.
22. F. A. Beach, *Horm. Behav.* 7:105 (1976).
23. M. J. Baum, B. J. Everitt, J. Herbert, and E. B. Keverne, *Arch. Sex. Behav.* 6:173 (1977).
24. R. W. Bonsall and R. P. Michael, *J. Reprod. Fertil.* 27:478 (1971).
25. D. A. Goldfoot, M. A. Kravetz, R. W. Goy, and S. K. Freeman, *Horm. Behav.* 7:1 (1976).
26. M. J. Rogel, *Psychol. Bull.* 85:810 (1978).
27. N. M. Morris and J. R. Udry, *Obstet. Gynecol.* 35:199 (1970).
28. J. R. Udry, N. M. Morris, and L. Waller, *Arch. Sex. Behav.* 2:205 (1973).

29. M. J. Russell, *Nature* 260:520 (1976).
30. R. L. Doty, M. M. Orndorff, J. L. Leyden, and A. Kligman, *Behav. Biol.* 23:373 (1978).
31. D. B. Adams, A. R. Gold, and A. D. Burt, *N. Engl. J. Med.* 299:1145 (1978).
32. H. Persky, H. I. Lief, D. Strauss, W. R. Miller, and C. P. O'Brien, *Arch. Sex. Behav.* 7:157 (1978).
33. A. Carney, J. Bancroft, and A. Mathews, *Br. J. Psychiatry* 133:339 (1978).
34. C. A. Smith, *J. Pediatr.* 30:229 (1947).
35. A. N. Antonov, *J. Pediatr.* 30:250 (1947).
36. A. Prange, Jr., Personal communication, 1974.
37. R. L. Moss and S. M. McCann, *Science* 181:177 (1973).
38. D. Apter, L. Viinikka, and R. Vihko, *J. Clin. Endocrinol. Metab.* 47:944 (1978).
39. J. W. Finkelstein, in *The Pediatric Clinics of North America* (I. Litt, ed.) Saunders, Philadelphia, 1980, p. 53.
40. J. J. Cowley, A. L. Johnson, and B. W. L. Brooksbank, *Psychoneuroendocrinology* 2:159 (1977).
41. J. LeMagnen, *J. Physiol. (Paris)* 45:285 (1953).
42. L. Keith, P. Stromberg, B. K. Krotoszynski, J. Shah, and A. Dravnieks, *Arch. Gynecol.* 220:1 (1975).

8 Sexual Behavior and the Menstrual Cycle

GREGORY D. WILLIAMS   Presbyterian-University of Pennsylvania Medical Center, Philadelphia, Pennsylvania

ANN MARIE WILLIAMS   Marriage Council of Philadelphia, Inc., Philadelphia, Pennsylvania

During the past half-century scientific interest in human sexual behavior has gradually been released from the shackles of Victorian morality and has taken its place as a legitimate subject of inquiry. More recently, interest in biological rhythms—circadian, circatrigintan, circannual—has blossomed. This chapter explores the interrelationships between these two subjects: human sexual activity and one of the most obvious human rhythms, the menstrual cycle.

This chapter assesses research done in an attempt to answer the following question: what is the effect of the menstrual cycle on sexual behavior? i.e., how do the hormonal and physiological changes which occur during the cycle affect sexual behavior? As one reviews the literature on this question, two related goals seem to be in the minds of the investigators. The first goal has been to determine in what way, if any, the various hormones, mainly the gonadal steroids, affect the frequency of sexual behavior. Another has been to shed light on the role of sexual behavior in human life. Is sex geared to the cycle in order to maximize procreation, or has the reproductive nature of sex been eclipsed by its sociocultural role? One might expect the frequency of coitus to be maximal near ovulation, since this is the case among almost all subhuman mammals. It is obvious, however, that procreation is not the sole purpose of sex, since men and women are both capable of being aroused to coitus and orgasm at *any* point in the woman's cycle. But how much of an evolutionary vestige is left in humans? Does any increased tendency for intercourse remain near ovulation?

I. Sexuality and the Menstrual Cycle

A. Retrospective Questionnaires

Most of the early research, and some of the more recent, has been based on data obtained from questionnaires. Davis (1929), using mailed questionnaires, received replies from 2200 women who reported both premenstrual and postmenstrual peaks in "sexual desire," with only 7.4% (unmarried women) to 11.1% (married women) reporting a midcycle peak.

Among Hamilton's (1929) 94 married couples giving complete replies, 37% reported a premenstrual peak in "desire," 49% claimed a postmenstrual peak, and none noted any midcycle change. Nineteen percent said they had no peak in desire at all, and two peaks in desire were reported by 21% of this sample.

Stopes (1931) questioned wives separated from their husbands who were in military service and they reported peaks of sexual desire both premenstrually and at midcycle.

In 1938, Terman received replies from 619 women who were asked questions similar to those in Davis' study. His findings supported those of Davis and Hamilton suggesting both pre- and postmenstrual rises in libido.

Van Emde Boas in 1955, while presenting his data from 246 married women, pointed to some of the methodologic problems in the work of previous authors. His major point was that there was no "typical" pattern of changing libido over the menstrual cycle. Some women (12.6%) reported *no* maximum sexual desire, others reported two or more maxima. As to the timing of maxima, one could find women reporting maximum desire at any point in the menstrual cycle. This does, as Van Emde Boas suggests, exclude a *predominant* hormonal influence on libido, but it does not exclude some type of hormonal influence. He showed that in each phase of the cycle there were women who reported a maximum and other women who reported a minimum; only two phases showed a significant excess of maxima, namely, the postmenstrual phase (46% reporting maxima and 4% reporting minima) and the "conception date" or fertile phase (26% maxima versus 6% minima). For the premenstrual phase 24% of the women reported maxima but 19% reported minima. Van Emde Boas also reminded his readers that some attention must be paid to the low points of sexual desire, and although there again was no homogeneity, in general, menses was the time of least sexual desire. Thus, Van Emde Boas has stressed that constructing an "average woman's libido curve" is very misleading.

Many of these studies have also not dealt with the risk of pregnancy. Certainly couples who are concentrating upon the midcycle phase because they *want* or do *not want* to conceive may reduce libido (by fulfillment through intercourse) or enhance it (by abstention). Hart (1960) looked at this issue in her report of 123 married women who were asking for contraceptive advice. Twenty-two percent of these women said they "felt more like having intercourse" just prior to menses. Another 22% said they felt that way just after menses and 8% named both periods as their time of maximum libido. Only 6% chose the midcycle. Fully 34% of this sample noted *no* particular time. Upon further questioning, it was found that only 47% of the women were aware of the "safe" period of their cycle. However, the proportion of women who said their libido was high around menses was similar whether they believed it to be a safe time or did not know when the safe time was. Hart concluded from this that knowledge of the safe period did not affect the reports about libido. On the contrary, the following study involving couples using the rhythm method of family planning suggests that concern about the safe period can markedly alter reported patterns of sexual desire.

Cavanaugh (1969) asked the following question of 580 Catholic wives using the rhythm method: "It has been said that woman's greatest sexual desire is at the time of ovulation, during the 'unsafe' period for those practicing rhythm. Was this true in your case?" Seventy-three percent said "yes," 8% said "sometimes," and only 18% said "no." Perhaps abstinence had intensified libido; more probably this was such a loaded question that the results were seriously biased toward an affirmative response.

In a study primarily focused on the incidence and severity of physical and emotional distress during the premenstrual and menstrual phases (Hamburg et al., 1968), 1100 wives of graduate students replied to a mailed questionnaire. Fifteen of these women, who were nulliparous and not currently using oral contraceptives, were studied intensively on eight occasions during two consecutive menstrual cycles (Moos et al., 1969). Sexual arousal, measured on a nine-point self-rated scale, was lowest during the menstrual flow (3.25 out of 9 points), showed an increase until about midcycle (5.59 out of 9 points), decreased slightly, then levelled off during the remainder of the cycle (about 4.75 out of 9 points). Seven of the women in this subgroup were chosen because on the mailed questionnaire they complained of high premenstrual tension. These women were contrasted with the remainder of the group who had reported low premenstrual tension. In addition, the authors concluded that the women with high premenstrual distress were lower in sexual arousal.

Shader et al. (1968) looked at the "characterological anxiety levels" associated with the premenstrual phase of the cycle. Based on the Taylor Manifest Anxiety Scale, the authors concluded that 30 of 76 female graduate students were highly anxious. Of these 30 young women, 11 reported marked changes in their premenstrual libido (nine reported an increase, two reported a decrease). In contrast, only seven of the 27 moderately anxious women reported premenstrual libido changes (six increases, 1 decrease), and only one of the 19 less anxious women reported an increase prior to menses. Thus, 16 of the 76 women, or 21.1%, reported increases in premenstrual libido which is comparable to the 22% figure described by Hart (1960). Only three women, or 4%, reported a decrease in desire during the premenstruum, leaving 75% of the entire group who apparently reported no change in libido at all.

Three more recent studies deserve only brief mention. Ferrero and LaPietra (1971) asked 1000 Italian wives when they experienced maximum libido. Fully 34.4% reported no particular time of the menstrual cycle. A premenstrual peak was noted by 25.6%, a postmenstrual peak by 24.4%, and a midcycle peak by 11.8%. Silbergeld et al. (1971) collected data on 120 symptom, mood, and behavior variables on only eight women for four cycles each. The three qualities that are relevant here—affectionate and sex arousal (from the Menstrual Distress Questionnaire) and sex aggressivity (from their Interview Rating Test)—showed only minor changes across the menstrual cycle. There was a tendency toward an increase in all three variables during the ovulatory phase and perhaps a small luteal decline. Oral contraceptives seemed to nullify these changes. Apparently none of these changes was statistically significant. The third study, by Genazzani et al. (1978), also used a retrospective questionnaire to study the female sexual response. Of 427 Sardinian women queried, many did not reply to the various questions. Among those who did reply to the three questions relevant here ("greatest desire for a partner," "facility in having sexual intercourse," and "ease in reaching orgasm"), their responses showed early follicular ("immediately after menstruation"), ovulatory ("in the midcycle, ovulatory period"), and premenstrual peaks. In contrast, erotic dreams showed only ovulatory and premenstrual highs. Similar peaks were found despite the use of oral contraceptives which casts serious doubt on the idea that hormonal changes were responsible for the variations reported.

By the late 1960s it became obvious to most researchers that no adequate answer to the question of sexual behavior and the menstrual cycle could be obtained through such retrospective questionnaire data. Several of the methodologic problems have already been mentioned. Several other comments should also be made. First, retrospective data are always of questionable validity. Many of the studies reported that 20 to 30% of the women had not noted *any* cyclic changes in sexual desire. There is no way of determining from retrospective data whether there was indeed no variation in desire or, rather, an observable pattern was not noticed. For example, the female author of this chapter became aware of some subtle variations in her dream content only after reviewing this literature.

Data collected through questionnaires or structured interviews risk suggesting that a woman *should* have observed patterns of variation in sexual desire, and she may feel that she ought to select one of the patterns suggested by the questions (e.g., Cavanaugh, 1969). Whenever clinical researchers fail to camouflage their hypotheses, the participants in the study are much more likely to help the researchers find the results they are looking for.

Another serious methodologic issue is the woman's ability to discern her own sexual arousal and report it objectively. When Heiman (1975) measured physiological response (vaginal photoplethysmography) to erotic stimuli, she found that some women were not accurately aware of their own degree of sexual arousal. Wincze et al. (1978) in a sex therapy outcome study, found that female clients reported improvement of their initially low sexual arousal despite the lack of objective change in the physiological measures of arousal to erotic stimuli (including vaginal plethysmography). Furthermore, some women may equate libido with sexual interest while others equate it with lust. Some women may not be willing to admit "arousal" unless it occurs in the context of coitus with their husbands.

There is also the methodologic problem of the timing of the menstrual cycle; every research design has to contend with cycles of varying length and with the variation in the time of ovulation. Most of these questionnaire studies have used only menses as a benchmark and have depended on the responding women to supply a definition of "just before menses," "midcycle," and "just after menses." But a woman with a 23 day cycle might well be ovulating 3 to 4 days after menses ends, and she might call this "just after menstruation" rather than midcycle.

Further, there is always the question of selective attention. Menses forces a woman to be aware of genital changes which she may interpret as arousing or unarousing depending on her learning history and cultural attitudes. At midcycle, less obvious genital changes may take place (e.g., passage of mucus; Billings, 1978), and again these may be variably interpreted by each woman.

Finally, no account has been taken of the man's response.

B. Dream Analysis

Before the recent relaxation of taboos against laboratory research on human sexual behavior, only *indirect* measures of sexual interest and activity were available for serious investigation. During the 1930s, when psychoanalysis was unsurpassed in popularity, dream analysis was heralded as a powerful tool for the exploration of the psychological determinants of sexual functioning. During the same period, daily vaginal smears and basal body temperatures were introduced for the intensive analysis of physiological changes occurring across the menstrual cycle, in particular, follicular maturation, ovulation, and the formation and degeneration of the corpus luteum in the absence of fertilization. A psychoanalyst and a physiologist, Therese Benedek and Boris Rubenstein (1939a,b; 1963) combined their respective tools, dream analysis, vaginal smears, and basal body temperatures, to explore the physiological and psychological correlates of the menstrual cycle. In the course of their painstaking study, daily verbatim transcripts were made of about 2000 dreams and free associations. Independently, the women in the study collected vaginal smears and recorded rectal temperatures each day. The results of each method were analyzed separately so that blind predictions could be made of phase of the cycle based solely on the psychoanalytic material.

The authors concluded that there were "no discrepancies in our correlations between hormone production and instinctual drives when the hormone levels were high" (1939a, p. 465). When the hormone production was low, however, they concluded that "the problems and conflicts of the individual cover over the underlying instinctual tendency" (p. 469). The 15 women undergoing daily psychoanalysis contributed records from 75 menstrual cycles. The fact that ovulation occurred in only 23 of these cycles was not felt significantly to alter the reliability or major patterns of the data. Benedek and Rubenstein (1939a) explained: "Even in the anovulatory cycles there was sufficient fluctuation of hormone production to define the characteristics of the cycle" (p. 250). In fact, the anovulatory cycles helped to delineate the impact of ovulation since the psychoanalytic material from these cycles "failed to show the psychological relation characteristic of ovulations" (p. 250).

This study remains a landmark because of the authors' thoroughness and attention to detail. Unlike subsequent reports which depended on administration of a single retrospective questionnaire or structured interview, the Benedek and Rubenstein study included longitudinal data: 11 of the 15 women contributed more than 6 months of daily records. Furthermore, ovulation was determined by relatively accurate methods (vaginal smears and basal body temperature) rather than being estimated by counting forwards or backwards from menses. Benedek (1963) later pointed out that "guesses" as to the time of ovulation would have jeopardized the high correlations found because of the menstrual irregularity and prevalence of anovulatory cycles in this group of seriously neurotic young women.

Another strength of this study is that several analysts and student analysts contributed case records in addition to those collected by the senior author. When these psychodynamic patterns were analyzed, the predictions of cycle phase were equally good so that the methodology could be considered independent of the personality and skill of the analyst as long as comprehensive notes were taken daily on dreams, fantasies, and free associations. Finally, unlike many subsequent studies which were limited to gross estimations of sexual behavior or interest (e.g., sexual intercourse did or did not occur) and rough approximations of hormonal functioning (e.g., luteal phase vs. follicular phase), their data correlated the *level* of hormone production (as reflected in the vaginal cytology) with the intensity of psychodynamic material (1939b, p. 463).

They reported that specific hormonal functions of the ovary were correlated with specific instinctual drives: (1) estrone production with heterosexual drive, and (2) progesterone production with passive receptivity and narcissism. Ovulation was associated with a brief period of relaxation, contentment, and a respite from neurotic symptoms. The premenstrual period showed a return of heterosexual interest which was attributed to two hormonal shifts. The first shift involves a rapidly decreasing progesterone level due to corpus luteum regression. The second shift involves increasing estrone levels secreted by a few newly developing follicles. In this way, Benedek and Rubenstein seem to have found psychodynamic and physiological evidence supporting what other studies refer to as the premenstrual increase in sexual desire and activity. They cautioned, however, that the analytic material was complicated by anticipation of menstruation with its associated negative cultural values and, in some cases, ambivalent feelings regarding the absence of pregnancy. Impending menstruation was signalled by psychoanalytic material associated with eliminative or excretory functions. The onset of menstrual flow was then characterized by the dramatic relief from the restlessness, hyperactivity, irritability, and oversensitiveness observed in the late premenstrual phase.

Unlike subsequent authors who averaged and combined data from large groups of women in order to draw a "normal" or "typical" female response pattern, Benedek and Rubenstein used the psychoanalytic material to define several premenstrual subtypes according to idiosyncratic progesterone/estrone ratios, both within a single patient (1939b, p. 474) and across a subgroup of patients. Since their data were collected from a clinical sample of disturbed women, it is not known whether the psychoanalytic patterns described would also be found in a reduced form in a nonclinical population, or if these variations over the menstrual cycle would be absent altogether. The authors felt that the intensity and complexity of the emotional reactions they observed, especially during the late premenstrual and menstrual phases, could *not* be attributed to the influence of hormones alone.

In 1968, Swanson and Foulkes attempted a "quasi-replication" of the Benedek and Rubenstein study using sleep laboratory equipment to pinpoint the occurrence of dream sleep. Each of their four participants was awakened and questioned during four dreams per night, one night per week, for 11 consecutive weeks. Unfortunately, the phase of menstrual cycle was designated by number of days since menses, one of the least reliable methods for studying physiological changes.

They found that dreams with high sexual content were associated with periods of low waking sexual desire ($P < 0.01$). For three of the young women, increased sexual dream content occurred during menses when waking sexual desire was lowest. For the fourth student, increased sexual desire occurred during postmenses when waking sexual desire was lowest for her. This fourth subject was unlike the other three subjects because of "her occasional unreliability in providing a date for the onset of last menses."

Methodologic flaws in this study, including the lack of physiological data on hormone levels and the occurrence or absence of ovulation, make interpretation of the results difficult. Presumably, the four university undergraduates were unmarried and nulliparous. There is no indication as to sexual experience in the past or to their sexual activity (e.g., intercourse, masturbation) during the 11 weeks of the study. Although two of the young women were referred to as "frequent daters," we do not know if they used oral contraceptives (which were very popular then) or if they were virgins. In all probability, specific questions regarding sexual experience and overt sexual activities did not pass the senior author's thesis committee. This is supported by the explanation given for their findings: "increased scores in manifest sexuality during menses are attributable

. . . to changes in the nature of interaction consummated with drive-relevant objects" (p. 362). Presumably, the authors were saying that the sexuality scores were affected by the type of sexual activity, if any, the women had with their boyfriends during menses.

Swanson and Foulkes concluded that their data were not supportive of Benedek and Rubenstein's findings regarding "direct hormonal regulation of arousal of the sexual drive in the human female" (1968, p. 362). In fact, the original Benedek and Rubenstein (1939a,b) reports had been entitled "The Correlations Between Ovarian Activity and Psychodynamic Processes," which does not imply that either process dominated or regulated the other (1939b, p. 478). Moreover, neither Benedek and Rubenstein nor Swanson and Foulkes could speak to the issue of "direct hormonal regulation of arousal" since they had not experimentally manipulated hormone levels in a double-blind study to establish a causal relationship between hormones and sexual drive.

Swanson and Foulkes did find that more heterosexuality was expressed in dreams during menses, but it is not known whether hormones could have played a *direct* role (e.g., very low progesterone levels with increasing estrogen production) or an *indirect* role (e.g., hormone decrease which precipitated menses which then led to sexual abstention and deprivation) or both.

A recent study of manifest dream content by Lewis and Burns (1975) claimed to confirm the principal results of Swanson and Foulkes. This later study used more stringent screening criteria. The subjects were not allowed to use oral contraceptives or other drugs, had to have regular menstrual cycles, had to have regular bedtimes, and were reported to be virgins. Of 35 volunteers, only two 19-year-old women were chosen. Time since onset of menses was used to estimate phase of the cycle. Two dreams were recorded during each of two sessions per week for 12 weeks.

The authors found the sexual content scores of 46 dreams each (92 dreams, total) to be highest during menses, lowest postmenstrually (days 7 to 12), and higher again in the postovulatory phase (days 13 to 18). They concluded that sexual dream content did vary with the phase of menstrual cycle, but they argued that their results "would not support the idea that there is a correlation between hormone levels during the menstrual cycle and dream content" (p. 377). As in the previous study, hormone levels were not actually measured and the presence of ovulation was not determined. Variation in dream content could not be attributed to abstention from intercourse only during menses because both subjects were virgins who abstained throughout the 12 weeks of the study. In order to conceal the purpose of the investigation, data on masturbation were not collected.

Lewis and Burns tried to explain the menstrual peak in dream content by saying that both young women were deprived of "feeling sexy" during their periods. The smaller postovulatory peak was not explained.

A variant of dream content analysis is the examination of thematic variations of the verbal content of 5-min. extemporaneous talks on "any memorable life experience." This method was used by Ivey and Bardwick (1968) to test for differences in anxiety level at ovulation vs. 2 to 3 days preceeding the onset of menses. Basal body temperatures were recorded for 3 or 4 days preceeding the anticipated ovulation of each subject (N = 26). Records were kept of ovulation symptoms and the observed onset of menses.

Ivey and Bardwick concluded that these data from a nonclinical population confirmed the earlier findings of Benedek and Rubenstein, especially regarding the higher premenstrual incidence of death, mutilation, and separation anxiety themes. Moreover, they also found a premenstrual increase in "yearning for love, anxiety about being separated from love, and a feeling of helplessness in dealing with the situation" (p. 341). This "yearning for love" may, in part, account for some of the reported increases in sexual desire and intercourse prior to menses. For women in satisfying dyadic relationships, these needs may be met through physical closeness, thus resulting in reports of greater receptivity or more initiation of sexual contact. For women in distressed relationships or women without a partner with whom they can be physically intimate, this increased need for physical contact may be frustrated resulting in restless hyperactivity akin to what traditionally has been labeled hysteria. Ivey and Bardwick suggested that some premenstrual symptoms may stem from psychosomatic conversion to preserve a psychological balance in a socially acceptable way (p. 344). In contrast, ovulation was associated with themes of self-satisfaction with success and confidence in one's ability to cope. These samples of verbal behavior were not analyzed for overt sexual fantasies or themes.

As a group, these four studies of dream and verbal content agreed that there were thematic variations across the phases of the menstrual cycle. However, only Benedek and Rubenstein (1939a,b) and Ivey and Bardwick (1968) related these psychoanalytic themes to endocrine changes. The former study was limited to a clinical sample, while the latter study used female college students.

The two studies which involved the immediate recall of interrupted dreams, recorded in a sleep laboratory, are flawed by a lack of accurate, reliable physiological measures of cyclic changes. They both reported that manifest sexual dream content was highest during menses when most studies report the lowest rate of sexual activity. There may also be an inverse relationship between waking sexual activity and sexual dream content. Thus, when intercourse frequency is low because of menstrual taboos, erotic dreams may increase.

C. Erotic Stimulation

Four studies have attempted to approach the central question of this chapter in a different way. They used sexual arousal of women at various stages in the menstrual cycle to investigate differences in degree of arousal across the cycle.

Bardwick and Behrman (1967) used erotic stimulation techniques to compare two groups of women: five women who were sexually anxious, passive, and neurotic, and five female medical staff who were not sexually anxious, were more assertive, and were not neurotic. Uterine contractions were measured in response to affect-arousing stimuli (erotic words, paintings, and cartoons and anxiety-producing intellectual tasks) during each of the four phases of the menstrual cycle. The phases were estimated from records of length of cycle and date of last menstrual period. No relationship between menstrual cycle phase and stress effect was noted: the uterus was found to respond to psychological sexual stimuli at *any* cycle phase. Differences in response were found between the anxious and nonanxious groups: anxious women extruded the intrauterine balloon in response to sexual stimuli. They were unaware of this action. Women with low anxiety levels had uterine spasms which were theorized to facilitate sperm intake.

Luschen and Pierce (1972) showed pictures of clothed men to women college seniors (ages 18 to 22) who then rated each slide from 1 to 5 to indicate how stimulating she felt it to be. Twenty-four women were assigned to each of two groups, a premenstrual group (3 to 5 days before expected menses), and an ovulatory group (15 days before the estimated onset of the next menses). An unspecified number of these women were on oral contraceptives but their results were not reported separately. The mean rating of the 27 slides was calculated for each woman, then the overall means for the premenstrual and ovulatory groups were compared. Although the difference between the means was small (2.56 vs. 3.00 on a five-point scale), it was said to be significant ($P < 0.01$). This supposedly suggests that premenstrual women are less sexually aroused than ovulatory women, but the subjectiveness of the ratings and the narrowness of the difference warrant caution. There was "a suggestion . . . of differences in arousability to sexual stimuli for pill-users and pill non-users," but there was not enough information presented to evaluate what effects, if any, the exogenous hormones may have had.

Three years later, Griffith and Walker (1975) reported showing slides of explicit human sexual behavior to 60 undergraduate women (modal age 21). The ratings were again subjective. A single questionnaire was used to determine each woman's menstrual cycle phase, and the subjects were then divided into six groups based on their cycle phases. Apparently, these phases were purposely varied in length from 3 to 6 days each so that an equal number of subjects were assigned to each group. No difference in arousability was found between any of the cycle phases. There was no mention of contraceptive use by these women. Interestingly, these authors, in their discussion, are reminiscent of Van Emde Boas' suggestion that, although hormonal changes may alter an individual woman's arousability across her cycle, they may do so idiosyncratically, according to the individual's own cultural history and expectations.

The third erotic stimulation study, by Abramson et al. (1976), involved 133 college women (mean age 19.2 years) who read an erotic story. Based on a questionnaire, the women were determined to be in the menstrual, follicular, luteal, or premenstrual phase of the cycle. The ovulatory phase was omitted as a category so that, presumably, women in that phase were averaged in with the follicular or luteal phase women. After reading the erotic story, the participants gave a subjective report of their degree of arousal and of genital sensations. The women who were not using contraceptive pills showed no change across cycle phase. However, the 28% who were using the pill reported the most arousal during menses and the least premenstrually.

The major shortcoming of all these studies is the lack of an objective measurement of arousal. Heiman's work (1975) showed that at least 4 .% of her sample incorrectly reported their degree of sexual arousal when compared with recordings of physiological changes (vaginal vasocongestion measured by photoplethysmograph). It is not surprising that very little effect was found. Moreover, the groups of women used in these studies make extrapolation difficult since they were all very young and apparently none were married. The quantity and quality of sexual experience among these women (29% of the participants in the latter study reported *no* intercourse experience) seems too incomplete to provide answers about mature human sexuality.

D. Daily Reports

No study can avoid all these problems, but the ones which come closest are those requiring daily reporting of clearly defined sexual events. Here, of course, different behaviors are being assessed. By and large among these studies, women are recording the occurrences of coitus and/or orgasm, whereas the previously mentioned studies purported to assess libido or sexual arousal. Limitations of the daily report studies are discussed below.

One of the most careful studies of daily reports was done more than 40 years ago. McCance et al. (1937) obtained daily recordings from 166 women on a standardized questionnaire covering many aspects of mood, feelings, physical symptoms, and behavior. These subjects were white, mostly educated middle-class; only 32 were nonworking. Data were obtained on 780 menstrual cycles. There were 110 single women whose ages ranged from 20 to 47 years (mean 29.2 years) and 56 married women whose ages ranged from 23 to 45 years (mean 30.6 years). The two measures of interest here are "sexual feeling" and intercourse. Both of these dependent variables rose rapidly from a menstrual phase (days 1 to 5) low and were maximal on day 8 of the averaged 28 day cycle. This was true for both the married and the single women. Following this peak, the frequencies declined but not very rapidly until days 15 to 17; there was a "shoulder" on the forward side of the peak at day 8. The rate then remained stable until it fell off dramatically at the onset of menses. However, frequency of sexual feeling rose slightly on days 26 to 28. These data are strong support for the concept of a postmenstrual peak in sexual activity, but they also suggest that the increase of sexual feeling and activity continues for most of the follicular phase. There is also moderate support for a premenstrual rise in libido but not for coitus. This is remarkably high quality research for the 1930s. Its only drawback is that it was done before a physiological measurement of ovulation was developed and made available (e.g., vaginal smears and basal body temperature).

More recently the major contributors to this field have been Richard Udry and Naomi Morris. In 1968 they reported two studies of the frequency of coitus and orgasm. The first study was of a group of 40 uneducated, black, working women, all of whom were married. Data from up to 115 menstrual cycles were recorded and collected daily. These workers charted the menstrual cycle by counted backward from the first day of menses (the "reverse cycle day" method). In so doing they found a "preovulatory" (days –14 to –17) maximum in the percentage of women reporting either coitus or orgasm. There was then a gradual luteal decline and another smaller peak on premenstrual day –3.

The other group of women reported by Udry and Morris (1968) were white, middle-class, and mostly college educated. Forty-eight women kept calendar records which were collected from them yearly or even less often. Up to 828 cycles were represented. These women had an overall higher frequency of coitus and orgasm compared with the lower-class sample. There was also much more stability in their frequency over the cycle. There was, however, a tendency toward a luteal phase decline, especially for orgasm, among the 37 married women. The graphs for the 13 single women showed marked variations over the cycle, expecially for coitus. The authors suggest that there is again a preovulatory peak (day –14) for both coitus and orgasm, but this peak is small for orgasm and there are three other, comparable peaks in coitus during the cycle (days –4, –10, and –20). Therefore, at least for the black women, the menstrual cycle does appear to account for some of the variability in frequency of intercourse. For white women similar changes occur but are less pronounced.

In a later study by these authors (Udry and Morris, 1970), daily records of intercourse and orgasm were obtained from 51 married women, mostly the wives of graduate students. Following a double-blind protocol, some of these women were given oral contraceptive agents during two of three cycles. In this report Udry and Morris plotted their data according to a standardized 28 day cycle, presumably compressing longer cycles and expanding shorter ones. For the women who received only a placebo, coital activity showed a broad maximum over days 13 to 15, but there were similar peaks on days 8, 18, and 24 to 26. There was also a tendency toward a luteal decline, day 22 being the lowest day of all excluding menstrual days. However, the most striking finding was that the birth control pills "erased" this luteal depression. The orgasm rates also showed the luteal depression (again, erased by the pill) and they showed a maximum at day 15, although this latter peak does not stand out strikingly against the fluctuations during the rest of the cycle. Thus, here again there seems to be clear evidence of hormonal effects on the incidence of sexual activity. Overall, the three groups of women studied by Udry and Morris showed similar findings: lowest rates of coitus and orgasm during menses, a decline in sexual activity during the luteal phase, a tendency toward a periovulatory maximum (reverse cycle days –14 to

-17 or standardized cycle days 13 to 15), and lastly, a smaller premenstrual peak (reverse cycle days -2 to -4, or standardized cycle day 24 to 26).

Udry et al. (1973) expanded their report on this latter group of women in an attempt to explain the effect of the contraceptive on the luteal phase slump in sexual activity. They did so by examining other information collected by the women during the three cycles studied. Because pedometer readings taken daily by the participants did not appear different between the pill and nonpill groups, they rejected the hypothesis that progesterone in the normal luteal phase had acted as a general activity depressant and hence had also depressed sexual activity.

Moreover, daily reports of general well-being allowed the authors to reject the suggestion that progesterone was acting as a general mood depressant, since there were no significant differences between the groups in these reports. However, the women on the pill said that their husbands desired intercourse more frequently during the luteal phase, whereas the nonpill women reported a decline in the frequency of their husband's sexual approaches. This suggests that, through some unidentified mediator, the husbands of women not on the pill found either that their wives were less sexually attractive or that their own libido had diminished.

In a subsequent study, Morris and Udry (1978) attempted to show that this mediator was a pheromone, i.e., a signal transmitted by odor. Work by Michael and Keverne (1968) had shown that pheromones did in fact exist and could function as mediators of sexual behavior among rhesus monkeys. Michael had identified the chemicals (short chain, volatile, aliphatic acids) in vaginal secretions of these monkeys. He further showed that a synthetic mixture of these acids acted as a sexual attractant. Indeed, these same chemicals had been found in the vaginal secretions of humans and even varied in concentration during a woman's cycle (Michael et al., 1975; Preti and Huggins, 1975; Doty et al., 1975). Thus it was reasonable to hypothesize that these substances varied in a normal woman's cycle so as to depress (or not enhance) sexual attractivity during the luteal phase. In contrast, women using contraceptives would have stable hormone levels and therefore no fluctuations in these vaginal substances.

With this hypothesis in mind, 62 couples (mean age 25 years) associated with a university were recruited. Each wife was asked to apply a solution to her chest at bedtime and to record daily what time coitus occurred, if at all. Four solutions (alcohol, a synthetic mixture of the aforementioned aliphatic acids in alcohol, water, and a perfume in alcohol) were used each night for three menstrual cycles. Each substance was used according to a randomized protocol. No effect of the "pheromone" could be demonstrated. Interestingly, this sample of couples did not show the expected luteal decline in coital activity. This was true whether the cycle was plotted by reverse cycle day or by standardized cycle day. These workers then tried to identify couples in this sample who *did* show the luteal decline, in order to see if this subgroup had been affected by the treatment. This analysis was done by singling out the couples who reported more sex during reverse cycle days –13 to –15 than during days –6 to –8. This subgroup did show a marginally significant effect of the synthetic pheromone. However, since this definition of luteal decline was so arbitrary, another subgroup (including only cycles during which basal body temperature records had shown clear evidence of ovulation) was examined. Even though these latter cycles showed great overlap with those of the first subgroup, the second group showed no treatment effect. These results are frustrating to researchers attempting to define the factors mediating the association of sexual behavior and the menstrual cycle. As is so often true, clarification awaits further research.

In the chronologic record of the daily report studies, the work of James (1971) followed soon after the Udry and Morris (1968) article. He was the first to approach the problem of combining data from cycles of different length (see below). He solved the problem by combining cycles only of the same length. Using this method he reanalyzed the data of McCance et al. (1937) and of Udry and Morris (1968) to which he added some data of his own. The resulting seven graphs for 25 day through 31 day cycles did not show a uniform pattern of coital rates. Six of the seven show the highest rates of intercourse postmenstrually with a sharp decline thereafter. Another six of the seven depict a midcycle rise, but the shorter cycles show this rise several days after the day of presumed ovulation (assuming a luteal phase of 14 days). All of the cycles show very low rates during the luteal phase (the menstrual flow days were excluded), and another six of the seven have a premenstrual rise during the final 2 to 5 days of the cycle. James was impressed only by the postmenstrual maximum, which he attributed to release from menstrual abstinence, and did not believe any of the other patterns was significant. Apparently no one had devised a statistical technique which would determine that a certain peak on a curve is unlikely to occur by chance alone, so the conclusions must be drawn by visual observation of the graphs.

James' conclusions were supported by Spitz et al. (1975) who collected daily recordings of sexual behavior from 24 undergraduate students aged 18 to 24. All were sexually experienced and were engaged in continuing heterosexual relationships, but none was married and an unknown number had more than one boyfriend. Thirteen were using oral contraceptives. The results of several aspects of sexuality (coitus, caressing, masturbation, the initiation of the experience, whether rejection occurred, and self-rated arousal) were plotted across the menstrual cycle in a novel way. The cycle was divided into seven unequal phases according to a theoretic model of events occurring during the cycle. Its purpose was to combine data from cycles of different lengths. The ovulatory period was defined as the four days surrounding the day of ovulation estimated from conception data (James, 1972). The luteal phase was defined as beginning 3 days after the basal body temperature rise and ending 3 days before menses began. Menses included the first 6 days of the cycle, so that the remaining periods, postmenstrual and postovulatory, were of variable length and filled the remaining gaps. When plotted this way, both pill and nonpill subjects had their lowest coital rates during menses and their highest rates in the postmenstrual phase. This was followed by a decline for the ovulatory phase and a leveling off for the remainder of the cycle. The self-ratings of sexual arousal correlated with the degree of sexual activity (coitus, caressing, or no contact) rather than with cycle phase. These workers concluded that sexual behavior in the human is minimally affected by hormonal factors since oral contraceptives made essentially no difference. They also felt that the postmenstrual peak was probably related to release from abstinence during menses.

Another report from the Morris and Udry research group (Morris et al., 1977) is indirectly related to this question. They attempted to find out if intercourse could trigger the midcycle luteinizing hormone (LH) surge and, hence, ovulation in the human female as it does in some animals. They documented a LH rise and a basal body temperature shift in 27 of 100 women who kept daily records of intercourse. All were married, their median age was 25, and they were not using an oral contraceptive or the rhythm method, although other types of contraception (condom, diaphragm, IUD) were being used. The incidence of coitus (or female orgasm) on the day before the LH surge was not significantly different from the frequency during the 2 weeks on either side of the surge; the incidence on the presurge day was lower than the average for the other days. This argues against a periovulatory enhancement of sexual behavior, although only one of the several fertile days was evaluated and there was such marked variability during the other cycle days that only a striking peak would have shown significance.

This was the state of the evidence when Udry and Morris (1977) directly addressed a serious methodologic problem which had challenged previous authors (e.g., James, 1971; Spitz et al., 1975). This problem was how to chart the menstrual cycle so that data from women with varying cycle lengths and varying times of ovulation could be combined to yield coherent results. Of course, the ideal method would yield a graph, each point of which represented women who were in exactly the same phase hormonally and physiologically. Only in this way could mild hormonal effects become sufficiently strong to be apparent.

Five basic methods of charting the menstrual cycle have been derived. The first and most obvious is to begin with the first day of menses as day 1 and count each day of the cycle forward from that day (forward cycle day method). Women would, of course, be most in phase with one another during the early follicular phase and become less so later in the cycle, making late cycle pooling of data less reliable. A second method again begins with menses but counts backward (reverse cycle day method), thus making the luteal phase most reliable. Another method is to standardize all cycles to a 28 day cycle by mathematically compressing longer cycles and expanding shorter ones; in this case, data on both sides of menses are most reliable but the midcycle, periovulatory phase is least reliable. The method of Spitz et al. was described above. One might disagree with their somewhat arbitrary definitions of menstrual, ovulatory, luteal, and premenstrual periods, but most women in each group will generally be in a similar physiological state. Furthermore, this method does not allow visualization of trends within a given phase. Finally, two related methods have been used to pinpoint ovulation more closely (the nadir of the basal body temperature curve or a rise in blood LH level) and they count both forward and backward from that point. Here, reliability will be greatest in the periovulatory period and decrease as one moves away from it in either direction.

Udry and Morris (1977) graphed data from 85 young married couples according to all five methods. The dependent variables were coitus, female orgasm, and wife's desire for intercourse. Their conclusions were: (1) the most consistent feature on all the plots was a rise in sexual behaviors about 6 days before presumed midcycle, (2) a luteal decline in sexual behavior was usually observed, (3) different conclusions might be drawn from the same data displayed in different ways, and (4) improvement in reliability could only come from direct assay of blood hormone levels and correlation with the behavioral records. They might have more clearly pointed out that each method has its own peculiar phase of maximum reliability and other phases on the same graph should be given less credence.

The most recent in this long list of work on sexual behavior is the report of Adams et al. (1978) who made an important conceptual advance. They hypothesized that menstrual cycle effects should be apparent only in female-initiated behaviors and that inclusion of male-initiated sexual events (as most previous studies had done) would obscure any cycle effect. Thus they asked 35 white, college-educated married women to record their sexual activities daily. These records included self-, husband-, and mutually initiated coitus and caressing, masturbation, fantasy, and arousal from any other source. The women were between 21 and 31 years of age. Twelve subjects were using oral contraceptives, 11 were using "nonintrusive" methods of contraception (IUD, vasectomy) and the remaining 12 used "intrusive" contraceptives (condom, foam, diaphragm). The data were collected for a total of 171 cycles (average 4.2 cycles per couple).

Wives who were not taking the pill showed definite ovulatory rises in both autosexual (masturbation as well as fantasy and other arousal) and female-initiated heterosexual activity (coitus and caressing), whereas those wives taking the pill showed no such ovulatory rise. For female initiated heterosexual behavior there were postmenstrual rises (days +4 to +9) for all three groups which were as great or nearly as great as the ovulatory rise. The nonpill couples using intrusive methods of contraception showed low luteal phase heterosexual activity as compated with couples using the pill or nonintrusive contraception who showed a luteal rise in heterosexual behavior. All groups showed a premenstrual rise (day −1 to −3). Male-initiated activity was more frequent on ovulatory days for both pill and nonintrusive, nonpill subjects and were less frequent on those days for the intrusive nonpill group.

In summary, Adams' group purported to show that there is a periovulatory rise in sexual behavior when female-initiated experiences are singled out. This was not seen in wives who took the pill, suggesting that the effect is due to hormonal changes. This is probably due to estrogen according to Adams et al., but Persky's group (1979) points out that testosterone may well be the important hormone here. Adams et al.'s results are quite interesting but suffer from a severe methodologic problem. Although they were interested in periovulatory events, they did not pinpoint ovulation by basal body temperature or blood LH surge; they counted 14 days backward from the onset of next menses and assumed that ovulation occurred on days –13 to –15. Their plot of the incidence of reported mittelschmerz vs. cycle days shows a broad peak from day –10 to –17; days –13 to –15 include only 49% of those reports. To the extent that mittleschmerz is an indicator of ovulation, many of these women ovulated on days other than those designated as ovulatory by the authors. It is not clear what effect this procedure might have had on their results; getting all the women exactly in phase might strengthen the ovulatory peak they found, thus strengthening their case. However, the results of such a reappraisal are unknown until the study is repeated using a better method of designating the fertile period.

II. Summary and Implications

What is the answer to the first question posed in the introduction? What effect does the menstrual cycle have on sexual behavior? In summarizing the data presented here, the reader should keep in mind that several different aspects of sexual behavior have been addressed. All of the retrospective studies were able to assess only libido. This is a difficult term to define and was defined differently by the various subjects. No conclusion may be drawn about libido since studies may be found to support postmenstrual, ovulatory, or premenstrual peaks. The work of Van Emde Boas (1955) stressed the great variability among women on this aspect of sexuality. Furthermore, the erotic stimulation studies were unable to show any change in arousability across the cycle. Thus, sexual desire as a segment of sexual behavior is too subjective to allow precise assessment. Moreover, it is much more susceptible to the visual and auditory sexual atimuli of our culture, so that any hormonal effects are largely submerged.

The incidence of coitus is a much more objective measure of sexual behavior. Assessments of this variable have also been recorded daily so that the data are also much more reliable. Most of this work has shown a peak in the incidence of intercourse in the follicular phase of the cycle. It is not agreed whether this is truly postmenstrual and thus likely to be the result of release from abstinence during menses or a broader peak covering most of the follicular phase (e.g., McCance et al., 1937). Part of this confusion has arisen from the several ways of plotting the menstrual cycle, as discussed above, so that data ascribed to this phase may be a mixture of women who are very early follicular physiologically (viz., women with short menstrual flows) and those who are near enough to ovulation to be fertile (viz., women with short cycle lengths). More recent work using methods of pinpointing ovulation (Udry and Morris, 1977; Morris and Udry, 1977, 1978) has found periovulatory rises in coital frequency. Additionally, most of the graphs presented in the papers reviewed have shown a small upswing of coital rates in the 3 to 4 days before menses, although it has been much smaller compared with other peaks and usually was not commented upon.

Finally, mention should be made of the lows in coital frequency across the cycle. Intercourse is least frequent during the menstrual flow, and all but one of Udry and Morris' reports (Morris and Udry, 1978) have tended to show a luteal decline in the rate of coitus. This is also apparent in the work of James (1971).

In general, coital frequency rises rapidly from its nadir during menses to a maximum during the follicular phase. It then gradually declines over the rest of the cycle, with perhaps another increase around ovulation. Just before menses there is another slight increase before falling again to the lowest rate during menses. The magnitude of these changes varies according to author but the follicular maximum is usually a 30- to 40-fold increase over the menstrual nadir and the luteal low may drop to about half the follicular peak rate. It must be emphasized that no such pattern would be evident in any individual woman.

What does this mean? Given that this is the "average" pattern, why is it this way? One would think first of hormone fluctuations, but sorting out such effects is extremely difficult. There is a large literature on the question of what effect each of the sex hormones (androgen, estrogen, progesterone) has on libido, but there is no consensus. Both estrogen and androgen have been implicated as "the libido hormone" in women; progesterone is generally felt to be a libido-depressant. It is beyond the scope of this chapter to evaluate this issue; however, (1) estrogen (unopposed by progesterone) could stimulate libido during the follicular phase, (2) androgen or estrogen may be responsible for the increased periovulatory coital rate (if it occurs), and (3) progesterone may cause the luteal depression in coital rates. The work of Benedek and Rubenstein (1939 a,b) is the most direct study of the correlation between sexual behavior and hormones although the hormones were not directly measured and the frequency of coitus was not directly assessed. They concluded that there was a relationship between hormone levels and the sexual content of dreams, but just how such dreams relate to waking sexual activity is not as clear. Finally, the data on the occurrence of sex according to phase of the cycle are not good enough to allow precise timing with cycle events. Principally, either the preovulatory rise in estrogen or the periovulatory rise in testosterone could account for the periovulatory rise in coital rates. But until more precise chronologic correlation between sexual activity and cycle events is made, these two possibilities cannot be distinguished.

Another contributing factor to variations of libido and intercourse during the cycle is the external physiological changes themselves. The menstrual flow itself probably results in a postmenstrual increased likelihood of sex because of the release from abstention and perhaps from an improvement in the feeling of physical well-being. Some couples might have sex more frequently a few days before menses because they know that deprivation is imminent. A woman might interpret the premenstrual genital congestive changes and/or the preovulatory increased mucus production as erotic and hence initiate or be receptive to more sexual contact when those changes are present. It would be of great interest to evaluate sexual behavior in women who are premenopausal but have had hysterectomies (ovaries left intact). Hormone measurements and basal body temperature recording could document the cycle, but the effect of the menstrual flow itself could be isolated.

Variation of mood during the cycle should also be mentioned, although it is probably an intervening variable between hormones or pelvic changes and sexual inclination.

Finally, there may be a role for human pheromones. To date, olfactory communication has not been conclusively demonstrated in humans, although the synchronization of menstrual cycles between women exposed to each other only via axillary odors is intriguing (Hopson, 1980). Vaginal (Michael et al., 1975; Preti and Huggins, 1975; and Doty et al., 1975) and oral (Tonzetich et al., 1978) odors have been shown to vary in women during the menstrual cycle, and some women have vaginal chemicals identical to those shown to be sex attractants in rhesus monkeys (Michael et al., 1975). The only attempt to identify human pheromones is that of Morris and Udry (1978) which failed to show a definite effect.

Thus, there does seem to be variation in the probability of sexual intercourse across the menstrual cycle. This variation is greatly overshadowed by social, cultural, and marital factors which have not been studied systematically. Moreover, there are several different ways (hormones, physical changes, moods, and pheromones) in which the changing physiology of the cycle could lead to variations in sexuality; much more work needs to be done to isolate and evaluate these factors independently.

References

Abramson, P. R., C. A. Repczynski, and L. R. Merrill (1976). The menstrual cycle and response to erotic literature. *J. Consult. Clin. Psychol.* 44:1018-1019.

Adams, D. B., A. R. Gold, and A. D. Burt (1978). Rise in female-initiated sexual activity at ovulation and its suppression by oral contraceptives. *N. Engl. J. Med.* 299:1145-1150.

Bardwick, J. M., and S. J. Behrman (1967). Investigation into the effects of anxiety, sexual arousal, and menstrual cycle phase on uterine contractions. *Psychosom. Med.* 29:468-482.

Benedek, T. (1963). An investigation of the sexual cycle in women. *Arch. Gen. Psychiatry* 8:25-36, 311-322.

Benedek, T., and B. B. Rubenstein (1939a). The correlations between ovarian activity and psychodynamic processes: I. The ovulative phase. *Psychosom. Med.* 1:245-270.

Benedek, T., and B. B. Rubenstein (1939b). The correlations between ovarian activity and psychodynamic processes: II. The menstrual phase. *Psychosom. Med.* 1:461-485.

Billings, J. J. (1978). *The Ovulation Method: Natural Family Planning,* 4th ed. Liturgical Press, Collegeville, MN.

Cavanaugh, J. R. (1969). Rhythm of sexual desire in women. *Med. Aspects of Hum. Sexuality* 3:29-39.

Davis, K. B. (1929). *Factors in the Sex Life of Twenty-Two Hundred Women.* Harper, New York.

Doty, R. L., M. Ford, G. Preti, and G. R. Huggins (1975). Changes in the intensity and pleasantness of human vaginal odors during the menstrual cycle. *Science* 190:1316-1318.

Ferrero, G., and O. LaPietra (1971). Libido fluctuations during the menstrual cycle. *Panminerva Med.* 13:407-409.

Genazzani, A. R., M. C. Devoto, C. Cianchetti, C. Pintor, F. Facchinetti, A. Mangoni, and P. Fioretti (1978). Menstrual cycle and sexual behavior in the human female. In *Clinical Psychoneuroendocrinology in Reproduction.* (L. Carenza, P. Pancheri, and L. Zichella, eds.). Proceedings of the Serono Symposia, vol. 22, pp. 419-436, Academic, London.

Griffith, M., and C. E. Walker (1975). Menstrual cycle phases and personality variables as related to response to erotic stimuli. *Arch. Sex. Behav.* 4:599-603.

Hamburg, D. A. R. H. Moos, and I. D. Yalom (1968). Studies of distress in the menstrual cycle and the postpartum period. In *Endocrinology and Human Behavior* (R. P. Michael, ed.). Oxford University Press, London.

Hamilton, G. V. (1929). *A Research in Marriage.* A. and C. Boni, New York.

Hart, R. D. (1960). Monthly rhythm of libido in married women. *Br. Med. J.* 1:1023-1024.

Heiman, J. R. (1975). Women's sexual arousal: The physiology of erotica. *Psychol. Today* 9:91-94.

Hopson, J. L. (1980). Scent and human behavior: olfaction or fiction? *Sci. News* 115:282-283.

Ivey, M. E., and J. M. Bardwick (1968). Patterns of affective fluctuation in the menstrual cycle. *Psychosom. Med.* 30:336-345.

James, W. H. (1971). The distribution of coitus within the human intermenstruum. *J. Biosoc. Sci.* 3:159-171.

James. W. H. (1972). Cycle day of ovulation. *J. Biosoc. Sci.* 4:371-378.

Lewis, S. A., and M. Burns (1975). Manifest dream content: changes with the menstrual cycle. *Br. J. Med. Psychol.* 48:375-377.

Luschen, M. E., and D. M. Pierce (1972). Effect of the menstrual cycle on mood and sexual arousability. *J. Sex. Res.* 8:41-47.

McCance, R. A., M. C. Luff, and E. E. Widdowson (1937). Physical and emotional periodicity in women. *J. Hygiene* 37:571-611.

Michael, R. P., R. W. Bonsall, and M. Kutner (1975). Volatile fatty acids, "copulins," in human vaginal secretions. *Psychoneuroendocrinology* 1:153-163.

Michael, R. P., and E. B. Keverne (1968). Pheromones in the communication of sexual status in primates. *Nature* 218:746-749.

Moos, R. H., B. S. Kopell, F. T. Melges, I. D. Yalom, D. T. Lunde, R. B. Clayton, and D. A. Hamburg (1969). Fluctuations in symptoms and moods during the menstrual cycle. *J. Psychosom. Res.* 13:37-44.

Morris, N. M., and J. R. Udry (1978). Pheromonal influences on human sexual behavior: an experimental search. *J. Biosoc. Sci.* 10:147-157.

Morris, N. M., J. R. Udry, and L. E. Underwood (1977). A study of the relationship between coitus and the luteinizing hormone surge. *Fertil. Steril.* 28:440-442.

Persky, H., C. P. O'Brien, H. I. Lief, D. Strauss, and W. R. Miller (1979). Female sexual activity at ovulation. Letter to the editor. *N. Engl. J. Med.* 300: 626.

Preti, G., and G. R. Huggins (1975). Cyclical changes in volatile acidic metabolites of human vaginal secretions and their relation to ovulation. *J. Chem. Ecol.* 1:361-376.

Shader, R. I., A. DiMascio, and J. Harmatz (1968). Characterological anxiety levels and premenstrual libido changes. *Psychosomatics* 9:197-198.

Silbergeld, S., N. Brast, and E. P. Noble (1971). The menstrual cycle: a double-blind study of symptoms, mood and behavior, and biochemical variables using Enovid and placebo. *Psychosom. Med.* 33:411-428.

Spitz, C. J., A. R. Gold, and D. B. Adams (1975). Cognitive and hormonal factors affecting coital frequency. *Arch. Sex. Behav.* 4:249-263.

Stopes, M. (1931). *Married Love.* Putnams, London.

Swanson, E. M., and D. Foulkes (1968). Dream content and the menstrual cycle. *J. Nerv. Ment. Dis.* 145:358-363.

Terman, L. M. (1938). *Psychological Factors in Marital Happiness.* McGraw-Hill, New York.

Tonzetich, J., G. Preti, and G. R. Huggins (1978). Changes in concentration of volatile sulphur compounds of mouth air during the menstrual cycle. *J. Int. Med. Res.* 6:245-254.

Udry, J. R., and N. M. Morris (1968). Distribution of coitus in the menstrual cycle. *Nature* 220:593-596.

Udry, J. R., and N. M. Morris (1970). Effect of contraceptive pills on the distribution of sexual activity in the menstrual cycle. *Nature* 227:502-503.

Udry, J. R., and N. M. Morris (1977). The distribution of events in the human menstrual cycle. *J. Reprod. Fertil. Control* 51:419-425.

Udry, J. R., N. M. Morris, and L. Waller (1973). Effect of contraceptive pills on sexual activity in the luteal phase of the human menstrual cycle. *Arch. Sex. Behav.* 2:205-214.

Van Emde Boas, C. (1955). Variations of libido during the menstrual cycle. *Int. J. Sexol.* 8:214-219.

Wincze, J. P., E. F. Hoon, and P. W. Hoon (1978). Multiple measure analysis of women experiencing low sexual arousal. *Behav. Res. Ther.* 16:43-49.

9 A Developmental Analysis of Menstrual Distress in Adolescence

DIANE N. RUBLE*   University of Toronto, Toronto, Ontario, Canada

JEANNE BROOKS-GUNN   Educational Testing Service, Princeton, New Jersey, and College of Physicians and Surgeons, Columbia University, New York, New York

A vast number and range of physical discomforts and emotional and behavioral changes have been associated with the menstrual and premenstrual phases of the menstrual cycle in adult women. Such symptoms are commonly believed to be debilitating for many women (cf. Ruble and Brooks-Gunn, 1979) and represent a source of concern about women's effectiveness and emotional stability (Bergsjo, 1979; New York Times, 1970; Delaney et al., 1976). Although there have been numerous theoretic and empiric attempts to describe the etiology of menstrual symptoms, such an understanding has remained elusive. Physiological factors such as varying hormone levels or sensitivity hormones are an obvious possible source of cyclic somatic or psychological changes. However, to date, all of the many theories concerning physiological mechanisms are inconclusive (Smith, 1975; Steiner and Carroll, 1977; Chap. 5). Numerous psychosocial theories have also been offered. In an early tradition, individual differences in personality variables such as degree of femininity or fear of sex have also been proposed (e.g., Heald et al., 1957), but as with the physiological studies, the data have been equivocal. It is important to note, however, that although definitive conclusions cannot be drawn from the data currently available, it is also not possible to rule out either a psychological or physiological explanation. Indeed, the obvious difficulties of supporting a single hypothesis have led most investigators working in

---

*Current affiliation: Department of Psychology, New York University, New York, New York.

this area to assume that a complex interaction of psychological and physiological factors underly menstrual symptoms.

More recently the psychosocial tradition has embraced a sociocultural rather than an individual personality approach. Specifically, menstrual symptoms are thought to represent, in part, a set of culturally influenced beliefs (Paige, 1973; Parlee, 1974; Ruble et al., 1980). For example, Parlee (1974) argued that self-reports of menstrual symptoms may reflect little more than cultural stereotypes, and subsequent research has supported this. For example, self-reports of menstrual symptoms have been found to be influenced by experimental manipulations of women's perceptions concerning the nature of the study, (Englander-Golden et al., 1978) and by manipulations of women's beliefs concerning whether they are in the premenstrual or intermenstrual phase of the cycle (Ruble, 1977). We suggested in a recent paper that such cultural beliefs may originate and be maintained by means of biases inherent in processing information about cyclic events (Ruble and Brooks-Gunn, 1979). This analysis led us to conclude that people may begin to perceive and continue to believe in associations between particular symptoms and cycle phases even in the absence of a true relationship. For example, a particular behavior or feeling may receive a different label (e.g., cramps vs. indigestion) depending on the cycle phase during which it is perceived to occur.

A focus on these sociocultural aspects of menstrual symptoms as well as the recognition that such symptoms must be viewed as reflections of interactions among multiple etiologic factors suggest the usefulness of studying the developmental and socialization processes associated with menstruation. Surprisingly, however, there has been little research on the early development of menstrual symptoms or the socialization processes that might be involved. Typically, research concerned with younger girls has addressed questions of physical maturation and factors determining the timing of menarche, not how girls themselves are perceiving and reacting to this biologic, psychological, and social milestone. This chapter will review the few developmental studies in adolescence relating to menstrual symptoms, focusing on the two types of symptoms most commonly associated with the menstrual cycle: dysmenorrhea and premenstrual tension. Our goals are: (1) to describe developmental changes in reports of dysmenorrhea and premenstrual tension in normative terms, and (2) to relate such changes to issues relevant to understanding the interaction of physiological and psychosocial factors in the etiology of "menstrual distress."

I. Developmental Analyses of Menstrual Distress

A. Value of a Developmental Approach

A developmental analysis of girls' reported experiences of menstrual symptoms and their acquisition of information about symptoms is important for several reasons. First, menarche, as the biologic symbol of a shift from child to woman, may represent a time of change in self-identity or self-definition. At a minimum, this event signals a need for the girl to determine what it means to be a menstruating woman: how the somatic and psychological changes she has heard about may translate into personal experiences. The definition of the experience established at this time may be difficult to change: subsequent experiences are perceived in terms of and may be distorted by this definition (Ruble and Brooks-Gunn, 1979). Thus, perceptions of and information received about the menstrual experience during menarche and shortly after may have a long-lasting impact. If such perceptions are negative, they may have unfortunate consequences for the subsequent experience of menstrual cycles. Furthermore, because of the intimate link between menstruation, womanhood, and sexuality, early experiences may have more general effects on a girl's identity as a woman and on her self-concept (Brooks-Gunn and Ruble, 1982).

Second, data on developmental changes in symptom reports are important because of popular assumptions that developmental variables, such as regularity, ovulation, and parity, are related to menstrual symptoms, even though the supporting data are equivocal (Dickey, 1976; Huffman, 1975). A developmental analysis is particularly useful in studying the relationship of symptoms to ovulation. It is commonly asserted that menstrual symptoms, such as dysmenorrhea or premenstrual tension, can only occur in oculatory cycles (e.g., Bickers, 1960; Dickey, 1976; Huffman, 1975; Sturgis, 1962). This is because of the assumption that menstrual symptoms are tied to hormonal shifts occurring during the second half of the cycle: the rapid rise and fall of progesterone and the ratio of progesterone to estrogens. Since progesterone shifts do not occur in anovulatory cycles, it is reasoned, menstrual-related somatic changes should not occur in them. Therefore, because ovulation does not commonly occur during the first few cycles after menarche and possibly not until 1 to 2 years later (Apter and Vihko, 1977; Lee et al., 1976; Penny et al., 1977; Vollman, 1977; Winter and Faiman, 1973), reports of menstrual symptoms would not be expected among early postmenarcheal girls. A normative/descriptive analysis of developmental changes in adolescents' reports of symptoms should provide valuable insights into this etiologic issue.

Surprisingly few studies have examined developmental changes in the experience of menstrual-related cyclic symptoms. Recently, however, two sets of investigators have been studying these issues in large samples of adolescent girls.

B. Developmental Samples

One set of developmental studies was conducted by a group of Finnish investigators (Kantero and Widholm, 1971; Widholm et al., 1967; Widholm and Kantero, 1971; Widholm, 1979). The main purpose of their research was to provide basic normative data concerning irregularity, dysmenorrhea, and other menstrual disorders in menstruating girls of different age groups. In their largest study, the menstrual patterns of 5485 adolescent girls (10 to 20 years of age) were examined. The sample was drawn from several different school districts and represented a reasonably broad cross-section of both inland and coastal districts of Finland. The questionnaire was administered to the girls' natural mothers as well as to the girls, thereby providing a sample of adult women with whom to make developmental comparisons. The responses of the girls were analyzed both in terms of chronologic age and gynecologic age (years after menarche).

We are conducting a second set of developmental studies in New Jersey (Brooks-Gunn and Ruble, 1979a,b, 1980, 1982; Clarke and Ruble, 1978). Our approach differs somewhat from that of the research described above, because the major focus has been on changes in perceptions of menstrual symptoms as a function of menarche. Consistent with our theoretic orientation described earlier, we view self-reports of menstrual symptoms as reflecting in part a set of cultural beliefs or learned expectations. For example, girls who report pain during menstruation may do so partly because of a physically based reality and partly because they have learned that pain is supposed to accompany menstruation (Ruble and Brooks-Gunn, 1979). Thus, in attempting to understand women's experience of menstrual symptoms, we believe it may be particularly informative to examine the expectations girls may have even before the onset of menstruation. By comparing pre- and postmenarcheal girls with age-controlled (in which physiological status varies but presumably sociocultural experiences do not), premenarcheal girls of differing ages (in which physiological status is similar but sociocultural experiences are not), and postmenarcheal girls of differing ages (in which physiological status of girls who have been menstruating several years should not vary systematically while sociocultural experiences will vary), the contribution of experience, culture, and physiology to reports of dysmenorrhea might be better elucidated. However, these comparisons are inferential as well as presupposing interactions among determinants, making it impossible to assess the precise contribution of physical and psychological variables.

Our largest study is a cross-sectional survey of 641 fifth to twelfth graders (a longitudinal sample is being surveyed). The girls were public school students, lived in central New Jersey, and were relatively heterogenous with respect to social class. Approximately 95% of the sample were white; one-half were first born and one-half later born. Forty percent of the sample were premenarcheal: 85% of the fifth to sixth graders, 33% of the seventh to eighth graders, and none of the eleventh to twelfth graders. A group of college women (N=154) attending one of three public colleges or universities in central New Jersey, was also surveyed for comparison purposes. These women were divided among the four college classes; somewhat more were in their freshman or sophomore year. The social class, race, and birth order of the college sample were the same as those of the adolescent sample.

Although these two studies address a wide range of issues relevant to girls' experiences of menstruation, we focus here on self-reports of the symptoms most commonly associated with menstrual distress: menstrual pain or dysmenorrhea, edema, and negative affect. For convenience (and because of a practice common in the literature), we have grouped the latter two together under the heading of "premenstrual tension." In the next two sections, we discuss results relevant to a developmental analysis of dysmenorrhea and premenstrual tension, respectively. The nature of these symptoms, their incidence, and their etiology have been discussed in several recent reviews (Abplanalp et al., 1980; Parlee, 1973, 1974; Ruble et al., 1980; Ruble and Brooks-Gunn, 1979; Sommer, 1978), and are not discussed in detail here. However, in each section, we will briefly describe some definitional and interpretational problems that are relevant to a developmental analysis of cyclic symptoms before beginning a detailed review of the adolescent studies.

II. Dysmenorrhea

A. Definitional Issues

A frequently reported physical discomfort is some type of pain accompanying menstruation. Pain, as it has been studied in the literature on the menstrual cycle, includes such symptoms as lower back pain, headache, and, most commonly, abdominal pain (cramps). Menstrual pain, known as dysmenorrhea, has been the subject of a great deal of attention and controversy, as researchers have sought to identify its incidence, etiology, and severity.

Surprisingly, researchers and practitioners do not even agree on a definition of dysmenorrhea, let alone on its prevalence or severity. For example, primary dysmenorrhea, which, unlike secondary dysmenorrhea, occurs in the absence of organic disorders in the pelvic region, usually includes abdominal, back, and upper leg pain and cramping associated with menstruation. However, headaches, nausea, irritability, and that most elusive of all symptoms, premenstrual tension, are sometimes subsumed under the label of dysmenorrhea. Even different types of dysmenorrhea have been proposed. The most popular distinction involves spasmodic and congestive dysmenorrhea (Dalton, 1969); the former referring to "spasms of pain similar to labor pain which begin the first day of menstruation," and the latter to "a symptom of the premenstrual syndrome with dull, aching pains accompanied by lethargy and depression prior to the onset of menstruation" (Chesney and Tasto, 1975a, p. 237). Dalton suggests that the two are distinguished physiologically by different hormone inbalances.

Recently, a Menstrual Symptom Questionnaire (MSQ) has been developed to distinguish between the two (Chesney and Tasto, 1975a). In support of Dalton's hypothesis, a factor analysis resulted in two distinct factors representing spasmodic and congestive symptoms, respectively. Furthermore, in other research, these authors showed that a behavior therapy involving relaxation and premenstrual imagery resulted in reduced reports of symptoms only for women suffering from spasmodic dysmenorrhea, not for those suffering from congestive dysmenorrhea. Thus, the results provided additional support for the validity of the distinction and also suggested the importance of psychological methods (e.g., relaxation) in the reduction of dysmenorrhea (Chesney and Tasto, 1975b).

The validity of conclusions on the two types of dysmenorrhea, however, has been questioned in a recent study (Webster, et al., 1979). In contrast with the results reported by Chesney and Tasto (1975a), a factor analysis of the MSQ based on a large sample failed to support the two-component model. Using a hypothesis-testing type of factor analysis, Webster et al. found support only for a spasmodic dysmenorrhea factor, not for the congestive type. Furthermore, an exploratory factor analysis resulted in seven factors rather than two. A major distinction appeared to exist between menstrual vs. premenstrual symptoms rather than a specific differentiated set of two types of dysmenorrhea symptoms. Finally, in direct contradiction to Dalton's original hypothesis, Webster et al. found a moderately high (0.56) *positive* correlation between the spasmodic and congestive item subscores, indicating that the self-reported experience of one symptom type does not preclude the experience of the other within individuals.

There are several possible explanations for the differences in the results of the two studies. One potentially important reason is that Chesney and Tasto used a selected sample: women who indicated a priori that they experienced menstrual discomfort. This procedure may have introduced an artifactual type of bias, as Webster et al. point out. Perhaps, however, a clear-cut distinction can emerge only among women with relatively severe menstrual discomfort. In a more normative sample, responses may be heavily influenced by stereotypic expectations of cyclic symptoms (Parlee, 1974; Ruble and Brooks-Gunn, 1979). Thus, whether or not there is a qualitative distinction (e.g., spasmodic) rather than a quantitative (e.g., severe) distinction across women may not be answered by existing research. In the two developmental studies described in this chapter, this kind of qualitative distinction was not assessed. If two types of dysmenorrhea exist, we have no information as to their developmental course.

B. Dysmenorrhea in Adolescents

1. The Finland Study

In this survey, the girls were asked to indicate how often their periods were painful (never, occasionally, always), and how soon the pain began after menarche. The percentages of girls reporting dysmenorrhea in the various groups as well as the responses of their mothers are shown in Table 1.

Just under 50% of the entire sample reported completely painless menstruation, while 38% and 13% reported pain occasionally and always, respectively. The analysis by chronologic age shows a jump in the incidence of dysmenorrhea

Table 1 Percentage of Girls and the Mothers Reporting Dysmenorrhea as a Function of Chronologic Age and Gynecologic Age

	Age (yrs)	No.	Never	Occasionally	Continuously
Chronologic age	up to 10.9	6	66.7	33.3	0.0
	11.0-11.9	99	63.6	32.3	3.0
	12.0-12.9	458	59.6	30.4	7.9
	13.0-13.9	1,027	55.8	33.6	7.9
	14.0-14.9	1,264	47.2	37.4	12.5
	15.0-15.9	931	45.8	37.0	16.0
	16.0-16.9	656	37.8	44.8	15.7
	17.0+	914	34.4	46.0	17.7
	Total	5,355	46.7	38.3	12.9
Gynecologic age	0.0-0.9	1,263	61.7	29.0	7.2
	1.0-1.9	1,200	50.7	36.7	10.5
	2.0-2.9	957	42.4	41.2	13.9
	3.0-3.9	600	37.2	43.3	17.7
	4.0-4.9	495	33.1	46.5	18.2
	5.0-8.9	640	30.0	46.1	25.6
	Total	5,155	46.0	38.5	13.2
Mothers		6,543	21.8	70.3	7.9

Source: Widholm and Kantero, 1971.

(as defined in this study as pain reported continuously) from 3 to 8% in girls under age 14 years to 16 to 18% in girls over 15 years. This analysis seems consistent with the assertion that the experience of dysmenorrhea is related to ovulation. In contrast, the analysis by gynecologic age shows a much more gradual increase from 7% during the first year after menarche to 26% after 5 years of menstruation. Interestingly, only 8% of the mothers report that they always experience pain during menstruation, although they also are less likely to report no pain at all. Unfortunately, the questionnaire did not include a measure of perceived severity, so that it is not clear to what extent incidence is perceived to be related and whether this relationship might change with age. It is also difficult to know if these developmental effects reflect true differences in the incidence of dysmenorrhea or if, for example, the different age groups have different definitions of what constitutes pain.

The question concerning the onset of pain yielded interesting results that seem somewhat inconsistent with the percentages reported in Table 1. Surprisingly, 75% of the girls reported that the pain began before the end of the first year after menarche, and 90% of these said the pain started with the earliest menstrual periods. The 75% figure is considerably higher than the percentage of girls reporting pain in the first year in Table 1 and may reflect a difference between prospective and retrospective self-reports. In this case, retrospective self-reporting seemed to result in an earlier recollection of when the pain began among girls who eventually reported experiencing painful menstruation. Nevertheless, it is important to note that whichever figure is used, the fact that pain is reported by many girls soon after menarche is in conflict with the assumption that dysmenorrhea does not occur until ovulatory menstrual cycles have begun, well after this time (e.g., Bickers, 1960; Dickey, 1976; Huffman, 1975; Sturgis, 1962). These findings led Widholm and Kantero (1971) to conclude that menstrual pain was not necessarily connected to ovulation. This is also supported by data in their earlier study (Widholm et al., 1967), in which vaginal smears from a large group of adolescent girls were used to determine estrogen balance. In contrast with the ovulation/ dysmenorrhea hypothesis, these authors reported an anovulatory cycle in 60% of the cases of dysmenorrhea (as well as vaginal hyperestrogenism), indicating that at least in these cases the pain was caused by some other factor.

In a more recent questionnaire study, developmental changes in other aspects of dysmenorrhea were examined: duration of pain, need for pain-relieving drugs, and absence from school (Widholm, 1979). The subjects were 331 girls aged 13 to 20 years. In response to a "yes-no" question concerning menstrual pain, the self-reported frequency increased from 36.1% at 13-14 years to 56.5% at 17 to 20 years, with an overall frequency of 47.1%. For most of these girls, the pain lasted 1 to 2 days, although 18% in the 17 to 20-year-old group reported experiencing pain for 3 or more days. Frequent absence from school due to menstrual pain was rare in this sample (2.7%), although 20.7% reported missing school sometimes for this reason. Both of the percentages increased with age. Finally, there was a marked developmental increase in percentages of girls who had consulted a doctor or taken drugs for menstrual pain. The percentage of 13 to 16-year-olds who had seen a doctor ranged from 3 to 7%, while 27% of 17 to 20-year-olds had. Very similar percentages are reported for use of drugs.

Thus, most indices used by this group of Finnish investigators indicate increases in symptoms of dysmenorrhea during the first several years after menarche. In contrast, older women (i.e., mothers) report less frequent symptoms. Unfortunately, it is very difficult to determine from these data how best to interpret such developmental trends. The absence of progesterone elevation due to anovulatory cycles in young girls does not appear to represent an adequate explanation, as discussed above, although other physiological changes may be involved. Psychological variables, such as learning about menstrual symptoms from girlfriends or changing definitions of pain, may be important.

Two other findings of interest to a developmental analysis have been reported by this group of investigators. First, body build (i.e., weight/height ratio) was shown to bear a relationship to incidence of dysmenorrhea (Widholm and Kantero, 1971). For both daughters and mothers, a pyknic or stout body build was related to a higher incidence of dysmenorrhea than either a normal or slender build. This supports earlier research from the same laboratory with smaller clinical samples showing that the obese are more likely to report dysmenorrhea (e.g., Frisk et al., 1965). The reasons for this relationship are unclear and require replication. From a developmental viewpoint, it is interesting to note that although the slender girls tended to reach menarche later than the other two groups, consistent with the critical weight hypothesis (Frisch, 1974), the girls of normal weight, not the overweight girls, began menstruating earliest, although the differences between these latter two groups were small. In contrast, Zacharias et al. (1970) report that the mean age of puberty decreases with increasing obesity. These authors suggest that such effects may be due to basic differences across groups in terms of the physiology of menarche.

The second incidental finding of developmental interest was a relationship between parity and dysmenorrhea observed among the mothers of the girls participating in the Widholm and Kantero (1971) study. The incidence in the multiparous group was only 6 to 8% as compared with 12% in the group with only one child. Whether this difference reflects a physical or psychological change is unknown.

2. New Jersey Study

In this study, postmenarcheal adolescents were asked whether or not they experienced cramps, how often they experienced pain, and how often they took medication for dysmenorrhea. More than three-quarters of the adolescents and college students reported menstrual cramps, and two-thirds experienced premenstrual cramps. Fewer seventh to eighth graders reported cramping than the younger and older students (but only 10% less). Of those who reported dysmenorrhea, two-thirds reported experiencing it every month, one-quarter every other month, and one-tenth every six months. The frequency of premenstrual cramps was the same as for menstrual pain. Ten percent more of the senior high school girls reported experiencing cramps every month than the younger and older students. The number of girls taking medication for cramping paralleled the incidence and frequency data, suggesting that girls take medication each time they experience pain, even though, as discussed next, the severity of cramping is generally rated as quite mild.

Severity of pain was determined by asking the girls to rate their experience (postmenarcheal) or expectations (premenarcheal) of symptoms during their intermenstrual, premenstrual, and menstrual cycle phases on a six-point scale (experience the symptom not at all to experience the symptom a lot). The symptoms were taken from the Moos (1968) Menstrual Distress Questionnaire (MDQ) but were modified by including more familiar adjectives (i.e., "crabby" as well as "irritable"). Only one of the eight factors generated by Moos (1968) is of interest here: pain. The main variable of interest was differences across the

Table 2 Report of Dysmenorrhea and Water Retention in Adolescents

	MDQ Factors								
	Pain			Water retention			Negative affect		
	M-I	P-I	M-P	M-I	P-I	M-P	M-I	P-I	M-P
Self Report									
Premenarcheal									
5-6 grade	0.69[a]	0.35[a]	0.34[a]	0.50[a]	0.40[a]	0.11	0.59[a]	0.33[a]	0.26[a]
7-8 grade	0.79[a]	0.74[a]	0.05	0.28[a]	0.26[a]	0.02	0.44[a]	0.30[a]	0.14
Postmenarcheal									
7-8 grade	0.65[a]	0.43[a]	0.22[a]	0.37[a]	0.28[a]	0.09	0.36[a]	0.26[a]	0.10
11-12 grade	1.13[a]	0.82[a]	0.31[a]	0.91[a]	0.92[a]	-0.01	0.64[a]	0.50[a]	0.14
College	1.12[a]	0.86[a]	0.26[a]	1.20[a]	1.31[a]	-0.10	0.86[a]	0.93[a]	0.17

M = menstrual; I = intermenstrual; P = premenstrual.
[a]Mean difference is statistically significant.
Source: Brooks-Gunn and Ruble, 1979a.

three phases of the cycle in ratings of severity. The left set of columns in Table 2 represent the mean difference in MDQ scores for each cycle phase comparison, as a function of the different age and menarcheal groups.

As in the majority of the adult studies, all groups of girls reported experiencing or anticipating cycle phase differences for the Pain Scale (all one-way ANOVAs were significant). In terms of pairwise comparisons, the menstrual-intermenstrual and premenstrual-intermenstrual differences were significant across age and menarcheal status. In addition, menstrual pain was reported to be more severe than premenstrual pain by most groups.

To examine age and menarcheal status effects, comparisons were made between the premenarcheal fifth to sixth and seventh to eighth graders, the premenarcheal and postmenarcheal seventh to eighth grades, and the postmenarcheal junior high school, senior high school, and college women. Among premenarcheal girls, there were no age differences in the expected experience of pain, suggesting that this belief is acquired quite early, i.e., by fifth grade. The premenarcheal seventh to eighth graders expected to experience *more* pain than the postmenarcheal junior high students actually reported experiencing themselves. Finally, the older postmenarcheal adolescent girls reported more severe pain than the younger postmenarcheal girls (differences significant in terms of subject status effects in two-way ANOVAs and specific comparisons with t figures). The college and senior high school women's symptom severity scores were similar.

Several aspects of these data merit highlighting. First, the expectation of menstrual pain is clearly present before the experience of it. An earlier but much smaller study also supported this conclusion for seventh and eighth graders and showed further that adolescent boys of the same age have similar expectations (Clarke and Ruble, 1978). Therefore, a girl's actual experience of menstrual pain as well as other symptoms may be substantially influenced by cultural beliefs, both because her own expectations may result in a self-fulfilling prophecy and because they are reinforced by peers. The nature and extent of this influence is difficult to estimate and requires, as a beginning, a longitudinal approach. Second, with increasing age, postmenarcheal adolescents report more severe symptoms which may be related to actual physical experience or to socialization. By late adolescence, severity seems to have stabilized, shown by the college and high school women's self-reports being the same. To examine further the fact that senior high school girls report more severe symptoms than their junior high school counterparts, we turn now to the relationship of the onset of dysmenorrhea to the onset of menarche.

In contrast with the belief that dysmenorrhea does not appear at menarche (presumably because early cycles are anovulatory), 80% of our postmenarcheal fifth to sixth graders report experiencing cramps, and the majority of these girls had been menstruating less than a year. These results are basically consistent with those reported by Widholm and Kantero (1971), as described earlier.

In a second relevant comparison, we examined the self-reports of dysmenorrhea in our adolescent sample in relation to how long they had been menstruating. We would expect those who have menstruated longer to report more severe or a higher incidence of dysmenorrhea than girls the same age who have menstruated a shorter time. The eleventh to twelfth grade girls were divided into those who have been menstruating more than 4 years (60%) and less than 4 years (40%), the seventh to eighth grade girls into those who had been menstruating more than 2 years (12%) and less than 2 years (88%). Mean difference scores on the MDQ Pain Scale were compared for an estimate of severity, and the number of subjects reporting cramps and using medication were compared for incidence estimates.

The senior high school girls who had been menstruating longer reported more severe pain both menstrually and premenstrually than those whose menarche was later (pain: P-I, 2.08 versus 1.48, $p < .05$ and M-I, 2.30 versus 1.57, $p < .02$). In the junior high school sample, no significant differences appeared (although girls with an earlier menarche reported somewhat more severe premenstrual pain, $p < .07$, than girls with a later menarche). In terms of incidence, more senior high school girls with earlier menarche reported menstrual cramps and taking medication for them than did those with later menarche ($p < .10$).

Thus, length of time menstruating affected dysmenorrhea more in the older adolescents, all who had been menstruating at least 2 years, than in the younger adolescents, none of whom had been menstruating more than 4 years. Since the onset of dysmenorrhea is believed to occur 12 to 18 months after the onset of menarche (e.g., Lennane and Lennane, 1973), the junior high school girls menstruating for more than 2 years should have experienced more pain and the differences in the senior high school girls should not have been as pronounced if the data were to support the dysmenorrhea-ovulation hypothesis.

Finally, the incidence of symptoms during the first menstrual period was examined retrospectively. Very few girls remembered experiencing any sumptoms; when asked about the number of menstrual symptoms experienced, 82% said "none," and the rest only said "one" or "two." When asked about the specific symptoms, cramps were only mentioned 10% of the time. Other symptoms were nausea (17%), moodiness or crabbiness (19%), laziness or fatigue (21%), and headache (10%). Thus, dysmenorrhea was not prevalent during the first period. Length of time since menarche did not seem to affect recall, as no differences were found between the junior high, the senior high girls or the few postmenarcheal elementary school girls. These data appear somewhat discrepant from the results of the Finnish study.

3. Comparison of the Two Samples

When summarized across the two sets of studies, the pattern of results show a remarkable degree of correspondence in spite of major differences in samples and measures. Both studies show increases with age among postmenarcheal girls in incidence, frequency, and use of medication for menstrual pain until at least the late teens. Similar increases are shown for reports of missing school and visits to a doctor in the Finland research and for ratings of severity in the New Jersey research. Interestingly, in both studies, there are indications of stabilization occurring after age 17 to 20 years in that mothers reported less frequent symptoms than the older adolescent girls in the Finland study and, among college girls in the New Jersey study, frequency was lower and severity leveled off relative to the senior high school girls. The major difference across studies on these measures was the level of overall incidence. Even though the age ranges were similar, overall, more than 75% of the girls in the New Jersey study reported experiencing menstrual pain in comparison with approximately 50% in the two Finnish studies. In addition, the increase over age (both chronologic and gynecologic) appeared to be substantially larger in the Finland than in the New Jersey samples.

The correspondence across studies is ambiguous on the issue of incidence of menstrual symptoms shortly after menarche. The high incidence of cramps among fifth to sixth grade girls in the New Jersey sample seems similar to the high incidence of *recall* of cramps during the first gynecologic year in the Finnish sample. However, when reporting on current experience of menstrual pain, the young Finnish girls reported a much lower incidence than did the young New Jersey girls. Also contradictory are the findings that very few New Jersey girls recalled experiencing cramps during their first menstrual period, while a substantial proportion of Finnish girls recalled experiencing pain during the first few periods after menarche.

It therefore appears that although there were increases with age in both samples, there was a higher incidence reported among young postmenarcheal girls in the New Jersey as compared with the Finnish sample. This difference, in turn, resulted in a lower rate of increase in the former sample. Furthermore, Finnish girls were more likely retrospectively to recall experiencing pain at a young age than the New Jersey girls. Such differences may be due to different socialization experiences in the two samples. The data on expectations among premenarcheal girls in the New Jersey sample suggests that much social learning about menstruation occurs before menarche. Although there are no comparable data available on the Finnish sample, the pattern of results suggests that such socialization may occur later for these girls.

III. Premenstrual Tension

A. Definitional Issues

Premenstrual tension or the "premenstrual syndrome" also refers to an unwieldy set of seemingly unrelated symptoms. These typically include negative mood or emotional characteristics (irritability, anxiety, depression) and edema (bloated feeling, weight gain, painful breasts), although various behavioral changes such as fatigue or altered concentration are also sometimes mentioned (cf. Abplanalp et al., 1980; Parlee, 1973; Ruble and Brooks-Gunn, 1979; Steiner and Carroll, 1977). A recent study of women with self-reported severe premenstrual tension identified irritability and bloating as being perceived as the worst symptoms (Haskett et al., 1980).

In addition to the lack of specificity of a symptom cluster to characterize premenstrual tension, an additional definitional problem is that, unlike the menstrual phase, exactly what days of the cycle constitute the premenstrual phase varies from a few days to a week or more before the onset of menstruation. According to most accounts, premenstrual symptoms are in some way related to a drop in estrogen and progesterone occurring several days before the first day of menstruation. However, data supporting this link and even the timing or simultaneity of the drop in hormones are, at best, weak. Recent evidence suggests that very large individual differences exist in the rate of fall of the hormones and even in the extent to which the two hormones are in phase (Abplanalp et al., 1980). Thus, it is not clear, at least with respect to hormonal explanations, how to define "premenstrual" either across studies or across individuals within studies.

Given the current definitional debates in the scientific literature, the responses of women participating in the studies may reflect similar levels of confusion when they are asked to report symptoms they experience premenstrually. It is not clear that reports of, for example, premenstrual swelling or weight gain necessarily reflect premenstrual symptoms as opposed to randomly occurring somatic symptoms that have become associated with the term "premenstrual" (Abplanalp et al., 1980; Ruble and Brooks-Gunn, 1979). Thus, the conclusion of Parlee's (1973) careful critique still seems relevant: "... as a scientific hypothesis the existence of a premenstrual syndrome has little other than face validity" (p. 463).

B. Premenstrual Tension in Adolescence

1. The Finland Study

In response to a question about whether they usually experience fatigue, swelling, and irritability before menstruation, a total of 67.5% of the girls in the Finnish sample reported having some kind of premenstrual symptom, with fatigue and irritability the first and second most commonly reported symptoms, respectively. The percentage of girls reporting "nervous" symptoms vs. edema as a function of chronologic and gynecologic age (as well as the percentage of their mothers who reported these) are shown in Table 3. There is an interesting discrepancy between the two types of symptoms in the extent to which incidence is age-related. The incidence of fatigue and/or irritability is relatively high, fluctuating in the 50 to 60% range at all age levels including mothers, and shows little relationship to either chronologic or gynecologic age. In contrast, the overall incidence of edema is relatively low (7.9%) but shows sharp increases for both developmental measures, reaching 16.5% after 5 years experience of menstruating, with the mothers

Table 3 Percentage of Girls and their Mothers Reporting Premenstrual Tension as a Function of Chronologic Age and Gynecologic Age

	Age (yrs)	No.	No tension	Fatigue and/or irritability	Edematous symptoms
Chronologic age	up to 11.9	104	40.4	54.8	4.8
	12.0-12.9	484	39.7	56.4	3.7
	13.0-13.9	1,037	35.6	59.5	4.8
	14.0-14.9	1,261	32.8	61.5	5.7
	15.0-15.9	914	32.3	59.1	8.6
	16.0-16.9	657	29.5	61.2	9.3
	17.0+	923	27.3	57.6	15.1
	Total	5,386	32.7	59.4	7.9
Gynecologic age	0.0-0.9	1,267	39.7	57.6	3.2
	1.0-1.9	1,198	34.6	60.3	4.7
	2.0-2.9	943	29.9	62.2	7.9
	3.0-3.9	602	28.9	60.1	10.0
	4.0-4.9	497	25.8	60.3	13.9
	5.0-5.9	650	24.5	59.0	16.5
	Total	5,164	32.1	60.1	7.8
Mothers		1,408	27.0	52.3	20.7

Source: Widholm and Kantero, 1971.

reporting the highest incidence (20.7%). Finally, in contrast with symptoms of dysmenorrhea, neither body type nor parity showed a significant relationship to reported premenstrual tension.

General support for these developmental findings were reported in the more recent study by Widholm (1979), although the overall incidence of edema was higher. In this sample, reports of edema increased from 12.5% in 13 to 14-year-olds to 46.7% in 17 to 20-year-olds, while headache and irritability were reported from the first years of menstruation onwards.

Two aspects of these findings are particularly noteworthy. First, the high incidence of reports of premenstrual fatigue and irritability during the first gynecologic year appears to contradict claims that premenstrual tension is "determined by ovulation and cannot occur in an anovulatory cycle" (Melody, 1961, p. 441). In contrast, edema does show age-related changes; however, the increase is so gradual (even continuing into adulthood), that regularity of ovulation occurring during the first year after menarche does not appear to be a likely explanation for this developmental change. The second finding of interest is that the incidence of premenstrual edema reported in these samples seems low compared with other research. For example, in a sample of adult Finnish women reported in a second study in the Widholm (1979) paper, 65.1% reported edema. The reasons for the discrepancies are not clear and are not discussed by Widholm. However, the possibility that such large differences may be due to either developmental differences or measurement differences is quite important and warrants careful scrutiny.

2. The New Jersey Study

In the New Jersey study, severity of symptoms associated with premenstrual tension were measured primarily by two scales on the Moos (1968) MDQ: water retention and negative affect. The middle and right set of columns in Table 2 represent the mean difference in MDQ scores for each cycle phase comparison as a function of group. As reported earlier for pain, all groups of girls reported experiencing or anticipating cycle phase differences on these two scales when menstrual and premenstrual scores were compared with the intermenstruum. Somewhat surprisingly, only the premenstrual fifth to sixth graders differentiated between premenstrual and menstrual negative affect. In contrast with the prevailing cultural stereotypes, they believed this symptom was more prevalent during menstruation. Apparently, they have not yet learned that premenstrual tension is believed to be at least as debilitating as menstrual tension.

When looking at the age and menarcheal status effects, the premenarcheal fifth to sixth graders expected to experience *more* water retention and negative affect than did the premenarcheal seventh to eighth graders. Thus, as with pain, it appears that beliefs regarding premenstrual tension are acquired quite early. However, unlike the findings for pain, the expectation of symptom severity decreased with age among premenarcheal girls, possibly because of the advent of junior high school health education classes. Again in contrast with the findings for pain, the premenarcheal and postmenarcheal seventh to eighth graders did not differ on these scales. Among postmenarcheal girls, the older girls reported more severe water retention and negative affect than did the younger girls, consistent with the developmental results reported for pain and for the edema symptoms in the Finland study. Finally, as with pain, most (79%) girls recalled no premenstrual symptoms associated with their first menstrual period.

3. Comparison of the Two Samples

An age-related increase among postmenarcheal girls in symptoms associated with premenstrual tension is seen in both investigations, and at least some of the symptoms are evident in quite young girls. However, developmental changes in negative affect differed across studies, and the incidence of reported edema seems relatively low in the Finnish as compared to New Jersey sample. Perhaps socialization mechanisms, as discussed earlier with respect to pain, may explain some of these differences.

C. Interpretations and Conclusions

Taken together, the findings of these two large studies of menstrual symptoms in adolescence raise some intriguing issues concerning the normative development of symptoms and the interaction of physiological and sociocultural factors influencing the nature of such developmental changes.

First, it is clear that girls are reporting some types of symptoms soon after menarche. At least superficially, these findings are inconsistent with the widely believed hypothesis that symptoms do not occur in anovulatory cycles. There are two alternative explanations, however. One is that only the girls who are ovulatory shortly after menarche are reporting symptoms. The fact that some percentage of girls at all stages exhibit signs of ovulation (Vollman, 1977) make this interpretation a possibility. Another possibility is related to the earlier suggestion that self-reports of symptoms may be heavily influenced by cultural beliefs or stereotypes concerning symptoms. Since most girls experience their first menstruation expecting to experience particular sets of symptoms, it may be difficult to detect a true influence of this physiological factor because it may be submerged by a stronger influence of cultural beliefs on paper-and-pencil measures of symptoms.

A second major pattern in the data concerns developmental changes. In both studies there were increases in most symptom reports with increasing age among postmenarcheal girls. Interestingly, however, age effects were also observed among premenarcheal girls in the New Jersey study for some of the symptoms, with younger girls reporting that they expected *more* severe symptoms than did older girls.

These developmental effects raise interesting questions about changes in the girls' socialization experiences. Although the postmenarcheal age effects may represent, in part, physiological influences (e.g., ovulation), it is difficult to explain the changes in premenarcheal girls' expectations in this way. One possible explanation is that the sources of information or the evaluative tone of the information being received may be age-related. For example, the youngest girls probably receive less specific information and their own expectations may be largely determined by negative images prevalent in the culture (e.g., as conveyed by mass media). In contrast, at the time of menarche, girls receive booklets and take health classes that may emphasize the more positive aspects of becoming a woman. We are currently investigating such possibilities.

Similar processes may be involved in both the developmental changes observed in postmenarcheal girls and the apparent cross-cultural differences observed. For example, as girls get older they may receive information about a

wider range of symptoms such as water retention, and as they increasingly talk
with peers the nature of the information may shift in a negative direction, emphasizing possible embarrassment or problems. Although caution must be exer-
cised in interpreting cross-cultural differences since different questions and procedures were used, the pattern of data suggests possibly striking differences in
the socialization of menarche-aged girls in Finland and the United States. In particular, the data suggest that Finnish girls may not learn much about menstrual
symptoms, except fatigue and irritability, until they have been menstruating for
a while. Interestingly, the perceptions about fatigue and irritability are very high
in young girls and show little age-related variation. In contrast, the U.S. girls
appear to know more about a wider range of symptoms at menarche, but seem to
find symptoms of pain more salient than either water retention or negative affect.
Although we have no direct evidence about such socialization differences across
the two cultures, studies in a number of different cultures indicate considerable
variation in the extent of advanced preparation for menarch and the nature of information transmitted (cf., Brooks-Gunn and Ruble, 1982). There is clearly
a need at this time for systematic longitudinal and cross-cultural analyses to
understand the nature, impact, and antecedents of developmental changes in
menstrual distress.

Acknowledgment

Preparation of this chapter and some of the reported research were supported
by Grants Nos. SOC-76 02137 and SOC-76 02129 from the National Science
Foundation and by the Educational Testing Service. We wish to thank Lesley
Biggs for bibliographic help and Linda Worcel for her invaluable assistance in all
aspects of the project.

References

Abplanalp, J. M., R. Haskett, and R. M. Rose (1980). The premenstrual syn-
    drome. *Adv. Psychoneuroendocrinol.* 3:324-347.
Apter, D., and R. Vihko (1977). Serum pregnenolone, progesterone, 17-hydroxy-
    progesterone, testerone, and 5-dihydrotestosterone during female puberty.
    J. Endocrinol. Metabol. 45:1039-1048.
Bergsjo, P. (1979). Socioeconomic implications of dysmenorrhea. *Acta Obstet.
    Gynecol. Scand. [Suppl.]* 87:67-68.
Bickers, W. (1960). Dysmenorrhea and menstrual disability. *Clin. Obstet.
    Gynecol.* 3:233-240.
Brooks-Gunn, J., and D. N. Ruble (1979a). Dysmenorrhea in adolescence. Paper
    presented at the Annual Meeting of the American Psychological Association,
    New York, September.
Brooks-Gunn, J., and D. N. Ruble (1979b). The social and psychological mean-

ing of menarche. A paper presented at the Society for Research in Child Development Meetings, San Francisco, March.

Brooks-Gunn, J., and D. N. Ruble (1980). The menstrual attitude questionnaire. *Psychosom. Med.* 42:503-512.

Brooks-Gunn, J., and D. N. Ruble (1982). Developmental processes in the experience of menarche. In *Handbook of Medical Psychology*, Vol. 2 (A. Baum and J. Singer, eds.). Erlbaum, Hillsdale, N.J.

Chesney, M., and D. Tasto (1975a). The development of the menstrual symptom questionnaire. *Behav. Res. Ther.* 13:237-244.

Chesney, M. A., and D. L. Tasto (1975b). The effectiveness of behaviour modification with spasmodic and congestive dysmenorrhea. *Behav. Res. Ther.* 13:245-253.

Clarke, A. E., and D. N. Ruble (1978). Young adolescents' beliefs concerning menstruation. *Child Dev.* 49:231-234.

Dalton, K. (1969). *The Menstrual Cycle*, Pantheon, New York.

Delaney, J., M. J. Lupton, and E. Toth (1976). *The Curse: A Cultural History of Menstruation.* Dutton, New York.

Dickey, R. P. (1976). Menstrual problems of the adolescent. *Postgrad. Med.* 60:183-187.

Englander-Golden, P., M. R. Whitmore, and R. A. Dienstbier (1978). Menstrual cycle as a focus of study and self-reports of moods and behaviors. *Motiv. Emot.* 2:75-86.

Frisch, R. E. (1974). Critical weight at menarche, initiation of the adolescent growth spurt and control of puberty. In *The Control of the Onset of Puberty* (M. M. Grumbach, G. D. Grave, and F. E. Mayer, eds.). John Wiley, New York.

Frisk, M., O. Widholm, and H. Hortline (1965). Dysmenorrhea—psyche and soma in teenagers. *Acta Obstet. Gynecol. Scand.* 44:339-347.

Haskett, R., M. Steiner, J. Osmun, and B. Carroll (1980). Severe premenstrual tension. Delineation of the syndrome. *Biol. Psychiatry* 15:121-139.

Heald, F. P., R. P. Musland, S. H. Sturgis, and J. R. Gallagher (1957). Dysmenorrhea in adolescence. *Pediatrics* 20:121-127.

Huffman, J. (1975). Principle of adolescent gynecology. *Obstet. Gynecol. Annu.* 4:287-308.

Kantero, R. L., and O. Widholm (1971). II. The age of menarche in Finnish girls in 1969. *Acta Obstet. Gynecol. Scand. [Suppl.]* 14:7-18.

Lee, P., T. Xenakis, J. Winer, and A. Matsenbaugh (1976). Puberty in girls correlation of senior levels of gonadotropins, prolactin, androgens, estrogens and progestins. *J. Clin. Endocrinol. Metab.* 43:775-784.

Lennane, M. B., and R. J. Lennane (1973). Alleged psychogenic disorders in women—a possible manifestation of sexual prejudice. *N. Engl. J. Med.* 288:288-292.

Melody, G. F. (1961). Behavioral implications of premenstrual tension. *Obstet. Gynecol.* 17:439-441.

Moos, R. H. (1968). The development of a menstrual distress questionnaire. *Psychosom. Med.* 30:853-867.

New York Times, July 26, 1970, p. 35.

Paige, K. E. (1973). Women learn to sing the menstrual blues. *Psychol. Today* 7:41-46.

Parlee, M. B. (1973). The premenstrual syndrome. *Psychol. Bull.* 80:454-465.

Parlee, M. B. (1974). Stereotypic beliefs about menstruation: a methodological note on the Moos Menstrual Distress Questionnaire. *Psychosom. Med.* 36: 229-240.

Penny, R., A. F. Parlow, N. O. Olambiwonnu, and S. D. Frasier (1977). Evolution of the menstrual pattern of gonadotropin and sex steroid concentrations in serum. *Acta Endocrinol.* 84:729-732.

Ruble, D. N. (1977). Premenstrual symptoms: a reinterpretation. *Science* 197: 291-292.

Ruble, D. N., and J. Brooks-Gunn (1979). Perceptions of menstrual symptoms: a social cognition analysis. *J. Behav. Med.* 2:171-194.

Ruble, D. N., J. Brooks-Gunn, and A. Clarke (1980). Research on menstrual-related psychological changes: alternative perspectives. In *The Psychology of Sex Differences and Sex Roles* (J. E. Parsons, ed.). Hemisphere, New York.

Smith, S. L. (1975). Mood and the menstrual cycle. In *Topics in Psychoendo-crinology* (E. J. Sachar, ed.). Grune & Stratton, New York.

Sommer, B. (1978). Stress and menstrual distress. *J. Hum. Stress* 4:5-10.

Steiner, M., and B. J. Carroll (1977). The psychobiology of premenstrual dys-phoria: a review of theories and treatments. *Psychoneuroendocrinology* 2: 321-335.

Sturgis, S. H. (1962). *The Gynecologic Patient: A Psychoendocrine Study.* Grune & Stratton, New York.

Vollman, R. F. (1977). *The Menstrual Cycle.* Saunders, Toronto.

Webster, S. K., H. J. Martin, D. Uchalich, and L. Gannon (1979). The menstrual symptom questionnaire as a spasmodic/congestive dysmenorrhea.Measure-ment of an invalid construction. *J. Behav. Med.* 2:1-19.

Widholm, O. (1979). Dysmenorrhea during adolescence. *Acta Obstet. Gynecol. Scand.* 87:61-66.

Widholm, O., M. Frisk, T. Tenhunen, and H. Hortling (1967). Gynecological findings in adolescence: a study of 514 patients. *Acta Obstet. Gynecol. Scand.* 46:1-27.

Widholm, O., and R. L. Kantero (1971). III: Menstrual pattern of adolescent girls according to chronological and gynecological ages. *Acta Obstet. Gynecol. Scand. [Suppl.]* 14:19-29.

Winter, J. S. D., and C. Faiman (1973). The development of cyclic pituitary and gonadal function in adolescent females. *J. Clin. Endocrinol. Metab.* 37:714.

Zacharias, L., R. Wurtman, and M. Schatzoff (1970). Sexual maturation in contemporary American girls. *Am. J. Obstet. Gynecol.* 108:833-846.

10 Dysmenorrhea and Dyspareunia

FRITZ FUCHS   The New York Hospital-Cornell Medical Center, New York, New York

Dysmenorrhea and *dyspareunia* are used to describe painful conditions associated with two important aspects of a woman's life: her menstrual flow and her sexual activity. Although different in cause, age distribution, and other features, they do have in common pelvic pain, a location of pain essentially limited to the female. Both can interfere with her family and social life and both are characterized by an organic substrate with a psychogenic superstructure. Each is a complex of symptoms and not a disease sui generis, and although the diagnosis and treatment of the underlying pathology is in the realm of gynecology, each must be recognized and understood by those who treat women. It is not customary to make symptoms, rather than disease entities, the subject of an extended discourse, but in the context of this book it was thought that dysmenorrhea and dyspareunia were of such importance in the life of women as to justify a deviation from the customary.

I. Dysmenorrhea

Dysmenorrhea is derived from the Greek and means difficult monthly flow; it now is used to describe painful menstruation. Dysmenorrhea is by far the most common gynecologic symptom complex; it has been estimated that at least one-half of all women have experienced menstrual pain at some time. The primary form, "essential dysmenorrhea," affects perhaps as many as 50% of postmenarchal women and is the dominant cause of absence from school or job. Until recently, there has been little understanding of etiology and pathophysiology of primary dysmenorrhea, and as a consequence, rational therapy has been lacking. Physicians have therefore taken a rather pessimistic approach to the problem or have overemphasized the psychogenic factors while neglecting the underlying pathophysiology. In spite of the substantial economic losses to society because of lost working hours of young women, surprisingly little scientific attention has been given to the etiology and rational therapy of this disorder until very recently.

A. Classification

Most women have some degree of pelvic discomfort at the onset of menstruation in ovulatory cycles. The discomfort is most often described as mild, cramplike pains which subside shortly after the beginning of the flow and do not interfere with normal activities. The differentiation between the "normal" and "abnormal" level of discomfort is difficult, partly because of the lack of objective yardsticks for assessing pain and partly because menstrual pain is so common that there is a gradual transition between the normal and the abnormal. To say that a woman does not have dysmenorrhea unless she seeks relief from her pain by self-medication or by consulting a physician ignores the great variations in pain tolerance. Less difficult is the distinction between primary and secondary dysmenorrhea. Dysmenorrhea is classified as *primary* (essential, idiopathic) if it begins early in the fertile life span and without any pelvic pathology, and *secondary* (acquired) if it occurs after years without menstrual discomfort and is associated with organic disease in the pelvis, such as endometriosis, adenomyosis, uterine myomas, chronic pelvic inflammatory disease, or use of intrauterine contraception.

B. Frequency of Primary Dysmenorrhea

Although the literature does contain statistical studies on fairly large groups of young women, there is no consensus about the incidence of primary dysmenorrhea. The correct figure is probably between 30 and 50% of adolescent and young nulliparous women, one-third of whom experience symptoms severe enough to incapacitate them occasionally or regularly. The great variations in incidence between published materials can be ascribed to differences in diagnostic criteria, and to ethnic, cultural, and geographical variations. No matter what the true incidence is, however, primary dysmenorrhea is both frequent and serious enough to merit scientific study and rational therapy.

C. Symptoms

Since primary dysmenorrhea occurs only in ovulatory cycles it is not surprising that there usually is an interval between the onset of menses and the appearance of menstrual discomfort. The cardinal symptom is cramplike, spasmodic pain deep in the pelvis, radiating to the lower abdomen, sacrum, and occasionally to the perineum and thighs. In the majority of dysmenorrheic women, pelvic pain is associated with systemic symptoms, including nausea, vomiting, diarrhea, headache, dizziness, nervousness, and fatigue. The symptoms usually begin a few hours before vaginal bleeding is observed, but can begin from as much as 24 h before to several hours after the onset of bleeding. The symptoms may last from a few hours to several days and are usually greatest on the first day of menstruation.

Some women experience a gradual alleviation of the menstrual discomfort with advancing age, but this is not as conspicuous as the effect of pregnancy and childbirth, after which the symptoms often disappear completely. These effects of body maturation and childbirth remain unexplained.

The diagnosis of primary dysmenorrhea is based on the history and the absence of abnormal findings on pelvic examination. The distinction between primary and secondary dysmenorrhea is important; if the symptoms appear after the age of 20, secondary dysmenorrhea must be suspected and if pelvic examination fails to reveal a cause, further work-up in the form of a hysterogram and laparoscopy should be considered.

D. Etiology of Primary Dysmenorrhea

Although psychogenic factors have been given great emphasis by many authors in the past, recent advances in uterine physiology have made it clear that the underlying cause is biochemical changes in the uterus at the onset of menstruation, and not psychogenic factors activated by the appearance of blood or the withdrawal of ovarian hormones. For this reason, we shall look at the physiology of menstruation first and consider the undisputed, associated psychogenic factors afterwards.

The crampy character of dysmenorrheic pain has drawn attention to the uterine contractile activity during menstruation. Although myometrial activity during the menstrual cycle has been studied mainly to learn more about its function during childbirth, these studies have provided considerable information about the cyclic variations in uterine contractility. From menarch to menopause, the uterine muscle is at rest only during pregnancy. The pattern of contractions during ovulatory cycles is quite consistent, with cyclic changes from low frequency and high amplitude contractions during menstruation to high frequency and low amplitude contractions at ovulation, with transitions in between [1,2]. The various contraction patterns are undoubtedly influenced by the ovarian steroids, but on any given day of the cycle they are far from constant, showing hourly and diurnal variations, variations from cycle to cycle, and variations from subject to subject [3]. Although the pattern of contractions is modulated by the cyclic variations in ovarian steroids, the contractions are not "spontaneous," not the contractions of a smooth muscle strip suspended in a bath in vitro. The contractions in vivo are stimulated by extrauterine factors, such as the neurohypophyseal hormones oxytocin and vasopressin, and intrauterine factors, such as prostaglandins synthesized in the endometrium. The precise role and interaction of these factors are not known, but that they do have a role is evident from the fact that inhibition of neurohypophyseal hormone secretion and prostaglandin synthesis both will inhibit the seemingly "spontaneous" contractions of the nonpregnant uterus, particularly during menstruation [4-6]. From a functional point of view, the strong contractions during menstruation are probably important for the removal of blood and necrotic endometrium from the uterine cavity.

While it is well-recognized that menstruation is caused by a withdrawal of estrogens and progesterone, the exact mechanisms by which this change in steroid levels causes ischemia, bleeding, necrosis, and shedding of the superficial layer of endometrium, and microclot formation and subsequent lysis of the menstrual blood, have not been fully elucidated. Undoubtedly various enzyme systems are activated by the withdrawal of steroids, but the lack of more detailed information of the mechanisms involved in such an important physiological event is surprising and regrettable.

One enzyme system in the endometrium activated during the luteal phase and thus dependent upon progesterone rather than progesterone withdrawal leads to the formation of arachidonic acid from various lipids and its transformation to prostaglandins (PGs), particularly of the E and F series. Analysis of endometrial biopsy specimens has shown increasing amounts of PGE_2 and $PGF_{2\alpha}$ as the time of menstruation approaches [7,8]. These prostaglandins may diffuse out of the endometrial cells before menstruation and be responsible, in part, for the changing pattern of myometrial contractions or be released at the onset of menstruation and amplify the contractions. Several authors maintain that the uterine contractions during menstruation in dysmenorrheic women have a greater amplitude and higher basal tonus than in nondysmenorrheic women and are the cause of the menstrual pain [9]. Whether exaggerated contractions are the cause of pain is debatable, but that dysmenorrhea is associated with elevated levels of PGs in the menstrual blood is now well-documented [10].

As early as 1957, Pickles demonstrated that acetone extracts of menstrual blood contained a substance which stimulated myometrial contractions and which he therefore called "menstrual stimulant" [11]. This menstrual stimulant subsequently proved to be a group of lipid-soluble substances including PGE and PGF [12]. Prostaglandins are derivates of prostanoic acid, a 20-carbon unsaturated fatty acid with a cyclopentane ring and two side chains. Many natural prostaglandins have been found and the most extensively studied are PGE_2 and $PGF_{2\alpha}$, both of which play a role in human reproductive processes.

Various lipids, such as phospholipids and cholesterol esters, can be converted to free fatty acids by enzymatic activity. Only free unsaturated fatty acids including arachidonic acid and eicosatrienoic acid can serve as precursors for prostaglandins. These essential fatty acids are converted via endoperoxides to PGE_2 and $PGF_{2\alpha}$. The factors regulating prostaglandin synthesis are not fully clarified, but the prostaglandins appear to be synthesized immediately prior to release and not stored in the tissues, the rate-limiting step being the availability of the precursor fatty acids. Cyclic AMP triggers prostaglandin synthesis by activation of a lipase to liberate these precursors. Consequently, the synthesis of prostaglandins can be initiated by hormones (including steroids, polypeptides, and adrenalin), the cellular action of which is mediated by cyclic AMP. Progesterone has an important regulatory role in the endometrial concentrations of PGE_2 and $PGF_{2\alpha}$ which increase markedly during the secretory phase [13]. Estrogens are also important, since all progesterone effects in the uterus depend on estrogen priming. Once removed from the site of synthesis, the PGs are rapidly metabolized to the 15-keto, 13,14-dihydro-metabolites of PGE_2 and $PGF_{2\alpha}$, mainly during their passage through the lungs with the circulating blood.

PGE_2 and $PGF_{2\alpha}$ can be demonstrated in the secretory endometrium, in jet washings of the uterine cavity, and in the menstrual blood [10,13,14]. In anovulatory cycles, the endometrium contains only 20% of the amount found on corresponding days of ovulatory cycles, confirming the importance of progesterone. Menstrual fluid, which is easier to collect than endometrium, may contain, in addition to prostaglandins of endometrial origin, PGs from the platelets participating in the intrauterine clotting of the menstrual blood. The increasing concentration of $PGF_{2\alpha}$ in the endometrium during the luteal phase is not reflected in the peripheral blood, undoubtedly due to the rapid metabolism during circulation [15].

Endogenous prostaglandins play a crucial role in the development of primary dysmenorrhea. Administration of PGE_2 and $PGF_{2\alpha}$ causes symptoms very similar to dysmenorrhea, including strong uterine contractions, nausea, vomiting, diarrhea, and backache. The bleeding following an anovulatory cycle is painless and the endometrial level of PGS remains low as does the content of PGs in the blood collected from the uterus at the time of bleeding. In contrast, subjects with primary dysmenorrhea have higher than normal concentrations of PGs in the endometrium, endometrial jet washings, and the menstrual fluid. Finally, administration of agents which inhibit prostaglandin syntheses and/or action provides marked releif of the symptoms of dysmenorrhea, including the systemic symptoms.

In a recent study of the relationship between uterine prostaglandins and dysmenorrhea [10], study subjects collected the total amount of menstrual fluid, using special vaginal tampons and saline-containing jars for collection of the tampons. This permitted the authors to measure both the total amount of menstrual fluid and the amount of PGs formed by unit time and during one whole menstrual flow. Five of the seven dysmenorrheic subjects had considerably higher amounts

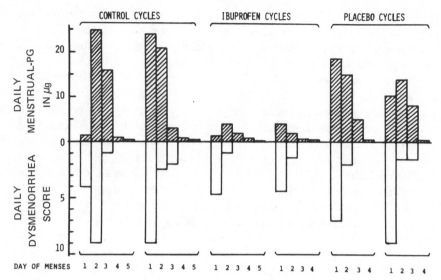

Figure 1 Relationship between severity of dysmenorrhea and levels of menstrual prostaglandin released in treatment and nontreatment cycles of a dysmenorrheic patient. Six cycles (two control, two ibuprofen treated, and two placebo) were studied. Double-blind cross-over procedures were followed in the treatment cycles. The open bars show the daily global assessment of dysmenorrheic symptoms by the patient, using a 10-point scale visual analog method. The hatched bars show the levels of menstrual PGs released during the corresponding period. (From Ref. 10, W. Y. Chan, M. Y. Dawood, and F. Fuchs, Relief of dysmenorrhea with the prostaglandin synthetase inhibitor ibuprofen: effect on prostaglandin levels in menstrual fluid, *Am. J. Obstet. Gynecol.* 135:105 (1979).)

of prostaglandins, as measured by a bioassay, than nondysmenorrheic controls. When given the prostaglandin synthetase inhibitor ibuprofen (Motrin, The Upjohn Co.), the prostaglandin levels were reduced markedly and good relief of the symptoms of dysmenorrhea was achieved (Fig. 1). Two subjects had low levels of PGs in the menstrual blood while on oral contraception; when they discontinued the medication, dysmenorrhea returned and with it high levels of PGs in the menstrual blood.

Prostaglandin synthetase inhibitors reduce the uterine activity both in dysmenorrheic and normal subjects. If primary dysmenorrhea is associated with exaggerated uterine contractions with high amplitudes and elevated tonus, as has been maintained by several investigators [16,17], the relief provided by prostaglandin synthetase inhibitors is easily explained. It follows, however, that other tocolytic agents, i.e., agents which inhibit uterine activity, should be equally useful for the treatment of dysmenorrhea. However, this is not necessarily so.

E. Psychological Factors

Given the strong evidence favoring a somatic etiology it is difficult, at least for a gynecologist, to accept psychogenic factors as causative in primary dysmenorrhea. But there is no doubt that psychogenic factors have a modulating influence on this symptom complex. It would indeed be strange if a physiological process, which is associated with so many societal and religious taboos, would not, when it is painful, be associated with a range of psychic symptoms. Pain in itself is a powerful stimulus of the psyche; so is menstruation, a period of neuroendocrine imbalance. Pain associated with a repetitive unsettling process that has strong sexual and societal implications must be even more powerful. That dysmenorrhea can be associated with depression, anxiety, neuroticism, severe guilt, rejection of femininity, negative peer group behavior, etc., is not surprising. Such psychogenic factors can undoubtedly influence the pain perception enormously and perhaps explain why, in the absence of a satisfactory somatic explanation, many psychiatrists and psychoanalysts in the past considered primary dysmenorrhea a primarily psychogenic disease. A rational therapy should go a long way, both to disprove psychogenic theories and to alleviate the psychogenic superstructure of primary dysmenorrhea.

F. Treatment of Dysmenorrhea

Many different forms of treatment have been used in the past to alleviate primary dysmenorrhea, from psychotherapy to surgery. Optimistic reports have not been lacking but none of the methods have been able to withstand the test of time. A constant problem has been the lack of a reliable method of assessment of pain and of the response to therapy. A multidimensional approach is necessary, and even then it is difficult to obtain numeric values that will permit statistical evaluation.

1. General Measures

A multitude of general measures has been applied, such as heat, exercises, diet changes, and changes of environment (school, job). While these may have an effect on the psychogenic superstructure, they rarely have much effect on the physical symptoms. Simple psychotherapy, which removes the fear of serious disease by explaining the nature of the problem, obviously can be very useful. Knowing that pregnancy and childbirth will cure the condition is reassuring but does not do much for the immediate problem, particularly for women to whom childbearing is not a primary goal.

2. Surgical Procedures

Stenosis of the cervical canal was once thought to be an etiologic factor in primary dysmenorrhea, by impeding the menstrual flow. Consequently, cervical dilatation, with or without curettage of the endometrium, was often performed for severe cases. The effect was usually only temporary and may have succeeded by facilitating the menstrual flow and more rapid elimination of the prostaglandin-containing menstrual fluid from the uterus.

Presacral neurectomy was sometimes used as a last resort. While usually effective when correctly performed, there was a high failure rate, due to partial resection, and a high complication rate. With the advent of rational pharmaco-therapy, there is no longer any place for surgical procedures.

3. Tocolytic Agents

If the immediate cause of menstrual cramps is uterine hyperactivity, tocolytic agents should provide relief of dysmenorrhea. These drugs are used primarily to arrest premature labor and include (1) betamimetic agents which inhibit uterine activity by stimulating beta-adrenergic receptors in the myometrium; (2) ethanol which inhibits uterine activity by blocking the secretion of neurohypophyseal hormones; (3) prostaglandin synthetase inhibitors; and (4) calcium antagonists which reduce the availability of intracellular calcium ions essential for muscular contraction. Progesterone is also assumed to reduce myometrial contractility but can hardly be classified as a tocolytic agent, since it takes 12 to 24 h for its effect on the myometrium to develop; furthermore, it stimulates prostaglandin synthesis. Dalton in England has claimed a beneficial effect from progesterone treatment prior to menstruation, but such therapy is controversial and does not seem rational in the light of present knowledge of the role of prostaglandins.

A number of betamimetic drugs have been used in primary dysmenorrhea. Isoxsuprine was the first to become available in the United States, but it has not been effective in dysmenorrhea [18] nor for the treatment of premature labor. Fenoterol, a newer German betamimetic, produced no significant effect in a placebo-controlled study [19]. Terbutaline, a Swedish preparation, now approved in the United States as a bronchodilator, did increase the myometrial blood flow and relieve the pain of dysmenorrhea, when administered intravenously. However, the side effects, such as tremor and palpitations, were too marked to render it clinically useful [20].

Many women have discovered that alcohol provides good relief in primary dysmenorrhea. The effect is achieved with amounts of alcohol which have little analgesic effect and there is no doubt that the effect is due to inhibition of the uterine activity, mediated through inhibition of the secretion of the neurohypo-physial hormones oxytocin and vasopressin [4,21]. The well-known side effects of alcohol preclude its practical use in young women with dysmenorrhea. However, the effect is interesting from a theoretic point of view because it supports the claim that dysmenorrhea is caused by strong uterine contractions. In this connection it would be important to know whether ethanol or betamimetic agents have any effect on the synthesis of prostaglandins in the uterus.

4. Prostaglandin Synthetase Inhibitors

Several authors have shown that nonsteroidal, antiinflammatory agents which inhibit prostaglandin synthesis and/or activity provide relief in primary dysmenorrhea [10,22-24]. An exception, strangely enough, is acetylsalicylic acid. Aspirin must have been used by the ton in the past to alleviate menstrual cramps, but usually with poor results, probably because the dose required to inhibit uterine prostaglandin formation is higher than the standard dose and is poorly tolerated.

Compounds shown to be effective include indomethacin (25 mg two or three times daily), various fenamates such as flufenamic acid, mefenamic acid (250 mg four times daily), ibuprofen (400 mg three or four times daily), and sodium naproxen (275 mg four times daily). In addition to their inhibition of prostaglandin synthetase activity, the fenamates have an antagonistic effect on the prostaglandin receptors. This explains why the compounds do not have to be taken before the onset of menstruation but can be initiated when the first symptoms of menstruation appear, as Chan et al. have found for ibuprofen [25]. Not all of the prostaglandin antagonists mentioned here, however, have been approved by the FDA for use in dysmenorrhea.

These drugs also have certain side effects. Indomethacin can cause blurred vision and other ocular symptoms, severe headache, gastrointestinal ulcerations occasionally resulting in perforations, and hematologic complications including aplastic anemia, agranulocytosis, or hemolytic anemia. Those agents which have been approved, including ibuprofen (Motrin, Upjohn), mefenamic acid (Ponstel, Parke-Davis), and sodium naproxen (Anaprox, Syntex) are much better tolerated in the doses recommended, but gastrointestinal symptoms, dizziness, drowsiness, headache, lightheadedness, rashes, and hematologic symptoms have nevertheless been described. However, the drugs of choice would be those which are effective even when given at the onset of menstruation. This eliminates the risk of taking drugs after a conception and also reduces the dosage taken each month.

One additional benefit of prostaglandin synthetase inhibitors is a reduction of the menstrual blood loss. These agents promise to revolutionize the approach to the treatment of primary dysmenorrhea while providing more insight into the mechanism of menstruation and the etiology of dysmenorrhea.

5. Inhibition of Ovulation

Even before the advent of oral contraception it was realized that dysmenorrhea is present only in ovulatory cycles. Large doses of estrogens were occasionally given in cases of severe dysmenorrhea and when successful probably acted to suppress ovulation. Oral contraception is more rational in this regard, because a regular cycle is maintained. Little is known about the prostaglandin content in the "menstrual" blood of oral contraceptive users. Chan et al. [25] found low levels in two cases studied; after discontinuing oral contraceptives the levels rose and dysmenorrhea returned.

G.   Secondary or Acquired Dysmenorrhea

While primary dysmenorrhea is a fairly distinct entity, secondary dysmenorrhea is clearly only a symptom, a manifestation of pelvic pathology of various kinds. The two most frequent causes of secondary dysmenorrhea are endometriosis and adenomyosis, two related disorders caused by ectopic development of endometrial tissue. Endometriosis is due to growth of endometriumlike tissue outside the uterus, in the tubes, on or in the ovaries, on the peritoneal surface of the pelvic and/or abdominal organs, in the sacrouterine ligaments, vagina and vaginal portion of the cervix, bladder, colon, scars in the perineum, and in the abdominal wall. Adenomyosis is caused by downgrowth of endometrial glands between the fibers of the myometrium. The ectopic endometrial tissues have retained the ability to respond to the cyclic variations of the ovarian steroids with proliferative and secretory changes, followed by necrosis and bleeding. Lacking the outlet of the uterine cavity, the tissue can only spread or grow in situ. The endometriotic foci stimulate fibroblast formation locally and thereby often get encapsulated, forming the so-called "chocolate cysts," containing old blood and blood pigment together with necrotic tissue residues and more or less functional endometrial tissue. The monthly breakdown of the tissue and bleeding causes the pain which, in contrast to primary dysmenorrhea, tends to worsen with time. Whether prostaglandin formation plays a role in the inflammatorylike response and fibroblast formation and in the causation of pain can only be surmised. The effect of prostaglandin synthetase inhibitors remains to be studied. When ectopic endometrium is found between the muscle fibers of the myometrium, the disorder is called adenomyosis. It is otherwise similar to endometriosis and the two types of ectopic endometrium are often found together. The treatment of endometriosis is directed against the disease itself and accomplished either with synthetic hormone preparations, such as Danazol, or by surgical removal.

Other, less frequent causes of secondary dysmenorrhea are fibroids, uterine synechia (scar formation in the uterine cavity), endometrial polyps, and carcinoma of the endometrium.

One iatrogenic cause is the use of intrauterine contraception. It has been postulated that the pressure on the endometrium and the leucocyte infiltration caused by the presence of an intrauterine contraceptive device (IUD) in the uterine cavity enhances the synthesis of prostaglandins. While increased prostaglandins have been demonstrated in IUD users, the exact mechanism is not known. Prostaglandin synthetase inhibitors do seem to have some effect in this type of dysmenorrhea, but further studies are required.

Some of the pathological conditions associated with secondary dysmenorrhea can also give rise to dyspareunia, thus providing another connection between the two symptom complexes.

II. Dyspareunia

Dyspareunia is used by American authors to describe pain or discomfort during
or after sexual intercourse. In European literature the use of the term has often
been different [26]. In Germany, Kehrer [27] has defined it as the lack of syn-
chronism between female and male orgasm, contrasting it with eupareunia. Such
confusion has led other European authors to use the term algopareunia [28].

Dyspareunia can be present in a large number of pathological conditions in
the internal and external genitalia. Unfortunately, it does not share with dysmenorrhea the excitement of new scientific discoveries about its etiology and
rational therapy. Dyspareunia can only be alleviated by treatment of the underlying pathology which is manifold and diverse. It is impossible to detail here
all the conditions of which dyspareunia can be a symptom.

That coitus, the ultimate expression of love and attraction between the sexes,
constitutes an important part of life for most adults, has always been *known,* but
only in our generation has it been *admitted* in medical textbooks, even in gynecology. Only now, when sexual dysfunction is becoming the preoccupation of
a whole new medical specialty, has a more systematic approach to the physical
causes of sexual dysfunction been applied. It is important to do so. The psychological consequences of dyspareunia can be both profound and durable, but unless the physical causes are diagnosed correctly and eliminated, no psychotherapy
can be expected to succeed.

A. Classification

Dyspareunia can be divided according to anatomy into external and internal dyspareunia, depending on the location of the underlying pathology in the genitalia.
It is also practical to distinguish between genital and extragenital causes of dyspareunia.

B. External Dyspareunia

1. Anatomic Abnormalities

After initial rupture of the hymen, the remainder of the membrane usually
shrinks to form small hymenal caruncles. Occasionally, healing is accompanied
by scar formation which can remain tender for a long time. Likewise, if a fibrous
hymen is too resistant to allow defloration and necessitates hymenotomy, a tender scar may form. Excision of the scar will resolve the problem.

Excessive length of the minor labia is rarely a problem, but surgical reduction
is occasionally required. Another rare cause of external dyspareunia is agglutina-
tion between the clitoris and its praeputium. During clitoral erection the praeputium may be stretched so much that it becomes painful. Once diagnosed, the

condition is easily corrected by separation of the praeputium from the clitoris, but general anesthesia may be required in some cases. Congenital malformations of the vagina, such as septa or cysts, are easily diagnosed by pelvic examinations.

Secondary anatomic problems can be caused by traumatic lesions of the vulva and vagina, including undiagnosed or poorly treated lesions during childbirth, and by surgical procedures, such as episiotomy and plastic procedures to correct a relaxed vaginal outlet.

2. Inflammatory Reactions

A number of infectious processes in and around the vulva and vagina often causes external dyspareunia, although other symptoms may dominate the picture. Vulvovaginitis caused by monilia, *trichomonas vaginalis,* or bacteria belong to this category, as do herpes genitalis, bartholinitis, and some of the less frequent venereal diseases. Once the inflammatory reaction has subsided under adequate treatment, the dyspareunia disappears. An important cause of vulvar and vaginal irritation is allergic reactions to such agents as perfumed soaps and deodorants, underwear made of synthetic materials or washed in synthetic detergents, spermicidal agents, and the rubber used in diaphragms and, occasionally, even condoms in spite of the relatively short exposure time. An often overlooked cause of vulvar lesions is cunnilingus; saliva contains digestive enzymes and prolonged or frequent exposure can caused marked reactions.

3. Vaginal Dryness

Inadequate lubrication due to lack of sexual stimulation, or to lack of response to sexual stimulation, can make sexual intercourse very painful. Women near or in the menopause often complain of reduced lubrication; estrogen treatment, either locally in the form of vaginal cream, or oral estrogen replacement therapy, usually provides prompt relief. However, the majority of women do not require estrogen replacement for adequate and completely satisfactory sexual function after the menopause, provided they have an active sexual life. Only when the sexual activity is interrupted for months or years does the ability of the vagina to function adequately gradually wane. Resumption of sexual activity after a prolonged period of inactivity can cause severe and occasionally intractable dyspareunia, although estrogens can provide relief. The vaginal epithelium is also very vulnerable and estrogen-deprived during the first 4 to 6 weeks postpartum.

4. Extragenital Causes

Pathologic conditions in the adjoining structures such as urethritis, carunculus urethrae, and diverticula of the urethra, can also cause external dyspareunia. Likewise, painful conditions of the rectum and anus, such as hemorrhoids, proctitis, and rectovaginal fistula can interfere with sexual activity. Therapy must be directed toward the underlying pathology.

C. Internal or Deep Dyspareunia

Internal dyspareunia is characterized by pain released by deep penile thrusts, while intromission and containment of the penis in the vagina are painless. Sometimes the pain is immediate and may require interruption of intercourse, sometimes the pain is delayed until after the penis has been withdrawn, possibly because sexual excitement reduces the immediate pain perception.

1. Cervicitis

Chronic cervicitis, an inflammatory process in the cervix which often involves the paracervical lymphatics, can cause marked tenderness of the cervix on motion and deep dyspareunia.

2. Endometritis, Parametritis, Salpingitis, Pelvic Inflammatory Disease

A common feature of the various types of pelvic inflammatory disease, acute as well as chronic, is marked tenderness of the adnexae and deep dyspareunia. Often the tenderness persists after the inflammatory process has subsided, probably due to the formation of adhesions between the pelvic organs. While early energetic treatment with adequate doses of antibiotics is essential, and usually curative, repeated courses of antibiotics do little for the more chronic forms, adding support to the suspicion that they represent sequelae rather than active inflammatory processes. Whenever an inflammatory process *is* present, it is clear that intercourse, apart from being painful, hardly promotes the healing.

3. Pelvic Congestion

Some patients with severe dyspareunia who are operated on after repeated conservative treatment for "chronic pelvic inflammatory disease" are found to have no signs of prior inflammatory processes but marked congestion of the pelvic organs with greatly dilated veins in the parametria, looking almost like varicose veins. Whether sexual stimulation without release can cause such chronic congestion is not known; that the condition is associated with deep dyspareunia I have observed repeatedly. Only hysterectomy seems to provide relief.

4. Malpositions of the Uterus

At the beginning of the century, the retroflexed uterus was considered pathological and the cause of many ills. This is no longer believed but occasionally a retroflexed uterus fixed in the cul-de-sac can be the only plausible explanation for complaints of deep dyspareunia. In such instances surgical correction is indicated.

5. Endometriosis and Adenomyosis

Endometriosis and adenomyosis, already described as frequent causes of second-ary dysmenorrhea, are also frequent causes of internal dyspareunia. When a patient complains of both secondary dysmenorrhea and deep dyspareunia, endo-metriosis is the most likely diagnosis.

6. Traumatic and Surgical Sequelae

Lesions in the vaginal vault and parametria can occur during childbirth, in spite of the great use of cesarean section to avoid traumatic deliveries. If these lesions are not adequately diagnosed and treated, the resulting scar formation can cause deep dyspareunia. Much more frequent, however, are the sequelae of pelvic sur-gery. *Any* surgical procedure in the pelvis can result in the formation of adhesions, and major procedures such as hysterectomy and salpingo-oophorectomy do result in some internal scar formation which can cause deep dyspareunia. Dyspareunia after total abdominal or vaginal hysterectomy is probably more frequent than most gynecologists admit, and should be borne in mind when the procedure is done for a benign condition. Good surgical techniques, including meticulous hemostasis, can reduce but not entirely eliminate the risk of the formation of a tender scar at the top of the vagina. When surgery is carried out for a malignant condition, it may be so extensive that scarring is unavoidable. Nevertheless, pre-servation of sexual function should be kept in mind whenever it can be done with-out compromising the results. Surgical treatment of genital malignancies is less likely to cause dyspareunia than radiation therapy, a fact that is of particular im-portance for the choice of therapy in younger women. Removal of the ovaries before the menopause results in immediate estrogen deprivation. Unless contra-indicated, estrogen replacement should be initiated early to avoid the dyspar-eunia that is seen after estrogen deprivation.

7. Extragenital Causes of Internal Dyspareunia

Pathologic processes in the rectum, colon, and bladder can occasionally cause deep dyspareunia. As usual, therapy must be directed toward the underlying pathology. A rare cause is muscular tension in the obturator muscles which may be encountered in dancers and gymnasts.

8. Chronic Pelvic Pain Without Obvious Pathology

Recently in Belgium, Renaer published a lengthy review of what he called "chronic pelvic pain without obvious pathology" (CPPWOP), a syndrome which he had studied for years [29]. This syndrome, of which deep dyspareunia is a frequent feature, baffles the gynecologist and has generated considerable litera-ture. Before this diagnosis can be applied, all the diagnostic methods available to the gynecologist, such as hysterosalpingography, ultrasonography, culdoscopy, and laparoscopy, must be utilized. In some cases, pelvic congestion will be found, either by culdoscopy or laparoscopy, or by explorative laparotomy. In other cases, one finds a depression or even a rent in the posterior leaf of the broad ligament, as described by Allen and Masters [30] and considered by them to indicate traumatic laceration of uterine support. Thus, a certain fraction of the patients have findings which will be considered pathological by some gynecologists, irrelevant by others. When the psychological characteristics of patients with CPPWOP are studied, it is evident that they cannot be reduced to a common denominator, although a tentative diagnosis of pelvic congestion is often temporarily associated with stressful life situations. The literature review by Renaer and his own studies makes it clear that patients with CPPWOP constitute a heterogeneous population presenting a spectrum of psychogenic and somatic conditions.

D. Sexual Dysfunction and Dyspareunia

Pain during and/or after intercourse is obviously a very important cause of sexual dysfunction, but sometimes the pain is used to hide other causes of sexual dysfunction, or the fear of pain rather than the pain itself becomes a factor. Pain, whether real or invented, is a very powerful component of sexual relations but its role can vary tremendously. In some women, dyspareunia can destroy a sexual relationship, and in others pain can heighten the sexual pleasure for both the woman and the man. It is not surprising, therefore, that elimination of the etiologic factors of dyspareunia does not always solve the problems. Analysis of the psychogenic factors is essential in such cases.

E. Symptomatic Treatment of Dyspareunia

Although a gynecologic history is not complete without information about the patient's sexual function, many patients tend to suppress important information and may not admit that they experience dyspareunia. Some women feel guilty that this symptom makes them inadequate as sexual partners, or they may have guilt feelings about a previous venereal disease or other "sins" for which they are now being "punished." To elicit a good sexual history it is necessary to gain the confidence of the patient. The problems should be discussed in private in the office, not while the patient is on the examining table, which women often find degrading, and not in the presence of the nurse.

Likewise, the results of the examination and the treatment are best discussed after the patient has dressed and returned to the office. When the cause of dyspareunia is an infectious process which can easily be cured, the patient should be reassured that her sexual dysfunction will disappear with the infection.

When internal dyspareunia is caused by pelvic endometriosis or other conditions of chronic nature, some advice about coital techniques can be very useful.

Since the dyspareunia is usually caused by deep penetration, the patient should be instructed in positions that prevent maximal penetration, such as adduction of her legs after intromission of the penis, or positions that permit her to control the degree of penetration, such as woman-superior positions. It is often useful if both sexual partners can participate in the consultation. Changes in sexual habits can often eliminate dyspareunia without compromising the pleasure and joy of sexual intercourse.

When dyspareunia is found in patients with both psychogenic and somatic pathology, and in patients with CPPWOP, psychotherapy becomes very important. The psychotherapist and the gynecologist must work together and have complete confidence in each other.

III. Concluding Remarks

Although mention was made in the introduction that both dysmenorrhea and dyspareunia have an organic basis and a psychogenic superstructure, the latter probably has not been given enough attention. Although the gynecologist must understand the psyche of women and be fully aware of the psychological impact of painful conditions, he or she is probably the wrong person to attempt an analysis of the psychogenic aspects of these painful conditions. Gynecologists should be aware, however, that removal of the causes of these conditions does not solve the problems in every instance. A relationship shattered by chronic dyspareunia cannot always be repaired by an operation for endometriosis. Dyspareunia and dysmenorrhea must always be given early attention and adequate treatment, to avoid their secondary psychogenic impacts, however insufficiently the latter have been described here.

References

1. E. M. Coutinho, Hormonal effects on the non-pregnant human uterus. *Excerpta Med. Int. Congr. Ser.* 184:945 (1968).
2. A. I. Csapo and C. R. Pintos-Dantas, The cyclic activity of the non-pregnant uterus. *Fertil. Steril.* 17:34 (1966).
3. C. H. Hendricks, Activity patterns in the non-pregnant human uterus, in *Muscle* (W. M. Paul, E. E. Daniel, E. M. Kay, and G. Monckton, eds.). Pergamon Press, Elmsford, New York, 1965, p. 349.
4. A.-R. Fuchs, E. M. Coutinho, R. Xavier, P. E. Bates, and F. Fuchs, Effect of ethanol on the activity of the nonpregnant human uterus and its reactivity to neurohypophyseal hormones. *Am. J. Obstet. Gynecol.* 101:997 (1968).
5. A.-R. Fuchs and E. M. Coutinho, Suppression of uterine activity during menstruation by expansion of the plasma volume. *Acta Endocrinol.* 66:183 (1971).

6. H. R. Lindner, U. Zor, S. Bauminger, A. Tsafriri, S. A. Lamprecht, Y. Koch, A. Antebi, and A. Schwartz, Use of prostaglandin synthetase inhibitors in analyzing the role of prostaglandins in reproductive physiology, in *Prostaglandin Synthetase Inhibitors* (H. J. Robinson and J. R. Vane, eds.). Raven Press, New York, 1974, pp. 271-287.

7. V. R. Pickles, Prostaglandins in the human endometrium. *Int. J. Fertil.* 12:335 (1967).

8. J. Downie, N. L. Poyser, and M. Wunderlich, Levels of prostaglandins in human endometrium during the normal menstrual cycle. *J. Physiol.* 236: 465 (1974).

9. W. Bickers, Uterine contractions in dysmenorrhea. *Am. J. Obstet. Gynecol.* 42:1023 (1941).

10. W. Y. Chan, M. Y. Dawood, and F. Fuchs, Relief of dysmenorrhea with the prostaglandin synthetase inhibitor ibuprofen: effect on prostaglandin levels in menstrual fluid. *Am. J. Obstet. Gynecol.* 135:102 (1979).

11. V. R. A. Pickles, A plain muscle stimulant in the menstruum. *Nature* 180: 1198 (1957).

12. V. R. Pickles, W. J. Hall, F. A. Best, and G. N. Smith, Prostaglandins in endometrium and menstrual fluid from normal and dysmenorrheic subjects. *Br. J. Obstet. Gynecol.* 72:185 (1965).

13. E. J. Singh, I. M. Baccarini, and F. P. Zuspan, Levels of prostaglandins F_{2a} and E_2 in human endometrium during menstrual cycle. *Am. J. Obstet. Gynecol.* 121:1003 (1975).

14. D. R. Halbert, L. M. Demers, J. Fontana, and D. E. Jones, Prostaglandin levels in endometrial jet wash specimens in patients with dysmenorrhea before and after indomethacin therapy. *Prostaglandins* 10:1047 (1975).

15. J. W. Wilks, A. C. Wentz, and G. S. Jones, Prostaglandin F_{2a} concentrations in the blood of women during normal menstrual cycles and dysmenorrhea. *J. Clin. Endocrinol. Metab.* 37:469 (1973).

16. A. I. Csapo, M. O. Pulkkinen, and M. R. Henzl, The effect of naproxen sodium on the intrauterine pressure and menstrual pain of dysmenorrheic patients. *Prostaglandins* 13:193 (1977).

17. V. Lundström, K. Gréen, and N. Wiqvist, Prostaglandin, indomethacin and dysmenorrhea. *Prostaglandins* 11:833 (1976).

18. B. I. Nesheim and L. Wallφe, The use of isoxsuprine in essential dysmenorrhea. A controlled clinical study. *Acta Obstet. Gynecol. Scand.* 55:315 (1976).

19. M. K. Hansen and N. J. Secher, Beta-receptor stimulation in essential dysmenorrhea. *Am. J. Obstet. Gynecol.* 121:566 (1975).

20. M. Åkerlund, K. E. Anderson, and I. Ingemarsson, Effects of terbutaline on myometrial activity, uterine blood flow, and lower abdominal pain in women with primary dysmenorrhea. *Br. J. Obstet. Gynaecol.* 83:673 (1976).

21. A.-R. Fuchs and F. Fuchs, The possible mechanisms of labor inhibition by ethanol, in *Uterine Contraction* (J. Josimovich, ed.). John Wiley, New York, 1973, p. 287.

22. A. Schwartz, U. Zor, H. R. Lindner, and S. Naor, Primary dysmenorrhea. Alleviation by an inhibition of prostaglandin synthesis and action. *Obstet. Gynecol.* 44:709 (1975).

23. V. Lundström, K. Gréen, and K. Svanborg, Endogenous prostaglandins in dysmenorrhea and the effect of prostaglandin synthetase inhibitors (PGSI) on uterine contractility. *Acta Obstet. Gynecol. Scand. [Suppl.]* 86:51 (1979).

24. P. W. Budoff, Use of mefenamic acid in the treatment of primary dysmenorrhea. *JAMA* 241:2713 (1979).

25. W. Y. Chan, M. Y. Dawood, and F. Fuchs, Prostaglandins in primary dysmenorrhea. Comparison of prophylactic and non-prophylactic treatment with ibuprofen and use of oral contraceptives. *Am. J. Med.* 70:535 (1981).

26. H. Lehfeldt, Dyspareunia in obstetric-gynecological practice, in *Dyspareunia: Aspects of Painful Coitus* (H. Musaph and A. A. Haspels, eds.). Bohn, Scheltema and Holkema, Utrecht, Holland, 1977, p. 63.

27. E. Kehrer, Die psychogenen gynaekologischen Krankheitsbilder und ihre Behandlung, *M. M. W.* 97:1091 (1955).

28. J. Raboch, Studien zur Sexualität der Frau, in *Die Sexualität der Frau* (Griese, Gebhard and Raboch, eds.). Rowohlt, Hamburg, 1968.

29. M. Renaer, Chronic pelvic pain without obvious pathology in women. Personal observations and a review of the problem. *Eur. J. Obstet. Gynaecol. Reprod. Biol.* 10:415 (1980).

30. W. M. Allen and W. H. Masters, Traumatic laceration of uterine support. *Am. J. Obstet. Gynecol.* 70:500 (1955).

11 Premenstrual Tension: An Overview

KATHARINA DALTON   University College Hospital, London, England

Frank in 1931 [1] is credited with the first paper on premenstrual tension in which he described a young unmarried woman with premenstrual epilepsy and another with premenstrual bronchial asthma. However, the treatment he advocated, irradiation of the ovaries, was considered too drastic, and it soon fell out of favor. In 1953 the term "premenstrual syndrome" was introduced to replace premenstrual tension, since "tension is only one of many symptoms of the syndrome. Its use has commonly led to a failure to recognise the disorder when tension is absent or overshadowed by a more serious complaint" [2].

Premenstrual syndrome covers a wide spectrum from normality to gross abnormality and its study belongs equally to behavior sceince and clinical medicine. Advances in our knowledge must come from mutual understanding and research by scientists and clinicians although their outlook, training, and aims are entirely different. The behavior scientist aims to understand the physiological and psychological variations which occur during the menstrual cycle in the normal healthy woman. The clinician aims to differentiate the normal from the abnormal, and hopes that by treating the abnormal diseased state, the woman may be restored to normality (Fig. 1). In medicine, premenstrual syndrome embraces the majority of specialities, but is mastered by none. Doctors are even accused of ignoring, ridiculing, or failing to recognize the symptoms of premenstrual syndrome. Inevitably these differences in approach by scientists and clinicians are reflected by the many authors of different chapters in this book.

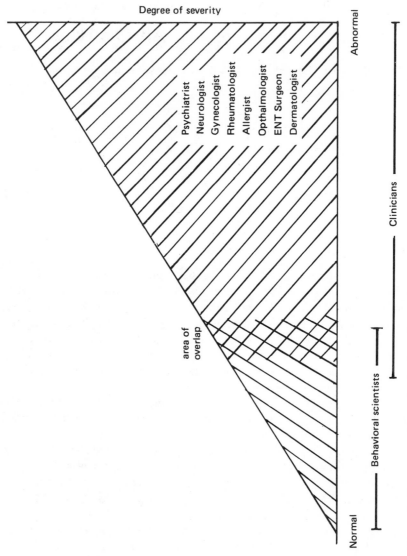

Figure 1 Spectrum of premenstrual syndrome.

I. Definition

There has been, and still is, considerable confusion over the definition of premenstrual syndrome. Failure to define the premenstrual syndrome adequately is responsible for much of the controversy and misunderstanding which surrounds the etiology and treatment.

Premenstrual syndrome is defined as: "The presence of symptoms which recur regularly at the same phase of each menstrual cycle, followed by a symptom free phase in each cycle" [3].

Premenstrual tension is similarly defined as: "The presence of psychological symptoms which recur regularly in the same phase of each menstrual cycle, followed by a symptom free phase in each cycle."

Thus, premenstrual tension is limited to psychological symptoms of which tension is the most frequent, while premenstrual syndrome includes both psychological and somatic symptoms. The somatic symptoms are of extraordinary diversity and form an almost endless list which includes such common presentations as epilepsy, asthma, rhinitis, boils, herpes, and conjunctivitis as well as the more unusual symptoms of uveitis, Behcet's syndrome, metatarsalgia, or enuresis.

The definitions of premenstrual syndrome and premenstrual tension, therefore, depend on the timing of symptoms in each menstrual cycle and not on the symptoms themselves which may occur equally in men, women, and children. There are no characteristic symptoms, although there may be common symptoms. The presence of symptoms alone is never diagnostic without a knowledge of their timing in the menstrual cycle. Furthermore, complete absence of symptoms during the postmenstruum or preovulatory phase is essential for the diagnosis of premenstrual syndrome or premenstrual tension. For research purposes, a complete absence of symptoms for a minimum of 7 consecutive days is required, although in practice nost women experiencing premenstrual syndrome have an interval of 2 or 3 weeks free from symptoms in each menstrual cycle.

The diagnosis of premenstrual syndrome also requires normal findings on full gynecologic examination. A bulky uterus or tenderness found on bimanual examination, as might occur in endometriosis or in the presence of an ovarian cyst, would exclude the diagnosis of premenstrual syndrome. Symptoms arising from the uterine or ovarian nerve distribution are also excluded, eliminating spasmodic dysmenorrhea and salpingitis.

"Menstrual distress," which is also known as "premenstrual distress' or "paramenstrual distress" must be differentiated from premenstrual syndrome and premenstrual tension. *Menstrual distress* is defined as: "Alteration in mood or symptoms in the menstrual cycle with deterioration during the premenstruum or menstruation."

Menstrual distress, therefore, denotes the mood swings and the alterations in severity of symptoms throughout the menstrual cycle, but does not demand a phase completely free from symptoms. It measures such items as the changes, day by day over the menstrual cycle, from happiness to sadness or calmness to anxiety.

The differentiation of premenstrual tension from menstrual distress is essential when considering the etiology and treatment of premenstrual tension. With appreciation of the differences between the two comes an understanding of many of the apparently confusing results described in literature. All too often one author is describing results in women with premenstrual tension and another group of workers find different results when they are discussing women who experience menstrual distress.

Within the definition of menstrual distress, premenstrual tension is included but also three other important subgroups (Fig. 2). The exacerbation of symptoms present throughout the month but become more marked as menstruation approaches, is included in menstrual distress. Thus the woman with depression throughout the menstrual cycle is likely to find an increase in her negative affect, which may even reach suicidal level, during the premenstruum. The patient with anxiety neurosis, or the "born worrier," is nervous and apprehensive at all times, but her phobias may increase during the premenstruum. Headaches present intermittently throughout the menstrual cycle are likely to occur with greater frequency and increased severity during the premenstruum or menstruation.

Spasmodic dysmenorrhea, or period pain, is also included in the definition of menstrual distress. Although the patient is completely normal and free drom symptoms during the premenstruum she develops cramps and spasmodic colicky pains in the lower abdomen, possibly accompanied by backache and pains in her upper legs, with the onset of the menstrual flow. She is likely to turn pale, sweat profusely, and may experience reflex vomiting or fainting at the height of the pains. Spasmodic dysmenorrhea only occurs during ovulatory cycles, so is usually absent for about the first 2 years after the menarche when menstruation is characteristically anovular. It is commonest in the late teens and early twenties and always ends after a full-term pregnancy. Treatment with estrogens or oral contraceptives is effective in eliminating the pain. Careful history-taking makes it easy to differentiate spasmodic dysmenorrhea from premenstrual tension, for the woman is free from symptoms during the premenstruum, but experiences the sudden onset of pain on the first day of menstruation.

Endometriosis is caused by misplaced endometrial cells which respond to the ever-changing levels of menstrual hormones and thus cause symptoms during the premenstruum or menstruation. The symptoms vary according to the position of the endometrial cell clusters in the pelvis, but the pain is always increased during the late premenstruum and early menstruation. The characteristic triad of symptoms includes dysmenorrhea, dyspareunia, and infertility. Vaginal examination usually shows a bulky uterus, and pain is experienced when the uterus is moved. There is a slow increase in symptoms over the years, which may start mildly with the first menstruation or may follow a pregnancy or abortion. Gynecologic treat-

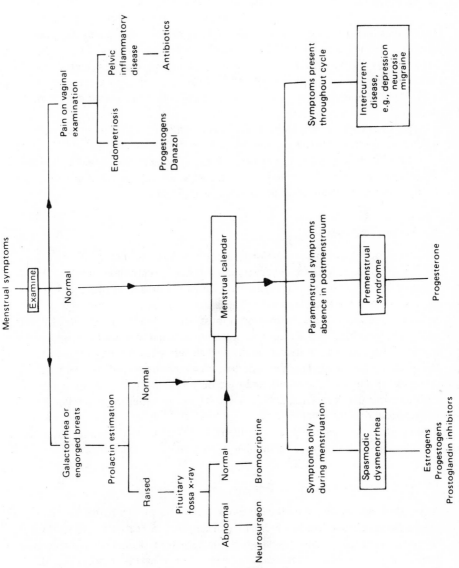

Figure 2 Flow chart for evaluation and differentiation of menstrual symptoms.

ment, and possibly surgical intervention, is required but in the early stages it responds to synthetic progestogens, often aimed at producing amenorrhea by giving continuous courses for 9 or 12 months.

The term *"premenstruum"* means "before menstruation" but in scientific and medical literature the term may be used in a multitude of ways. Asso [4] reviewed 36 studies on arousal in the premenstrual phase and noted the wide variation covered by the term which included periods of 1, 2, 3, 4, and 7 days before menstruation; the "luteal phase;" "from ovulation to 1 day premenstrually;" "late secretory phase;" and "1 day premenstrual and the first day of menstruation."

"Paramenstruum" meaning "around menstruation" is a term limited to the 4 days before menstruation and the first 4 days of menstruation [3].

Until the definitions of premenstrual tension, premenstrual symdrome, menstrual distress, and premenstruum are used uniformly, the comparability of studies is impossible and our advances in knowledge are slowed.

II. Sociologic Surveys

A series of sociologic surveys in North London demonstrating the influence of menstruation on various critical events showed a remarkable correlation with a range of 45 to 52% of incidents occurring during the paramenstruum (strictly 4 days before and the first four days of menstruation) compared with an expected incidence of 29% (Table 1). However, it must be stressed that this is a reflection of the incidence of menstrual distress, not premenstrual tension, for it is not known if, for instance, those who attempted suicide were depressed throughout the whole month or whether the prisoners convicted for shoplifting had been doing this throughout the month and were only apprehended when they were in their lethargic paramenstruum. Nor may it be assumed that the general incidence of menstrual distress is between the range of 45 and 52% as each event dealt with a different population group, e.g., accidents were limited to those who were admitted to hospital and the total number of women at risk is unknown.

III. Diagnosis of Premenstrual Tension

As yet there are no simple biologic diagnostic tests for premenstrual tension, or indeed for menstrual distress. Premenstrual tension can best be diagnosed by the use of a menstrual calendar on which the patient marks the days of menstruation and the dates when symptoms are present, for at least 2 months (Fig. 3). Thus "X" might denote the days of aggression, weeping, frustration, or panic, and "x" when the symptoms were present but mild. The investigator should then make sure that the symptoms occur in the same phase of each menstrual cycle and that there is an interval exceeding 7 days completely without

Table 1 Incidents Occurring During the Paramenstruum; from Sociologic Surveys in North London

Schoolgirls' punishments [5]	45
Industrial employees' sickness [6]	45
Acute psychiatric admission [7]	46
Prisoners commit crimes [8]	49
Acute hospital admissions [6]	49
Eye symptoms in glaucoma [9]	49
Mothers of children admitted to hospital as emergencies [10]	49
Accident admissions [11]	52
Pyrexia in women requiring home visits [3]	52
Visits to doctors' offices by women with sick children [6]	53
Attempted suicides [7]	53

symptoms. If these conditions are fulfilled, the diagnosis of premenstrual tension can be made.

There are a few rare instances when cases of aggressive outbursts or suicidal attempts can be diagnosed retrospectively by examination of police or prison records, hospital admission notes, or school attendance records, for these are always carefully documented. For example, a 28-year-old nulliparous barmaid was convicted of manslaughter. She had 26 previous convictions and had served several prison sentences. While in prison she was described by the medical officers as "pleasant and co-operative apart from episodes of attention-seeking behaviour," even while in prison she was noted to have outbursts of bizarre behavior (Fig. 4) and searching through her records revealed that 25 episodes of violence occurred at intervals of 29.55 ± 1.45 days or multiples of this. Similarly the intervals between the last episode of violent behavior prior to discharge from prison and her next offence, leading to another admission, showed an average length of 29.04 ± 1.47 days. She was diagnosed as having premenstrual tension, based on the normality of behavior during most of the month and the monthly episodes of bizarre behavior, although the exact date of menstruation was only known on two occasions. She was successfully treated with progesterone and released from prison [12].

At the Premenstrual Syndrome Clinic, University College Hospital, London,

Calendar 1 (left):

Day	Jan.	Feb.	Mar.	Apr.
1				
2				
3				
4				X
5				M
6				M
7				M
8				M
9			XM	
10			M	
11		X	M	
12		M	M	
13		M		
14		M		
15	X	M		
16	M	M		
17	M			
18	M			
19	M			
20				
21				
22				
23				
24				
25				
26				
27				
28				
29				
30				
31				

Calendar 2 (middle):

Day	Jan.	Feb.	Mar.	Apr.
1				
2				
3				
4				
5				
6				
7				
8	x			
9	x			
10	X			
11	X			
12	X	x		
13	XM	x		
14	xM	X		
15	M	X		
16	M	X	x	
17		X		
18		xM		
19		M	x	
20		M	X	
21		M	X	x
22			X	x
23			M	x
24			M	X
25			M	xM
26				M
27				M
28				M
29				
30				
31				

Calendar 3 (right):

Day	Jan.	Feb.	Mar.	Apr.
1				x
2				x
3		x		x
4	x	x		x
5	x	x		x
6	x	x	x	X
7	X	x	x	X
8	x	x	x	X
9	x	X	X	X
10	x	X	X	X
11	x	X	X	X
12	x	X	X	X
13	X	X	X	M
14	X	X	X	M
15	X	Mx	x	M
16	Mx	M	M	M
17	Mx	M	M	M
18	M	M	Mx	M
19	M	M	M	M
20	M	M	M	
21	M		M	
22				
23				
24				
25				
26				
27				
28				
29				
30				
31				

Figure 3 Menstrual calendars showing premenstrual syndrome M = menstruation, x = mild symptoms, X = severe symptoms.

it is found that only about 50% of newly referred patients are finally diagnosed as having premenstrual syndrome after inspection of their menstrual calendars, and this figure is echoed by another clinic in a nearby London teaching hospital. Wood and Jakubowicz [13], on a commercial radio program, invited volunteers for trials of mefenamic acid in premenstrual symptoms. The authors stated "the telephone conversations ensured that the volunteers had premenstrual complaints," but after daily recording of symptoms only three women had premenstrual symptoms alone and 34 had premenstrual and menstrual symptoms.

For patients who state that their symptoms always occur premenstrually and are anxious for immediate treatment, although they do not have an accurate record of the timing of symptoms in relation to menstruation, some helpful diagnostic pointers may assist in the assessment of an individual patient. These should not, however, be used instead of a menstrual calendar in studies into the etiology, pathology, and treatment of premenstrual tension.

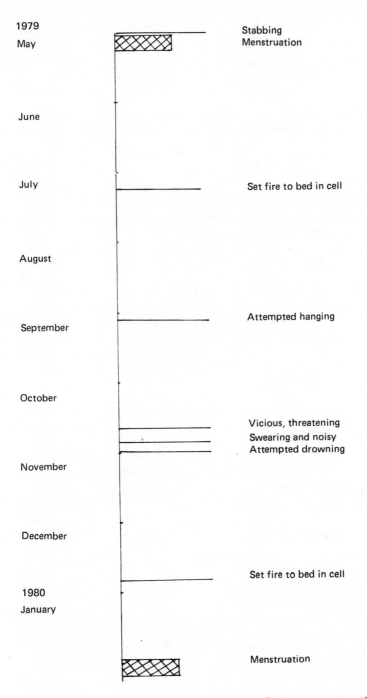

Figure 4 Timing of offences while in prison relative to menstruation.

A. Diagnostic Pointers in Premenstrual Tension

1. Time of Onset

Premenstrual tension tends to start at puberty, after pregnancy, during or after stopping the pill, or after a spell of amenorrhea as may occur with anorexia nervosa [3].

2. Time of Increased Severity

Although mild symptoms may have been present for some years the patient may note a marked increase in symptoms following a pregnancy, on stopping the pill, after amenorrhea, or after sterilization [3].

3. Painless Menstruation

This is characteristic of premenstrual syndrome [3]. The very normality of menstruation is the reason many women fail to notice the correlation of their bizarre behavior, epilepsy, or asthma with menstruation. Some women have congestive dysmenorrhea, with heaviness of the lower abdomen during the premenstruum increasing until the onset of menstruation, in addition to their other premenstrual symptoms, but if menstrual cramps or pain is the presenting symptom then premenstrual tension is an unlikely diagnosis.

4. Increase in Libido During the Premenstruum

Patients experiencing depression note a decrease in libido as their depression deepens, however the reverse may occur in premenstrual tension with an increased libido in the premenstruum. Israel [14] was the first to record nymphomania occurring in the premenstruum, and Gray [15] noted it in 13 of his 38 patients.

5. History of Threatened Abortion

Bleeding in the early months of pregnancy followed by a successful pregnancy is relatively common in premenstrual syndrome.

6. History of Preeclampsia

An 87% incidence of premenstrual syndrome was noted among 153 women hospitalized for preeclampsia during pregnancy. Their diagnosis of premenstrual syndrome was subsequently confirmed by a 3 month calendar [16].

7. History of Postnatal Depression

The depression must have been of sufficient severity to require psychiatric treatment or hospital admission. An incidence of 90% was reported in one London hospital series [3].

8. Inability to Tolerate the Oral Contraceptive Pill

Women with premenstrual tension experience weight gain, depression, headaches, and other side effects from oral contraceptives. This is in marked contrast with those experiencing spasmodic dysmenorrhea who then experience good symptomatic relief from oral contraceptives [3].

9. Weight Fluctuations

Not only do patients experience monthly weight swings of 3 to 4 kg, but over the years weight swings of 12 kg (28 lbs) are common. Comparison of the highest-ever weight (excluding pregnancy) with the lowest-ever weight should be included in the medical history.

10. Altered Hunger Tolerance During the Menstrual Cycle

This may cause food cravings and binges in the premenstruum [3]. The onset of acute symptoms (violence, panics, migraine) occur after long food gaps, exceeding 5 hours by day or 13 hours overnight.

11. Altered Tolerance to Alcohol During the Menstrual Cycle

This may be accompanied by premenstrual cravings and intoxication [3]. The patient may find that whereas she can tolerate a definite amount of her favorite drink on most days, during the premenstruum she becomes intoxicated on half the usual amount.

B. Diagnostic Checklist

When a reliable 2 month menstrual calendar is not immediately available or is ambiguous a checklist such as that in Table 2 is useful. Items are scored "not relevant," "positive," or "negative." Items, which would be marked "not relevant," would include the effect of the pill in a nonuser, the complications of pregnancy in nulliparous women, and the altered tolerance to libido, hunger, and alcohol in those who have not previously considered this possibility. The total positive scores are multiplied by 100 and divided by the sum of positive and negative scores to give a percentage. Women with symptoms who have scores exceeding 66% may be expected subsequently to produce a menstrual calendar confirming premenstrual syndrome.

C. Biochemical Diagnosis

A low level of sex hormone binding globulin (SHBG) below 50 nmol DHT/liter was shown to occur in 50 women with severe premenstrual syndrome in comparison with 50 women who specifically denied premenstrual symptoms [17]. However, the SHBG must be tested while the women are free of all medication, including the pill, sedatives, and analgesics. Altered SHBG levels also

Table 2 Diagnostic Checklist

	Not relevant	Positive	Negative
Time of onset (puberty, pill, pregnancy, amenorrhea)			
Time of increased severity (pill, pregnancy, amenorrhea, and sterilization)			
Painless menstruation (Score 2 negatives if period pain is presenting symptom)			
Increased libido in premenstruum			
Threatened abortion			
Preeclampsia			
Postnatal depression			
Side effects with oral contraceptives			
Weight fluctuations in adult life exceeding 12 kg			
Altered hunger tolerance in premenstruum			
Altered alcohol tolerance in premenstruum			

occur in obese women, those with thyroid disease, hirsutism, and in some women in the hirsute races.

D. Diagnostic Criteria for Clinical Studies

For scientific studies into a group of premenstrual tension sufferers, definite diagnostic criteria for inclusion must be decided upon, and should be clearly stated in the text. As premenstrual tension varies in severity from normality to abnormality it also becomes necessary to define the cut-off point. For instance, in the studies into the incidence of premenstrual syndrome in the general population of North London [16], patients were only included if they satisfied the following three criteria

1. Symptoms present in each of the three preceding cycles, thus eliminating any chance occurrence
2. Severity sufficient to demand relief with medication or seeking medical advice

3. Occurrence at a specific phase of the cycle confirmed by calendar.

However, different criteria are used today in Premenstrual Tension Clinics. For instance, Kerr and his colleagues [18] in their treatment studies of premenstrual syndrome included only patients satisfying the following:

1. Symptoms were sufficiently marked to cause personal distress or handicap in working or social life.
2. Symptoms were occurring in a regular cyclical manner in each menstrual cycle (28 ± 2 days). If symptoms were seen in the first half of the cycle or persisted for more than 2 days after the start of menstruation the patients were excluded.
3. No psychotropic, diuretic, or other medication was being taken.

IV. Diagnosis of Menstrual Distress

The diagnosis of menstrual distress depends on the day-to-day variation in mood and severity of the symptoms in relation to menstruation. Unlike premenstrual tension, it is not dependent on the absence of symptoms in the postmenstruum. The diagnosis of menstrual distress is made by frequent self-assessment of mood or symptoms. The Moos Menstrual Distress Questionnaire (MMDQ) is a useful diagnostic tool for menstrual distress, for which it was designed, but not for premenstrual tension. In the questionnaire, the woman is asked to rate on a six-point scale some 47 symptoms; the symptom scale ranges from "no experience" to "disturbing experience" [19]. Moos differentiated eight symptom clusters in the questionnaire in the areas of pain, concentration, behavior change, autonomic reactions, water retention, affect, arousal, and control. The pain cluster includes muscle stiffness, headache, cramps, backache, fatigue, and general aches and pains, so it does not relate specifically to spasmodic dysmenorrhea or endometriosis. Sampson and Jenner [20] have described a method of analyzing the data from the questionnaire by using sine waves to assess quantitatively the complaints associated with menstruation. However, this also fails to differentiate menstrual distress from premenstrual tension.

Another method of diagnosis of menstrual distress is by frequent assessment of mood using visual analog scales [21], from which the premenstrual mood index (PMI) may be calculated. Women are asked to mark on a 100 mm lineal scale their appropriate mood for the day in terms of depression, sadness, tension, bloatedness, loss of libido, aggression, lethargy, and anxiety. The score is measured by the distance along the line and a total score is obtained for each day. The difference in value of the preovulatory from the premenstrual score gives the Premenstrual Mood Index for the month. It should be noted that a decrease in libido is calculated as a positive symptom of menstrual distress, although patients with premenstrual tension may well experience an increase.

The success of a self-assessment questionnaire depends on the diligence of the woman completing it. Sampson [22], in her double-blind controlled treatment trials, requested her volunteers to rate the 47 symptoms on a six-point scale each evening for a total of 5 months. Thus the findings were only relevant for highly motivated or obsessional women, and there was always the possibility that a woman might forget or only complete it some days later, or even give a false answer. Furthermore, these questionnaires cannot be used by those with a poor command of the language. The visual analog scale also requires intelligence to enable a woman to differentiate sadness from depression and anxiety from tension each day; to many people these words are synonymous.

V. Timing of Symptoms of Premenstrual Tension

The diagnostic criteria for premenstrual tension demand careful attention to the timing of the symptoms, although there can be considerable variations. In some, especially epileptics, the symptoms are very short-lived possibly lasting only minutes and occurring on the day immediately before the onset of menstruation, or heralding menstruation. Others have increasing severity of symptoms for 4 to 7 days before with a sudden end accompanying the onset of menstruation. Yet other women have mild short-lived symptoms at ovulation, followed by a few days free from symptoms and then a gradual onset of symptoms reaching a crescendo on the last premenstrual day and slowly easing throughout menstruation, so that full relief only occurs at the end of menstruation. Some women are conscious of the onset of symptoms occurring simultaneously with ovulation and find symptoms increase until menstruation and then end suddenly at the beginning of, or gradually during, menstruation (Fig. 5). However symptoms will never occur for more than 14 days before menstruation and one must beware of the woman who states "symptoms used to be present only for a few days premenstrually, then it lasted as long as 2 weeks, and now it goes on for 3 or more weeks before menstruation." She may even add that her cycles are prolonged to 5 or 6 weeks, but even so symptoms will not last longer than 14 days before the onset of menstruation, i.e., from ovulation to menstruation and then may possibly last for the first few days of menstruation.

VI. Severity of Symptoms of Premenstrual Tension

It is difficult to quantify the severity of symptoms of premenstrual tension. Herve, quoted by Cerutti [23], suggested a classification based on the duration and the number of different symptoms. Thus, mild premenstrual tension required only 2 or 3 days of symptoms and only a few different symptoms; medium severity described patients with a duration of 7 to 8 days and with many symptoms; and severe premenstrual tension was limited to patients who had

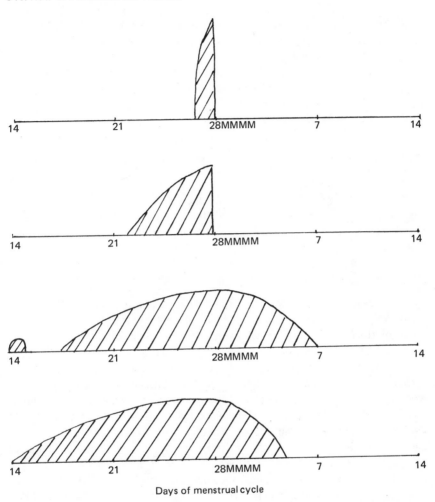

Days of menstrual cycle

Figure 5 Variation in timing of premenstrual symptoms M = day of menstruation.

symptoms for 8 to 14 days, disappearing only after the beginning of menstruation, or even lasting until the end, with numerous severe symptoms.

However, as noted, the barmaid only had bizarre behavior for a few hours each month, but the disturbance was severe with confusion and amnesia, so neither the duration or symptoms nor the number of different symptoms can be used as a measure. Clinically, it is convenient to classify the severity as:

Severe when life-threatening, thus including the parasuicides, patients subject to
    outbursts, child abusers, and alcoholics, and also where the recurrent and un-
    controllable symptoms interfere with employability and marital stability
Moderate when recurrent symptoms interfere with employment or with the en-
    joyment and satisfaction of personal, social, or family life
Mild when symptoms are present and are a nuisance but do not prevent the wo-
    man from leading a normal life

VII. Problems Encountered with Surveys of Premenstrual Tension

Apart from the vital differentiation of premenstrual tension from menstrual distress, many other problems are frequently encountered by researchers in this
area. These need careful consideration if studies are to add fresh knowledge to
the subject and be comparable to the findings of other workers. The following
factors may cause difficulties

A. Variations in the Length of the Menstrual Cycle

A normal cycle may range between 21 and 35 days and may vary by 4 days
month to month. This variation must be known and appreciated when considering the performance of any special investigation designed for a specific day such
as blood test, completion of questionnaire, or weighing. If it is to be performed
on day 28, this day may not be reached by a large proportion of the sample whose
cycle is 27 days or shorter. Ovulation would theoretically occur on day 14 in the
woman with a 28 day cycle, but day 14 may, in fact, be in the premenstruum in
one with a short cycle, or in the preovulatory phase in one with a long cycle. At
interview many women claim a precise 28 day cycle which is a rarity unless they
are receiving hormone treatment. In these women, it is wise to ask which day of
the week menstruation starts; a precise cycle of 28 days will always start on the
same day of the week, and it will only be one day early, by date, year by year (2
days in leap year). Coppen and Kessel [24], in a survey of 500 South London
women, noted that 16% did not know when their next menstruation was due. A
woman whose menstrual cycle is outside the range of 21 to 35 days should not
be included in a study of normal women, since there is a strong possibility that
her cycles are anovular.

B. Variation in Menstrual Flow

The duration of menstruation in normal women may vary from 2 to 8 days, being
longer but with a lighter loss in the teenager. The pattern of flow also varies from
a heavy loss initially for 1 or 2 days, to a slight loss for up to 7 days (especially
in those of high parity and with an intact intrauterine device) followed by the
full menstrual flow. It is usual for the symptoms of premenstrual tension to ease

with the onset of the full menstrual flow. Thus those with an initial scanty loss may not have relief of symptoms until a few days after menstruation has started. If the bleeding is slight, the problem remains; should it be recorded as the first day of menstruation or not?

C. Stress

An individual's menstrual pattern can be altered by stress, which may either shorten or lengthen the cycle, or the duration of the flow. In a survey of 91 British boarding school girls taking their O-level examination at age 16 years, just under half experienced an alteration of their normal menstrual pattern [25]. The usual menstrual pattern may be altered by both happy and sad events such as weddings, holidays, surgery, accidents, moving house, or loss of employment, and considerations must be given to these events in observations that last several months.

D. Age

Premenstrual tension tends to increase in incidence with age, indeed Lloyd [26] suggested that the syndrome should be designated "mid-thirties syndrome" because of its high incidence in that age group. In contrast, spasmodic dysmenorrhea is common in the late teens and early twenties, after which the incidence decreases rapidly and it is rare after the age of 30. Many workers select volunteers from hospitals and universities. These subjects tend to be young nurses and students, who are in an age group with a high incidence of spasmodic dysmenorrhea and a lower incidence of premenstrual syndrome.

E. Parity

Premenstrual syndrome often starts after a pregnancy, especially when complicated by preeclampsia or puerperal depression, and the incidence increases with increasing parity [16]. Yet, all too often, volunteers are nulliparous and not representative of the usual premenstrual syndrome patient. Many studies fail to mention the parity of the subjects studied, or to consider parity in the selection of their matched controls.

F. Hormonal State

Women who have recently or are currently receiving hormonal treatment or oral contraceptives should be excluded from studies. Recent work by Radwanska et al. [27] has shown that women who have undergone a tubal ligation are liable to develop progesterone deficiency, suggesting that those who have had tubal sterilization should be excluded from surveys.

G. Biased Selection of Subjects

Not all patients with premenstrual tension or menstrual distress seek medical help either from their general practitioner, gynecologist, or specialized clinic, so studies of those attending hospital are biased sample. This bias is increased if women are selected from a special clinic within the hospital, as occurred with the study of Benedek-Jaszmann and Hearn-Sturtevant [28] who studied the prolactin levels of patients with premenstrual syndrome attending their infertility clinic.

H. General Health

Subjects for studies into premenstrual tension or menstrual distress should be free from other diseases. One controlled evaluation of lithium in the treatment of premenstrual tension selected a series of 19 subjects, who included five with schizophrenia, four with neurosis, and three with affective psychosis [29]. Women whose premenstrual tension is severe or life-threatening should not be studied in controlled trials, but given immediate treatment.

I. Collection of Blood Samples

Those studies entailing the collection of blood samples for hormonal estimations must have the sample taken at the same time of day on each occasion since some hormones, e.g., prolactin, have a diurnal variation. Other medication and oral contraceptives must be stopped, thus premenstrual epileptics on anticonvulsants are automatically excluded. It is necessary to inquire specifically if a patient is taking sleeping pills since, very often, patients who have been taking them for years do not consider them medication.

J. Contraception

Daily self-assessment questionnaires should be evaluated with the knowledge that, in the premenstruum, there will be a natural anxiety in women who are not using secure contraception but are anxious to avoid conception; their mood will improve with the onset of menstruation. On the other hand, those trying to conceive will be depressed when their hopes are dashed by the onset of menstruation. Women most suitable for study are contraceptively secure and use noninvasive techniques, but the limitation of subjects and controls to such women in some populations may itself represent a selection bias.

K. Controls

Ideally, control subjects should be selected from healthy volunteers of the same population as patients with premenstrual tension and menstrual distress, and be matched for age and parity, be free from medication and oral contraceptives, not sterilized, and in good health. Curious selections of controls are to be found in some studies. One study into the minor psychiatric and physical symptoms during the menstrual cycle [30] selected as controls seven women who had undergone hysterectomy with conservation of their ovaries 1 to 5 years previously, on the assumption that their hormonal function continued normally without a uterus. No mention was made as to the reason for the hysterectomy, which may have been due to hormonal imbalance.

VIII. Extrapolation of Results

In considering the findings of reported studies in literature, it is important to appreciate the problems associated with extrapolation of results. In studies relating to premenstrual tension, the following factors are relevant.

A. Differential Diagnosis of Premenstrual Tension and Menstrual Distress

The findings in one cannot necessarily be applied to the other. For instance, in a study of progesterone, fluid, and electrolytes in women with menstrual distress, diagnosed by the use of visual analog scales, O'Brien et al. [31] found plasma progesterone concentration was higher in women with symptoms in the post-ovulatory phase of the cycle and their peak progesterone concentration appeared earlier. They also noted that the mood symptoms occurred after the changes in progesterone and electrolyte concentrations. From these studies on menstrual distress they falsely concluded that "progesterone deficiency is probably not the cause of premenstrual syndrome and treatment with progesterone is probably illigical unless a deficiency is detected." Conversely, the findings in a study of premenstrual tension cannot be extrapolated to cover menstrual distress.

B. Species Differences

These must be appreciated with the recognition that estrus in animals is not the same as menstruation in humans. The function of progesterone also differs in various species.

C. Like Must Be Compared with Like

This is especially true in hormonal studies. The absorption and metabolism of oral progesterone was studied in five women who had experienced a normal menopause 2 to 5 years previously [32]. The metabolism of this group of women with low estrogen and raised follicle stimulating hormone is not, however, necessarily the same as in those with functioning ovaries and regular menstruation. The same comment applies to Oelkers, et al. [33] who studied the effect of progesterone and four synthetic progestogens on sodium balance and the renin-aldosterone system in 20 male medical students.

IX. Etiology of Premenstrual Tension

Chapter 19 covers this subject, so it only remains here to consider a few points for the reader to bear in mind. A psychological etiology has been postulated, suggesting that the symptoms result from the woman's conflict with her feminine role, her cultural dissatisfaction, maladjustment to the trauma of her first menstruation, or frustration at her own failure to modify the conflict between professional life and childbearing. For any such stress to be manifested as somatic symptoms, a chemical, biochemical, or more precisely hormonal factor would need to be implicated. When the exact hormonal fault is located it can be corrected. This is likely to prove infinitely easier and quicker to remedy than by the time-consuming process of attempting to placate the psychological conflicts.

By definition, the time in the menstrual cycle when premenstrual tension occurs corresponds to the days when a discernable level of progesterone is present in the peripheral blood, while the days when symptoms are absent correspond to those days when no progesterone is discernable in the peripheral blood. This suggests that progesterone may play an important part in the etiology of premenstrual tension. In contrast, patients with menstrual distress experience symptoms throughout the menstrual cycle with deterioration of mood in the premenstruum. The etiology of menstrual distress is more likely to be related to the ever-changing levels of all the hormones which vary throughout the menstrual cycle, including those of the hypothalamic-pituitary-ovarian axis, the renin-aldosterone system, the adrenal steroids, and those which regulate glucose metabolism.

In considering the etiology of premenstrual tension and the possible part played by progesterone either alone or in relation to estrogen, it must be appreciated that at present our measurements of progesterone by radioimmunoassay estimate the total progesterone. It may well be that the free progesterone and free estrogen, as opposed to the bound portions of the hormones, are of significance in precipitating the symptoms [17]. Endocrinologists recognize that the free levels of other hormones are of importance and not the total levels, e.g., thyroid. Interesting work is underway in the estimation of free progesterone and estrogen. Also, progesterone receptors are present in the brain and are known to be highly specific. This may account for the difference in effect when natural progesterone is administered compared with the synthetic progestogens, which have a different formula, and are not utilized by the progesterone receptors [34]. In both these fields one may expect dramatic advances in the next few years.

X. Differences Between Progesterone and Progestogens

The vital differences between natural progesterone and synthetic progestogens need to be fully appreciated when considering both the etiology and treatment of premenstrual tension. Unfortunately, when progesterone is administered orally it is metabolized by the progesterone receptors in the liver before it reaches the systemic circulation, and in particular the brain, so oral use is of no value for the relief of premenstrual tension. Also when progesterone is administered intramuscularly the effect lasts only 24 to 48 h, so biochemists searched for a substitute which could be given orally or by long-term injections. They developed a series of compounds which, like progesterone, could cause vaginal bleeding in estrogen-primed ovarectomized rabbits and which could be given orally or by long-term injections. These compounds, mainly analogs of testosterone, were called "progestogens" or "progestins" and included nor-ethisterone, norgesterol, medroxyprogesterone and hydroxyprogesterone caproate, and dydrogesterone, which have proved of great value in the field of contraception and gynecology. Their action in women, however, is quite different from the studies in animals and from natural progesterone. When progesterone is given intramuscularly, rectally, or vaginally, it causes a rise in the plasma progesterone level [35], whereas the progestogens cause a drop in progesterone level [36]. Recently dydrogesterone, which is a noncontraceptive progestogen, has also been shown to lower the plasma progesterone level [16]. The effect of natural progesterone is to cause proliferation of the endometrium, whereas the synthetic progestogens cause an initial proliferation followed by atrophy of the endometrium. Progesterone is excreted as pregnanediol, whereas the progestogens are excreted either unchanged or partially metabolized, but never as pregnanediol. Progesterone is thermogenic, progestogens are not. Progesterone is not estrogenic, anabolic, nor androgenic whereas some progestogens have these qualities. If progestogens are administered during the early weeks of pregnancy there is a risk of masculinization of the female fetus, while if progesterone is administered, masculinization does not occur, and the intellectual potential may be enhanced [37].

XI. Progesterone Treatment for Premenstrual Tension

Since 1953, when treatment with progesterone was first reported [2], it has continued to be the drug of choice in well-diagnosed and moderate to severe cases of premenstrual tension. Over the years, the value of other treatments has been assessed but none has given such consistently good and prolonged results. Some patients have been continuously receiving progesterone therapy each month with benefit for 20 years and longer.

In severe cases requiring daily supervision, such as suicide risks, alcoholics, child abusers, and those likely to be violent, progesterone 50 to 100 mg intramuscularly is given daily from midcycle to menstruation. The injections ensure full absorption and some women can benefit from alternate day instead of daily injections. Other patients are treated with progesterone suppositories or pessaries 200 or 400 mg usually used once or twice daily, but doses of up to 400 mg every 4 h may be needed. Parous women need, on average, double the dose of nulliparous women and those with a history of preeclampsia or puerperal depression require high levels of progesterone. The dosage needs to be individually tailored in accordance with the timing of symptoms and menstrual pattern as shown on patients' menstrual calendars. There are no contraindications, although in the presence of monilial infection, there may be a recurrence, and in those with a history of colitis it is wisest to use progesterone vaginally. Overdose causes euphoria and spasmodic dysmenorrhea in the nulliparous woman, but as parous women have experienced sustained high progesterone levels during pregnancy, it is virtually impossible to give an overdose.

Progesterone is not effective in menstrual distress, which is the reason for repeatedly emphasizing the importance of correct diagnosis. Progesterone can also increase the pain in patients with spasmodic dysmenorrhea. In double-blind controlled trials of progesterone and premenstrual syndrome, Sampson [22] found progesterone to be of no value. However, her patients in fact proved to be suffering from menstrual distress and not premenstrual syndrome.

Progesterone administered by suppository raises the blood progesterone level within 1 h of administration and its action lasts for 12 to 24 h [35]. This explains why women need to use the suppositories at least daily, if not twice daily. Smith [38], in controlled trials, gave progesterone suppositories 200 mg on alternate days from day 19 to 26 of the cycle and was surprised when it proved ineffective. If progesterone is to be used, it needs to be given in an effective dose and with the necessary frequency, at least once daily, but often twice a day.

In Britain, progesterone suppositories and pessaries are freely available; they have been licensed by the Committee of Safety of Medicines and can be prescribed by the general practitioner under the National Health Scheme. During 1981 more than two million progesterone suppositories were used in Britain. These are undergoing clinical trials in America, although pharmacists may prepare them for individual patients [39].

XII. Other Treatments for Premenstrual Tension

Numerous trials of various progestogens have been reported over the last 20 years, with poor results and marked placebo effects of between 30 and 50%. Kerr and his co-workers [18] cleverly overcame the difficulty of placebo response by adding the 51% improvement which was noted during the placebo and active treatment months, to the 21% of women who reported improvement on active treatment only, and thus claimed 72% of patients improved on treatment with dydrogesterone.

Bromocriptine is effective in those with a raised prolactin level who have breast tenderness and abdominal bloatedness [28], but it is not universally effective for premenstrual tension [40].

Numerous diuretics have been tried from ammonium chloride, used by Greenhill and Freed [41], to the newer and much more effective diuretics used today. Diuretics are only helpful in those women with water retention, and not all patients with premenstrual tension have premenstrual water retention. However, these women have water and sodium retention with potassium depletion and, unfortunately, diuretics, while increasing water and sodium excretion, tend to increase the potassium depletion causing excessive lethargy. If diuretics are used, the potassium level needs to be checked constantly, and potassium supplements given if necessary. Another hazard is that of addiction to diuretics, initially prescribed for the luteal phase only, but used continuously, sometimes for years. This may then present as idiopathic edema, which MacGregor and colleagues [42] found to be the result of excessive diuretic use, abetted in some patients by self-imposed fluctuations of sodium and carbohydrate intake.

Spironolactone, the aldosterone antagonist, is advocated by those who believe the cause of premenstrual tension lies in an abnormality of the renin-angiotensin-aldosterone system, but its effectiveness may be due to its diuretic action [43].

Vitamin B has been advocated since 1943 [44]. It fell into disfavor but has recently been revived, as pyridoxine (B6) is involved in tryptophan metabolism. It is effective in some women who become depressed on oral contraceptives. Since it is completely harmless, it is worth prescribing in doses of 50 mg three times daily for 4 weeks as a therapeutic trial, and continued if found to be effective. About one in 10 men and women find pyridoxine helpful for mild depression but its use is not specific to premenstrual tension.

The search continues for cheaper, simpler, and equally effective treatments which will require controlled clinical trials to evaluate their safety and efficacy. However, in premenstrual tension, controlled trials present insuperable difficulties due to the fixed criteria which need to be imposed. There must be a definite day in the cycle fixed for starting and ending treatment, irrespective of the timing of symptoms or usual length of menstrual cycle. A standard dose of the drug must be used irrespective of the type or severity of symptoms, parity, gynecologic history, or age, yet all these factors are of improtance in treating an individual patient.

The resolution of the many problems posed in this chapter requires the close collaboration of many disciplines. The harrassed mother, the violent prisoner, and distressed epileptic as seen by the clinician are in a different category from the healthy young volunteers in the university studied by the psychologist. Narrow views must not impede the overall view of premenstrual tension. The time has come to leave our entrenched position and critically and analytically look afresh at all the evidence presented.

References

1.   R. T. Frank, The hormonal causes of premenstrual tension. *Arch. Neurol. Psychiatry* 26:2053-2057 (1931).

2. R. Greene and K. Dalton, The premenstrual syndrome. *Br. Med. J.* 1:1007-1-14 (1953).

3. K. Dalton, *The Premenstrual Syndrome and Progesterone Therapy.* Heinemann, London, 1977.

4. D. Asso, Levels of arousal in the premenstrual phase. *Br. J. Soc. Clin. Psychol.* 17:47-55 (1978).

5. K. Dalton, Schoolgirls' behaviour and menstruation. *Br. Med. J.* 2:1647-1649 (1960).

6. K. Dalton, The influence of menstruation in health and disease. *Proc. R. Soc. Med.* 57:262-264 (1964).

7. K. Dalton, Menstruation and acute psychiatric illnesses. *Br. Med. J.* 1:148-149 (1959).

8. K. Dalton, Menstruation and crime. *Br. Med. J.* 2:1752-1753 (1961).

9. K. Dalton, The influence of menstruation on glaucoma. *Br. J. Ophthalmol.* 51:692-695 (1967).

10. K. Dalton, Children's hospital admissions and mothers' menstruation. *Br. Med. J.* 2:27-28 (1970).

11. K. Dalton, Menstruation and accidents. *Br. Med. J.* 2:1425-1427 (1960).

12. K. Dalton, Cyclical criminal acts in premenstrual syndrome. *Lancet* 2:1070-1071 (1980).

13. C. Wood and D. Jakubowicz, The treatment of premenstrual symptoms with mefanamic acid. *Br. J. Obstet. Gynaecol.* 87:627-630 (1980).

14. S. L. Israel, Premenstrual tension. *JAMA* 110:1721-1723 (1938).

15. L. A. Gray, The use of progesterone in nervous tension states. *South. Med. J.* 34:1004-1006 (1941).

16. K. Dalton, Similarity of symptomatology of premenstrual syndrome and toxaemia of pregnancy and their response to progesterone. *Br. Med. J.* 2:1071-1075 (1954).

17. M. E. Dalton, Sex hormone binding globulin concentrations in women with severe premenstrual syndrome. *Postgrad. Med. J.* 57:560-561 (1981).

18. G. D. Kerr, J. B. Day, M. R. Munday, M. G. Brush, M. Watson, and R. W. Taylor, Dydrogesterone in the treatment of the premenstrual syndrome. *Practitioner* 224:852-855 (1980).

19. R. H. Moos, Typology of menstrual cycle symptoms. *Am. J. Obstet. Gynecol.* 103:390-402 (1969).

20. G. A. Sampson and F. A. Jenner, Studies of daily recordings from the Moos Menstrual Distress Questionnaire. *Br. J. Psychiatry* 130:265-271 (1977).

21. R. C. B. Aitken, Measurement of feelings using visual analogue scales. *Proc. R. Soc. Med.* 62:989-993 (1969).

22. G. A. Sampson, Premenstrual syndrome: a double-blind controlled trial of progesterone and placebo. *Br. J. Psychiatry* 135:209-215 (1979).

23. R. Cerutti, The premenstrual syndrome. 6th International Congress of Psychosomatic Obstetrics and Gynaecology Aug. 1980, p. 3.

24. A. Coppen and N. Kessel, Menstruation and personality. *Br. J. Psychiatry* 109:711-721 (1963).

25. K. Dalton, Menstruation and examinations. *Lancet* 2:1386-1388 (1968).

26. T. S. Lloyd, The mid-thirties syndrome. *Virginia Med. Monthly* 90:51-52 (1963).

27. E. Radwanska, G. S. Berger, and J. Hammond, Luteal deficiency among women with normal menstrual cycles, requesting reversal of tubal sterilisation. *Obstet. Gynecol.* 54:789-792 (1979).

28. L. J. Benedek-Jaszmann and M. D. Hearn-Sturtevant, Premenstrual tension and functional infertility—aetiology and treatment. *Lancet* 1:1095-1098 (1976).

29. K. Singer, R. Cheng, and M. Schou, A controlled experiment of lithium in the premenstrual tension syndrome. *Br. J. Psychiatry* 124:50-51 (1974).

30. P. J. V. Beaumont, D. H. Richard, and M. G. Golder, A study of minor psychiatric and physical symptoms during the menstrual cycle. *Br. J. Psychiatry* 126:431-434 (1975).

31. P. M. S. O'Brien, C. Selby, and E. H. Symonds, Progesterone, fluid and electrolytes in premenstrual syndrome. *Br. Med. J.* 280:1161-1163 (1980).

32. M. I. Whithead, P. T. Townsend, D. K. Gill, W. P. Collins, and S. Campbell, Absorption and metabolism of oral progesterone. *Br. Med. J.* 280:826-828 (1980).

33. W. Oelkers, Schöneshöfer, and A. Blümel, Effects of progesterone and four synthetic progestogens on sodium and sodium balance and the renin-aldosterone system in man. *J. Clin. Endocrinol. Metab.* 39:882-889 (1974).

34. H. Al-Khouri and B. D. Greenstein, Role of corticosteroid binding globulin in interaction of corticosterone with uterine and brain progesterone receptors. *Nature* 287:58-60 (1980).

35. S. J. Nillius and E. D. B. Johanssen, Plasma levels of progesterone after vaginal, rectal and intramuscular injection of progesterone. *J. Obstet. Gynecol. St. Louis* 110:470-477 (1971).

36. E. D. B. Johanssen, Depression of progesterone levels in women treated with synthetic gestogens after ovulation. *Acta Endocrinol.* 68:779-792 (1971).

37. K. Dalton, Prenatal progesterone and educational attainments. *Br. J. Psychiatry* 129:438-442 (1976).

38. S. L. Smith, in *Topics in Endocrinology* (E. J. Sachar, ed.). New York, Raven Press, 1975, pp. 19-59.

39. B. D. Roffe, R. A. Zimmer, and H. J. Derewicz, Preparation of progesterone suppositories. *Am. J. Hosp. Pharm.* 34:1344-1346 (1977).

40. K. Ghose and A. Coppen, Bromocriptine and premenstrual syndrome: controlled study. *Br. Med. J.* 1:147-148 (1977).

41. J. D. Greenhill and S. C. Freed, The mechanism and treatment of premenstrual distress with ammonium chloride. *Endocrinology* 26:529-531 (1940).

42. G. A. Macgregor, N. D. Markanda, J. E. Roulston, J. C. Jones, and H. E. De Wardener, Is 'idiopathic oedema' idiopathic? *Lancet* 1:397-400 (1979).
43. P. M. S. O'Brien, D. Craven, S. Selby, and E. M. Symonds, Treatment of premenstrual syndrome by spironolactone. *Br. J. Obstet. Gynaecol.* 86: 142-147 (1979).
44. M. S. Biskind, Nutritional deficiency in the etiology of menorrhagia, metrorrhagia, cystic mastitis and premenstrual tension. Treatment with vitamin B complex. *J. Clin. Endocrinol.* 3:227-237 (1943).

12 Classification of Premenstrual Syndromes

URIEL HALBREICH   Albert Einstein College of Medicine, Bronx, New York

JEAN ENDICOTT   College of Physicians and Surgeons, Columbia University, New York, New York, and New York State Psychiatric Institute, New York, New York

Many women experience changes in their physical condition and/or mood and behavior during the premenstrual period. The significance of such changes premenstrually and many unanswered questions about their correlates have been discussed at length in recent reviews of the literature [1-5] and recent papers by these authors [6-8]. The changes may at times be sufficiently severe to warrant medical attention because of great physical or emotional discomfort or even disability [9-15]. Furthermore, certain "events" such as child abuse, accidents, crimes, admissions to psychiatric facilities, and suicide attempts have been reported to occur with increased frequency during the paramenstruum [12,13,16-19].

I. Need for Better Definition of Subtypes of Premenstrual Change

Reports of the prevalence of premenstrual changes have ranged from 20 to 100% [1-5]. One of the major reasons for this wide disparity and for other inconsistencies in findings is that many different kinds of somatic, mood, and behavioral features are often lumped together into a single "premenstrual syndrome." Furthermore, the features included vary considerably from study to study, and are of undefined severity. Different samples of women may also manifest different subtypes of change [20-24].

Since premenstrual phenomenologic changes recur cyclically and regularly within a limited period of time and in combination with hormonal, physiological, and biochemical changes, there have been many efforts to relate these two types of change to each other. The results of such studies are often not replicable. Frequently they have had major methodologic problems, including a tendency to fail to take into account the great variability in types of premenstrual change as well as in the levels, rate, and degree of change of interrelated biologic substances.

II. Evidence of the Value of Subtyping Premenstrual Features

As in the case of studies of mental and physical disorders, there has been more recognition recently of the need for better definition and discrimination among the many subtypes of premenstrual changes manifested. Reliable differentiation is needed to investigate better the correlates of and possible contributions to specific subtypes of change [1,3,20-24]. Failure to differentiate among the different patterns of change or different syndromes may obscure relationships with other variables. The possible importance of a delineation of subtypes of premenstrual change is illustrated by studies which have separated affective changes from physical changes [20-25].

Kashiwagi et al. [20] demonstrated a relationship between a premenstrual "affective syndrome" (defined to include both worse mood and better mood) and a life-time diagnosis of an affective disorder. The rates of the "affective syndrome" in women attending a headache clinic and grouped by different diagnoses were: affective disorder (65%); nonaffective mental disorder (14%); no mental disorder (21%). In contrast, the three groups did not differ in the prevalence of a "somatic" premenstrual syndrome. When more severe criteria were used for the "affective syndrome" (moderate to severe interference with functioning), 51% of the affective disorder group and 0% of the women in the nonaffective mental disorder group met the criteria. Wetzel et al. [21] found that college students who reported a premenstrual "affective syndrome" were more likely to seek psychiatric help than those without such a syndrome (20% vs. 14%) and were also more likely to be diagnosed as having an affective disorder during the following 4 years (18% vs. 10%). Diamond et al. [22] also found higher premenstrual affective symptoms in women with primary affective disorder as compared with nonill controls, but no difference in premenstrual somatic symptoms.

These studies did not differentiate between premenstrual depressive and "hypomanic" affective features. It has been reported that women who experience better mood and other changes similar to those of hypomanic episodes during the premenstrual period are likely to have a family or personal history of bipolar affective disorder [22,24]. Systematic studies of this relationship have not been made, nor have attempts been made to relate other specific features of premenstrual affective changes to similar features during episodes of affective disorder (i.e., hypersomnia vs. insomnia).

Some subtypes of premenstrual changes should be differentiated because they may not be related to affective disorder even when combined with affective

features (e.g., those with psychotic features) [25]. No systematic efforts have
been made to determine which, if any, subtypes of mental disorder are differentially associated with such severe premenstrual changes.

The potential importance of differentiation, even at the single-dimension
level, has come from studies such as that of the presence or absence of premenstrual irritability [26]. Unfortunately too few studies have attempted to relate
biologic variables or treatment outcome with different subtypes of premenstrual
changes.

III. Different Procedures for Subtyping Clinical Features

When faced with the task of describing or subtyping individuals so as to commu-
nicate key clinical features to others, two major approaches are available for developing criteria: the categorical and dimensional [27,28]. Clinicians are most
familiar and most comfortable with the categorical approach whereby one deter-
mines whether or not criteria for a particular "type" are met. After considering
the clinical features one then subtypes the subjects as belonging in the category
or not (e.g., having congestive heart failure, a manic disorder). The dimensional
approach involves describing a subject either by level of severity on one or more
dimensions of interest (e.g., energy level, judgment, euphoria) or by determining
the degree to which the "profile" on these dimensions "fits" a particular subtype
pattern.

The criteria for a typologic category may be simple or complicated, specific
or relatively vague. The specification of criteria is usually guided by clinical experience coupled, when possible, with research evidence of the differential significance of a particular combination of clinical features. Categorical criteria usually
include rules for both inclusion and exclusion. A typological category is usually intended for a purpose beyond that of simple clinical description, (e.g., prediction
of treatment response, relationship to biologic changes, etiology, evidence of
genetic transmission). Such criteria are often evolving, particularly in research
settings, but at times there is consensus that a particular cluster of features at a
particular level of severity represents a "type" worth differentiating from other
"types" of similar phenomena (e.g., panic disorder vs. generalized anxiety disorder, cluster headache vs. migraine headache).

The dimensional approach may also be very simple (e.g., a score on irritability)
or complicated (e.g., a set of rules by which subjects' dimensional scores are compared with those derived from cluster or discriminant function analyses). In general, the more dimensions involved, the more difficult the assignement to subtype by dimensional rules.

There is some controversy as to which approach is best for different purposes
and most investigators use both approaches to subtyping. One of the advantages of
the typologic approach is that it facilitates the selection of subjects for studies in
which the entire range of phenomena are not to be included. It also facilitates

description which is clinically recognizable and can be easily applied. The typology often uses criteria based evidence of the differential significance of a clinical feature depending on the context in which it occurs. For example, fever with cough and chest pain and fever with painful urination usually have a different etiology and respond to different treatments.

IV. Subtyping of Premenstrual Features

An investigator or a clinician who wishes to focus on specific subtypes of premenstrual change will find that most of the procedures used to evaluate premenstrual features are not suitable for sensitive and reliable differential subtyping. Although they may have coverage suitable for a simple physical vs. mood and behavior subtyping, they do not have sufficiently broad coverage, specificity of item description, or differentiation of severity levels to provide reliable criteria for more detailed subclassification of premenstrual features.

The Premenstrual Assessment Form (PAF) was developed by the authors and their colleagues in an effort to provide a new procedure for initial evaluation and selection of subjects with a number of different subtypes of premenstrual change. A description of the development of the PAF and the psychometric properties of the items and dimensional summary scoring systems is given elsewhere [6]. A companion procedure, the PAF-Time Chart, was developed for daily ratings so that retrospective reports of selected premenstrual changes can be confirmed.

In this chapter, we will describe the PAF criteria for typological categories for classifying premenstrual changes, the rationale for their selection, preliminary evidence concerning their interrelationships and differential frequencies, as well as evidence of differential correlates.

A. Initial Development of Premenstrual Assessment Form (PAF) Criteria

During the development of the PAF, steps were taken to assure coverage of the many different clinical changes seen premenstrually to allow detailed description and categorization. Although they have been reported to occur premenstrually, the major area not covered in the PAF is symptoms indicative of psychosis. The authors decided that, if present, these are best evaluated by clinicians rather than by self-report.

The PAF contains 95 items descriptive of specific types of change in mood, behavior, and physical condition (Table 1). Each item is rated to indicate the degree of change from the woman's usual "nonpremenstrual state" during the three premenstrual periods prior to evaluation. The following descriptive levels are used:

Table 1 Examples of Items from the Premenstrual Assessment Form[a]

Have rapid changes in mood (e.g., laughing, crying, angry, happy) all within the same day

Have decreased energy or tend to fatigue easily

Have decreased ability to coordinate fine movements, poor motor coordination, or clumsiness

Feel anxious or more anxious

Sleep too much or have difficulty getting up in the morning or from naps

Have a feeling of malaise (i.e., general, nonspecific bad feeling or vague sense of mental or physical ill health)

Feel jittery or restless

Have loss of appetite

Have pain, tenderness, enlargement or swelling of breasts

Have headaches or migraines

Be more easily distracted (i.e., attention shifts easily and rapidly)

Tend to have accidents, fall, cut self, or break things unintentionally

Have nausea or vomiting

Show physical agitation (e.g., fidgeting, hand wringing, pacing, can't sit still)

[a]95 items are rated as to the degree of premenstrual change usually present, compared with usual nonpremenstrual state

1. Not applicable (e.g., "missed work," if not employed) *or* no change (feature not present at all or did not change in severity)
2. Minimal change (only slightly apparent to you; others would probably not be aware of change)
3. Mild change (definitely apparent to you and/or others who know you well)
4. Moderate change (clearly apparent to you and/or others who know you well)
5. Severe change (very apparent to you and/or others who know you well)
6. Extreme change (the degree of change or severity is so different from your usual state that is is very apparent to you OR even people who do not know you well)

The rationale for this approach, which differs from that of other procedures used to evaluate premenstrual features and is reported to be more sensitive to differences in severity of change, is discussed in detail elsewhere [6].

The PAF developmental sample consisted of 154 women who were students or employed at the Columbia-Presbyterian Medical Center. They were selected on the basis of their willingness to complete the PAF. Details of the selection procedure and other characteristics of the sample are described elsewhere [6]. Data from this sample were used in the development of the typological criteria, since differentiation among a relatively "average" sample of women would be a more stringent test for subtyping premenstrual changes than differentiation among women who were seeking treatment for severe syndromes.

B.   Initial Grouping of Item Sets to Develop Subtype Criteria

The authors initially grouped the PAF items to reflect selected clinical syndromes observed by them to occur premenstrually, or found in patients with mental or physical disorders. The specific items in a set were selected on the basis of similarity to syndromes of change in mood, behavior, and physical condition and evidence that such phenomena occurred premenstrually. The intercorrelations among the items in the sets and with items in other sets were used to determine whether they covaried during the premenstrual period in a syndromal fashion. Some items did not "assort" in the expected fashion and were not included in the final subtype criteria. Items were used in the criteria for subtyping only if their major correlates were among the other items in the time set and their inclusion would not result in misclassifying a significant number of subjects (see detailed discussion below).

C.   Description of PAF Criteria for Classifying Premenstrual Changes

Criteria were developed for 18 syndromal categories. Their names and the degree to which they are mutually exclusive or are subtypes of other categories are indicated in Table 2. As can be seen, the categories of PAF major and minor depressive syndrome are mutually exclusive and with the categories of anxiety and angry/irritable. There are six subtypes of PAF major depressive syndrome (five of which are also used for subtyping PAF minor depressive syndrome). These subtypes of depressive syndrome are not mutually exclusive with the exception of endogenous depressive features and atypical depressive features. None of the remaining clinical categories are mutually exclusive. The inclusion and exclusion criteria for each of these ways of subtyping premenstrual changes are discussed in detail below.

Table 2 Decision Tree for Premenstrual Assessment Form Typological Classification

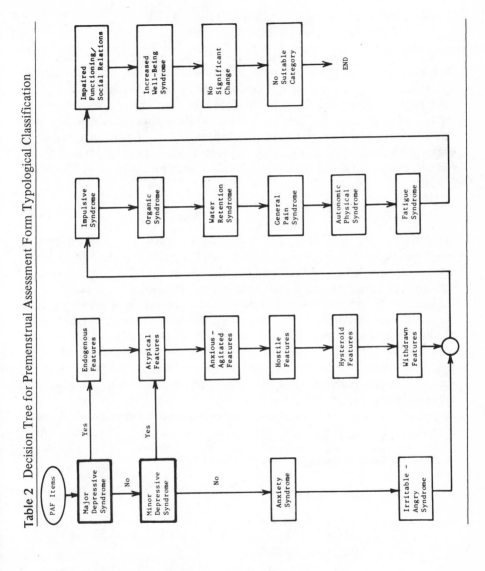

D. Classification of Premenstrual Changes Associated with
    Depressed Mood or Loss of Interest and Pleasure

Depressed mood and loss of interest and pleasure are among the most prevalent
changes in mood reported to occur premenstrually. These changes are associated
with other changes in sleep, appetite, activity, etc., generally considered part of
a depressive syndrome. Criteria were developed for many different ways of subtyping these changes so that they can be used singularly or in a combined fashion.
These include: PAF major and minor depressive syndrome, further subtyped as
having endogenous features (PAF major depressive syndrome only), atypical features, hysteroid features, agitated/angry features, hostile features, or withdrawn
features.

1. Criteria for PAF Major and Minor Depressive Syndrome

The criteria for the categories of PAF major and minor depressive syndromes are
based to a great extent on those of the Research Diagnostic Criteria (RDC) for
major and minor depressive disorders [29,30]. The RDC were developed to provide criteria to classify selected syndromes of mental *disorders* and as such have
requirements of impairment in functioning and duration that are too stringent to
use for premenstrual depressive features, hence the use of the term "syndrome."
The PAF criteria for depressive syndromes are similar in clinical features to those
of the RDC but differ in that impaired functioning or treatment-seeking behavior
is *not* required and the duration may be less than a week. Differentiation was
made into major and minor rather than a single depressive syndrome, because
the two categories represent what is often thought of as a "full" vs. "partial"
depressive syndrome, and because past research has suggested that more stringent
criteria lead to greater association with affective disorder [20]. The specific PAF
criteria are presented here, using item abbreviations. (As shown in Table 1, the
items themselves are longer and more specific.)

2. Criteria for PAF Major Depressive Syndrome

A.   1. Depressed or low mood: *one* of the following five items must be rated as
         at least mild (rated 3 to 6): Feel depressed *or* Feel sad or blue *or* Feel
         lonely *or* Pessimistic outlook.
  or 2. Loss of interest or pleasure: *all* of the following four items must be
         rated as at least mild (rated 3 to 6): Less sexual interest *and* Avoid
         social activities *and* Want to be alone *and* Less leisure activities.
  or 3. Irritable: *one* of the following two items must be rated as at least mild
         (rated 3 to 6): Outbursts of irritability *or* Feel "at war"
B.   If depressed: at least four of the following eight items, or item scales,
         must be rated as at least mild (rated 3 to 6): If irritable or loss of in-
         terest or pleasure only, at least five of the eight items must be rated as
         at least mild (rated 3 to 6):

1. Appetite change: Loss of appetite *or* Weight gain *or* Increased appetire
2. Sleep change: Hypersomnia *or* Trouble sleeping
3. Decreased energy
4. Psychomotor change: Physical agitation *or* Less desire to talk/move
5. Less interest: Less sexual interest *or* Avoid social activities *or* Want to be alone *or* Less leisure activities
6. Self-deprecation: Guilt feelings *or* Decrease in self-esteem
7. Concentration difficulties
8. Suicidal ideation

3. Criteria for PAF Minor Depressive Syndrome

A. Does not meet criteria for major depressive syndrome
B. Depressed mood: *one* of the following five items must be rated as at least mild (rated 3 to 6): Feel depressed *or* Feel "empty" *or* Feel sad *or* blue *or* Feel lonely *or* Pessimistic outlook
C. Associated Features: At least two of the following 13 items or item sets must be rated as at least mild (rated 3 to 6):
    1. Appetite change: Loss of appetite *or* Weight gain *or* Increased appetite
    2. Sleep change: Hypersomnia *or* Trouble sleeping
    3. Decreased energy
    4. Psychomotor change: Physical agitation *or* Less desire to talk/move
    5. Less interest: Less sexual interest *or* Avoid social activities *or* Want to be alone *or* Less leisure activities
    6. Self-deprecation: Guilt feelings *or* Decrease in self-esteem
    7. Concentration difficulties
    8. Suicidal ideation
    9. Feel tearful
    10. Brood over events
    11. Feel insecure
    12. Irritability/Hostility: Tend to nag *or* Violent *or* Outbursts of irritability *or* Feel "at war" *or* Intolerant/Impatient
    13. Dependency: Feel passive *or* More childlike *or* Seek advice

E. Criteria for Subtypes of Depressive Syndrome

Research on depressive disorders has tended to focus upon subjects with a "classic" depressive syndrome characterized by "endogenous" features (insomnia, loss of appetite, lack of reactivity of mood, guilt, etc.). Recently there has been an increase in the recognition that periods of depression can be quite severe without a syndrome of "endogenous features" and an increase of interest in subtyping severe and mild depressive syndromes according to other clinical features. It has been noted that while most people who are depressed manifest features of the "endogenous" syndrome, many do not have the full syndrome and are primarily irritable, anxious, or have "atypical" depressive features [31]. Since all of these features are also sometimes present premenstrually, criteria were developed for subtyping depressive premenstrual features.

1. Endogenous Depressive Features

Over the years, criteria have been derived for classifying depressed patients as endogenous or nonendogenous. Although the weight given to individual features varies, there is a fairly general consensus regarding the core features. These features are used in the RDC criteria for an endogenous subtype of major depressive disorder, and those of the PAF for major depressive syndrome with endogenous features are similar to those of the RDC.

The PAF criteria for endogenous depressive features are applied to data for subjects who meet criteria for PAF major depressive syndrome only. As far as possible, they employ item descriptions of the features of an endogenous syndrome suitable for a self-report format. No effort was made to evaluate "distinct quality of mood."

F. Criteria for PAF Endogenous Depressive Features

A. Meets criteria for major depressive syndrome
B. Loss of interest and pleasure defined as:
    1. More enjoyment/excitement (rated as absent, less than 2)
    2. Less sexual interest (rated as at least mild, i.e., 3 or more)
    3. Less leisure activities (rated as at least mild)
    4. Avoid social activities (rated as at least mild)
    5. Want to be alone (rated as at least mild)
C. At least two of the following features rated as at least mild:
    1. Feel worse in morning
    2. Guilt feelings
    3. Trouble sleeping
    4. Terminal insomnia
    5. Physical agitation
    6. Less desire to talk/move
    7. Loss of appetite
    8. Become constipated
D. No strong "atypical" features: *None* of the following rated as at least mild (rated 3 to 6):
    1. Hypersomnia
    2. Crave specific foods
    3. Increased appetite

G. Atypical Depressive Features

Some investigators have rejected the study of premenstrual affective changes as a model for other periods of affective change because of the relative lack of a classic endogenous syndromal cluster of premenstrual features (e.g., loss of sleep at least mild: 22%; loss of appetite at least mild: 13%). On the contrary, it is far more common for women to have premenstrual depressive features often referred to as "atypical" in the sense that they are the opposite of the classic "endogenous" features (e.g., hypersomnia at least mild: 36%, increase in appetite at least mild: 50%, and reactivity of mood at least mild: 49%). The more commonly used procedures for the evaluation of premenstrual features (or for depression in general) do not have items suitable for the classification of the syndrome according to these atypical features.

The PAF criteria are based on those used clinically and in studies [31-34]. One clinical feature, an increase in sexual interest and activity, which has been noted by some [31] to occur with the other atypical features, although highly correlated with the other PAF "atypical" features, was not included in the criteria. It was also highly correlated with items in the criteria for increased well-being and therefore lost any differential significance.

1. Criteria for PAF Atypical Depressive Features

A. Meets criteria for major or minor depressive syndrome
B. At least two of the following four items rated as at least mild (rated 3 to 6)
   1. Hypersomnia
   2. Feel sleepy
   3. Crave specific foods
   4. Increased appetite

H. Hysteroid Depressive Features

One subtype of depressive periods proposed in recent years is "hysteroid dysphoria" [32]. The clinical criteria include atypical depressive features coupled with rejection sensitivity, an increased need for contact with others, and somewhat theatrical behavior. Since some women display similar features premenstrually (but far fewer than manifest the atypical depression features), PAF criteria were developed for hysteroid depressive features apart from those of atypical depressive features.

1. Criteria for PAF Hysteroid Depressive Features

A. Meets criteria for major *or* minor depressive syndrome *and* atypical depressive features
B. Becomes hysterical if upset: rated as at least mild (rated 3 to 6)
C. At least three of the following four items rated as at least mild (rated 3 to 6)
   1. Dissatisfaction with appearance
   2. More childlike
   3. Self-indulgent
   4. Sensitive to rejection

I. Anxious-Agitated Depressive Features

Much of the research on premenstrual features has focused on "premenstrual tension" and the description, when given, has often included a mixture of depressed mood and prominent anxiety. A recent procedure and criteria developed for a single premenstrual syndrome reflect this focus [35]. Furthermore, in studies of depressive disorders, the presence or absence of prominent and severe anxiety is often noted. Since anxiety is frequently present to some degree in people with depressed mood, whether premenstrually or at other times, the criteria for categorization of the syndrome generally require that the level of anxiety be relatively high and that the anxious features be prominent. The PAF criteria reflect this in the requirement that the anxiety levels must reflect at least a moderate change from the usual levels experienced by the subject. (Most of the PAF criteria involve at least a mild degree of change.)

1. Criteria for PAF Anxious-Agitated Depressive Features

A. Meets criteria for major or minor depressive syndrome
B. At least two of the following four items rated as at least moderate (rated 4 to 6)
    1. Feel anxious
    2. Feel jittery or restless
    3. Physically agitated
    4. Pick skin/bite nails

J. Withdrawn Depressive Features

In contrast with those who seek help or seek out others when depressed, some people withdraw from social contact. Although it is not a subtype of depressive syndrome often mentioned, clinically it is a distinction that receives attention because of its relationship to social impairment. This tendency is also characteristic of some women during the premenstrual period.

1. Criteria for PAF Withdrawn Depressive Features

A. Meets criteria for major or minor depressive syndrome
B. At least three of the following four items rated as at least mild (rated 3 to 6)
    1. Less desire to talk/move
    2. Stay at home
    3. Avoid social activities
    4. Want to be alone

K. Hostile Depressive Features

The distinction between depressive syndromes characterized by prominent anger and hostility and those without obvious irritability or anger has been recognized clinically and in studies of depression, although they are not in the formal sets of diagnostic criteria. Since premenstrual irritability is sometimes strikingly present and has been found to be differentially related to premenstrual biologic changes in at least one study [26], PAF criteria were developed for this distinction.

1. Criteria for PAF Hostile Depressive Features

A. Meets criteria for major or minor depressive syndrome
B. At least three of the following six items rated as at least mild (rated 3 to 6)
    1. Violent
    2. Outburst of irritability
    3. Feel "at war"
    4. Act spiteful
    5. Intolerant
    6. Blames others

L. Classification of Other Types of Dysphoric Premenstrual Changes

Two additional sets of PAF criteria were developed for subtyping premenstrual syndromes characterized by anxiety or irritability in the absence of a depressive syndrome. These are clinical distinctions thought to be important under other circumstances and, although the "pure" syndromes may be rarely seen premenstrually (because of the frequent association with depressive features), they were included for their heuristic value. The criteria for the PAF anxiety syndrome are based on those of the RDC for generalized anxiety disorder, differing primarily in that there is no requirement for impairment and the duration may be less than a week. Those of the irritable/angry syndrome are based on clinical descriptions.

1. Criteria for PAF Anxiety Syndrome

A. *Not* major or minor depressive syndrome
B. At least one of the following two items rated as at least mild (rated 3 to 6)
    1. Feel anxious
    2. Feel jittery or restless
C. At least one of the following six items rated as at least mild (rated 3 to 6)
    1. Physical agitation
    2. Dizziness, faintness, vertigo
    3. Sense of unreality
    4. Rapid heartbeat
    5. Pick skin/bite nails
    6. Trouble sleeping, but *not* Terminal insomnia

2. Criteria for PAF Irritable/Angry Syndrome

A. Not major or minor depressive syndrome

B. At least three of the following six items rated as at least mild (rated 3 to 6)
    1. Violent
    2. Outbursts of irritability
    3. Feel "at war"
    4. Act spiteful
    5. Intolerant/impatient
    6. Blames others

M. Classification of Premenstrual Increase in Well-Being and Impulsiveness

As previously mentioned, some women have increased feelings of well-being, are
more efficient, and have more energy during the premenstrual period. These features may appear alone or may alternate with those of depression at that time. In
view of the possible differential relationship with bipolar affective disorder, PAF
criteria are provided for categorizing such affective changes separately from other
affective changes. Two clinical features of a "hypomanic" syndrome which were
not included, overtalkativeness and increase in sexual interest and activity, were
not used in the criteria because both were also highly correlated with some of
the items in criteria for subtypes of depressive syndromes.

Separate PAF criteria are also provided for subtyping those premenstrual
changes characterized by impulsive behavior, since there are many reports of a
higher premenstrual incidence of events which might be attributed to impulsive
behavior.

1. Criteria for PAF Increased Well-Being Syndrome

A. At least two of the following four items rated as at least mild (rated 3 to 6)
    1. More enjoyment/excitement
    2. Increased well-being
    3. Increased activity/efficiency
    4. Bursts of energy

2. Criteria for PAF Impulsive Syndrome

A. At least two of the following four items rated as at least mild (rated 3 to 6)
    1. Violent
    2. Lack self-control
    3. Impulsive behavior
    4. Outbursts of irritability

N. Classification of Changes in Physical Condition

Many different kinds of physical changes have been reported to occur premenstrually. During the development of the PAF many more items descriptive of

physical changes were included than are usually included in measures of premenstrual features. Criteria were developed for four subtypes of premenstrual physical changes: water retention syndrome, general discomfort syndrome, autonomic physical changes syndrome, and fatigue syndrome. These types of changes demonstrated syndromal clustering. The other physical changes appeared to represent individualized exacerbations of physical symptoms, or individualized development of physical changes, rather than syndromes.

1. Criteria for PAF Water Retention Syndrome

A. At least three of the following six items as at least mild (rated 3 to 6)
  1. Breast pain or swelling
  2. Urinate less
  3. Weight gain
  4. Abdominal discomfort/pain
  5. Water retention signs
  6. Feel bloated

2. Criteria for PAF General Discomfort Syndrome

A. At least one of the following three items rated as at least mild (rated 3 to 6)
  1. Headaches or migraine
  2. Backaches/joint/muscle pains
  3. Abdominal discomfort/pain

3. Criteria for PAF Autonomic Physical Changes Syndrome

A. At least three of the following seven items rated as at least mild (rated 3 to 6)
  1. Nausea or vomiting
  2. Dizziness, faintness, vertigo
  3. Rapid heartbeat
  4. Urinate frequently
  5. Become constipated
  6. Urinate less
  7. Feel cold

4. Criteria for PAF Fatigue Syndrome

A. At least three of the following four items rated as at least mild (rated 3 to 6)
  1. Decreased energy
  2. Feeling of malaise
  3. Feelings of weakness
  4. Tired legs

O. Criteria for Impairment in Functioning

Since many women develop premenstrual syndromal changes in mood, behavior, and physical condition without impairment in functioning, the PAF criteria for impairment were separated to facilitate the study of the syndromes with and without impairment in functioning, and to separate the possible "causes" of the impairment from the impairment itself. With so many different types of changes occurring concomitantly, it would be difficult to know if such behavior as missing time at work were due to any specific change (e.g., headache or desire to be alone).

Reports of impaired functioning tend to take two forms: those involving social relations and obligations and those involving mental and physical functioning. Therefore, criteria were developed for PAF impairment in social functioning and PAF "organic" mental syndrome.

1. Criteria for PAF Impairment in Social Functioning

A. At least three of the following 11 items rated as at least mild (rated 3 to 6)
    1. Tend to nag
    2. Decreased judgment
    3. Family notes mood
    4. Stay at home
    5. Avoid social activities
    6. Lowered performance/efficiency
    7. Miss time at work
    8. Lack of inspiration
    9. Less attention to appearance
    10. Less housework
    11. Less leisure activities

2. Criteria for PAF "Organic" Mental Syndrome

A. At least four of the following six items rated as at least mild (rated 3 to 6)
    1. Poor motor coordination
    2. Tend to have accidents
    3. More forgetful
    4. Easily distracted
    5. Concentration difficulties
    6. Feel confused

P. Criteria for No Significant Change in Mood, Behavior, or
    Physical Condition

Finally, some women may have premenstrual changes but may not meet any of the PAF criteria for particular syndromes of change. Criteria were developed for identifying those women who show no significant changes, as distinct from those who have changes but for whom there is no suitable subtype.

The criteria for this category are: (1) no items rated as at least mild (rated 3 to 6); (2) no more than three items rated as present (rated 2 to 6); and (3) did not meet criteria for any specified PAF subtypes.

V. Frequencies of Subtypes of Premenstrual Change and Joint Frequencies of Occurrence

Tables 3 and 4 indicate the relative frequencies and the joint frequencies of occurrence of the PAF categories of premenstrual change within the developmental sample. These frequencies are presented to illustrate the great diversity shown within an "average" sample of women but not as representative of expected relative frequencies or of "norms." Data from other samples of women evaluated with the PAF indicate that the patterns of changes may vary considerably depending upon the selection process.

Table 4 indicates that the joint classification of any two categories, i.e., the degree of overlap within subjects, is dependent on the category with which one starts. For example, 100% of subjects who meet PAF criteria for "organic" mental syndrome also meet PAF criteria for major depressive syndrome, while only 26 percent of those with major depressive syndrome meet criteria for "organic" mental syndrome. Attention to such overlap is important in obtaining a relatively homogeneous sample of subjects or contrasting groups of subjects who differ only on one set of criteria.

Tables 3 and 4 indicate that while some subtypes of premenstrual change are relatively common, e.g., physical discomfort, the degree of differentiation is most impressive. Certainly there is no evidence here for one basic "premenstrual syndrome." Furthermore, such diversity in syndromal patterns suggests that stereotypic concepts are not the major source of the endorsement of the items as has been suggested by some authors [36]. The degree of differentiation shown in Tables 3 and 4 is not an artifact of the typological criteria since similar diversity was shown in the scores on the summary bipolar dimensional scales and bipolar continua [6].

Many clinicians and investigators would wish to specify further the characteristics of any sample of subjects or of any individual subtype by using the summary dimensional scales to further index severity of the specific clinical features, degree of social impairment, etc. Those who wish to use more stringent criteria may also choose to combine syndromal subtypes (e.g., major depressive syndrome subtypes with that of social impairment: 67% of those with PAF major depressive syndrome met both).

Table 3 Frequency with which Subjects Met Criteria for
Premenstrual Assessment Form Typological Categories
(N = 154)

	N	%
Change in mood and behavior		
Major depressive syndrome	70	45
Minor depressive syndrome	29	19
Subtypes of depressive syndrome		
Endogenous features	0	0
Atypical features	54	35
Hysteroid features	8	5
Agitated-anxious features	31	20
Hostile features	44	29
Withdrawn features	17	17
Anxious syndrome (not depressed)	1	1
Irritable syndrome (not depressed)	1	1
Impulsive syndrome	41	27
Increased well-being syndrome	26	17
Change in physical condition		
General discomfort syndrome	105	68
Water retention syndrome	95	62
Fatigue syndrome	54	35
Autonomic physical syndrome	33	22
Changes in functioning		
Impaired social functioning	53	17
"Organic" mental features	18	12
No significant changes	4	3
No suitable PAF subtype	18	12

VI. Possible Relationship of PAF Subtypes and Subtypes of Mental Disorder

Previous research relating a premenstrual depressive syndrome to a life-time diagnosis of affective disorders was discussed in the introduction. In addition to those studies, others indicate that at times there are premenstrual exacerbations of mental disorders.

Table 4 Joint Classifications of Premenstrual Assessment Form (PAF) Typological Categories (%)[a]

	Major depression	Minor depression	Atypical dep. feat.	Hysteroid feat.	Agitated/anxious	Hostile feat.	Withdrawn feat.	Anxiety (not dep.)	Irritability (not dep.)	Impulsivity	Organic mental feat.	Signs of water reten.	General discomfort	Autonomic phys. feat.	Fatigue	Impaired soc. funct.	Increased well-being
Major depression (70)[b]	—	0	63	11	40	50	37	0	0	46	26	90	93	40	67	67	24
Minor depression (29)	0	—	35	0	10	31	0	0	0	17	0	66	62	3	21	17	10
Atypical dep. feat. (54)	82	19	—	15	35	50	33	0	0	41	20	87	91	39	72	57	20
Hysteroid feat. (8)	100	0	100	—	63	75	50	0	0	75	25	100	100	50	75	100	38
Agitated/anxious feat. (31)	90	10	61	16	—	68	32	0	0	52	29	94	90	42	71	68	23
Hostile feat. (44)	80	21	61	14	48	—	34	0	0	61	18	86	84	32	61	77	25
Withdrawn feat. (26)	100	0	69	15	39	58	—	0	0	46	50	89	92	39	73	96	27
Anxiety (not depressed) (1)	0	0	0	0	0	0	0	—	0	0	0	0	100	0	0	0	0
Irritability (not depressed) (1)	0	0	0	0	0	0	0	0	—	100	0	100	100	0	0	0	0
Impulsivity (41)	78	12	54	15	39	66	29	0	2	—	15	81	83	29	61	63	22
Organic mental feat. (18)	100	0	61	11	50	44	72	0	0	33	—	100	100	44	72	83	39
Signs of water retention (95)	66	20	50	8	31	40	24	0	1	35	19	—	86	33	51	51	20
General discomfort (105)	62	17	47	8	27	35	23	1	1	32	17	78	—	31	47	46	21
Autonomic physical feat. (33)	85	3	64	12	39	42	30	0	0	36	24	94	97	—	61	58	27
Fatigue (54)	87	11	72	11	41	50	35	0	0	46	24	89	91	37	—	65	22
Impaired social funct. (53)	89	9	59	15	40	64	47	0	0	49	28	91	91	36	66	—	23
Increased wellbeing (26)	66	12	42	12	27	42	27	0	0	35	27	73	85	35	46	46	—

[a] N = 154 medical center staff. The table should be read across, not down (e.g., 63% of those meeting criteria for PAF major depressive syndrome met criteria for atypical depressive features).
[b] Number meeting criteria.

There is also preliminary evidence of a differential relationship between the PAF subtypes of major and minor depressive syndrome and the presence or absecne of a life-time RDC diagnosis of affective disorder. Reports of a PAF depressive syndrome are related positively to the presence of affective disorder (54 percent) vs. no affective disorder (0 percent) in a sample of 30 women. The PAF subtypes of physical discomfort (58 percent vs. 75 percent) or impaired social functioning (34 percent vs. 25 percent) did not show such a differential association.

Other studies are underway to determine if the subtypes of premenstrual change characterized by prominent anxiety are related differentially to a life-time diagnosis of an anxiety disorder.

VII. Possible Advantages for Subtyping of Premenstrual Changes for Clinical and Research Use

Clinicians as well as research investigators who wish to evaluate premenstrual changes in individuals or groups of women will find that the broad and sensitive coverage of the PAF provides an easy-to-use initial procedure for such an evaluation. Since it has been noted that the retrospective reports of premenstrual change are sometimes not confirmed by daily ratings across the menstrual cycle, one might wish to obtain such ratings for one or more cycles. The PAF-Time Chart is designed for such use with focus on target changes of interest.

The use of the PAF has confirmed the clinical impression of diversity of syndromal changes premenstrually. As has been the case with research on affective disorders, such diversity undoubtedly accounts for some of the conflicting findings with regard to treatment response, relationship to biologic changes, and incidence. Evaluation of premenstrual changes should take this diversity into account until there is persuasive evidence that it is not of importance.

The results of previous studies as well as preliminary PAF data showing a statistical relationship between a life-time diagnosis of affective disorder and premenstrual depressive features suggest that there may be some common denominator. This conclusion can be drawn in spite of the lack of the development of a clear cut endogenous depressive syndrome.

The PAF data to date agree with those of previous studies in that none of the women had a sufficient number and severity of endogenous clinical features to be considered as having an endogenous syndrome. However, many of the women met the PAF criteria for an "atypical" or "anxious-agitated" or a "hostile" depressive syndrome, all clinical syndromes of increasing interest to both clinicians and investigators. Given that endogenous features are not that clearly separated from the "nonendogenous" features just listed, it seems premature to conclude, as have some investigators, that premenstrual affective changes cannot serve as a model for affective changes at other times.

The availability of specific inclusion and exclusion criteria for categories of affective change should lead to the selection of subjects which will provide more focused and stringent tests of the possible relationship between such premenstrual features and affective changes at other times.

The same specificity of subtyping should also lead to more clear-cut and replicable research in the genetics and epidemiology of types of premenstrual change. Furthermore, genetic and epidemiologic studies of mental disorder might include the assessment of premenstrual changes for (1) to avoid confusion between changes limited to the premenstrual period and changes that take place at other times, and (2) to account partially for male-female differences in point-prevalence of individual items descriptive of mood, behavior, or impairment which might be dependent on the woman's menstrual status at time of evaluation.

A procedure that reflects the recognition of the diversity in patterns and severity of premenstrual change and is sensitive to such, as well as the availability of specific criteria for subtyping such changes, should lead to more specific (and thus better) research. This should result in better understanding and treatment of severe premenstrual changes.

References

1. J. M. Abplanalp, R. F. Haskett, and R. M. Rose, The premenstrual syndrome. *Psychiatr. Clin. North Am.* 3:327-347 (1980).
2. M. Brown-Parlee, The premenstrual syndrome. *Psychol. Bull.* 80:454-465 (1973).
3. L. Dennerstein and G. Burrows, Affect and the menstrual cycle. *J. Affect. Dis.* 1:77-79 (1979).
4. M. Steiner and B. Carroll, The psychology of premenstrual dysphoria: Review of theories and treatments. *Psychoneuroendocrinology* 2:321-335 (1977).
5. C. M. Tonks, Premenstrual tension in contemporary psychiatry. *Br. J. Psychiatry Spec. Publ.* 9:399-408 (1975).
6. U. Halbreich, J. Endicott, S. Schacht, and J. Nee, The diversity of premenstrual changes as reflected in the premenstrual assessment form. *Acta Psychiatr. Scand.* 65:46-65 (1982).
7. U. Halbreich and J. Endicott, Possible involvement of endorphin withdrawal or imbalance in specific premenstrual syndromes and postpartum depression. *Med. Hypotheses* 7:1045-1050 (1982).
8. J. Endicott, U. Halbreich, S. Schacht, and J. Nee, Premenstrual changes and affective disorders. *Psychosom. Med.* 43:519-529 (1981).
9. A. W. Clare, The treatment of premenstrual symptoms. *Br. J. Psychiatry* 135:576-579 (1979).

10. V. M. Pennington, Meprobromate in premenstrual tension. *JAMA* 164:638-640 (1957).

11. L. Rees, The premenstrual tension syndrome and its treatment. *Br. Med. J.* 1:1014-1016 (1953).

12. K. Dalton, *The Premenstrual Syndrome.* Chas. C Thomas, Springfield, Illinois, 1964.

13. K. Dalton, Influence of mother's menstruation on her child. *Proc. R. Soc. Med.* 59:1014 (1966).

14. R. H. Tuch, The relationship between a mother's menstrual status and her response to illness in the child. *Psychosom. Med.* 37:388-394 (1975).

15. H. Sutherland and I. Stewart, A critical analysis of the premenstrual syndrome. *Lancet* 1:1180-1183 (1965).

16. D. Pallis and I. Holderg, The menstrual cycle and suicidal intent. *J. Biosoc. Sci.* 8:27-33 (1976).

17. N. Lisky, Accidents: rhythmic threat to females. *Accident Anal. Prev.* 4:1-11 (1972).

18. J. Horney, Menstrual cycles and criminal responsibility. *Law Hum. Behav.* 2:25-36 (1980).

19. J. Birtchnell and S. Floyd, Further menstrual characteristics of suicide intendors. *J. Psychosom. Res.* 19:81-85 (1975).

20. J. Kashiwagi, J. J. McClure, and R. D. Wetzel, Premenstrual affective syndrome and psychiatric disorder. 127:219-221 (1976).

21. R. D. Wetzel, T. Reich, J. M. McClure, and I. Wald, Premenstrual affective syndrome and affective disorder. *Br. J. Psychiatry* 127:219-221 (1975).

22. S. Diamond, A. Rubinstein, D. Dunner, and R. Fieve, Menstrual problems in women with primary affective disease. *Compr. Psychiatry* 17:541-548 (1976).

23. M. A. Schuckit, V. Daly, G. Herrman, and S. Wiseman, Premenstrual symptoms and depression in a female university population. *Dis. Nerv. Syst.* 36:516-517 (1975).

24. J. N. McClure, T. Reich, and R. D. Wetzel, Premenstrual symptoms as an indicator of bipolar affective disorder. *Br. J. Psychiatry* 119:527-528 (1971).

25. M. Endo, M. Daiguji, Y. Asano, I. Yamashita, and S. Takahashi, Periodic psychosis recurring in association with menstrual cycle. *J. Clin. Psychiatry* 39:456-466 (1978).

26. J. Cullberg, Mood changes and menstrual symptoms with different gestagen/estrogen combinations. *Acta Psychiatr. Scand. [Suppl.]* 236:3-74 (1972).

27. A. E. Maxwell, Difficulties in a dimensional description of symptomatology. *Br. J. Psychiatry* 121:19-26 (1972).

28. J. L. Fleiss, Classification of the depressive disorders by numerical typology. *J. Psychiatr. Res.* 9:141-153 (1972).

29. R. L. Spitzer, J. Endicott, and E. Robins, *Research Diagnostic Criteria (RDC) for a Selected Group of Functional Disorders,* 3rd ed. N.Y.S. Psychiatric Institute, New York, 1978.

30. R. L. Spitzer, J. Endicott, and E. Robins, Research Diagnostic Criteria: rationale and reliability. *Arch. Gen. Psychiatry* 35:773-782 (1978).

31. J. Davidson, C. Turnbull, R. Miller, and J. Sullivan, Atypical vegetative symptoms and atypical depression. (Manuscript submitted for publication, 1980).

32. M. R. Liebowitz and D. F. Klein, Hysteroid dysphoria. *Psychiatr. Clin. North Am.* 2:555-575 (1979).

33. D. J. Kupfer and T. P. Detre, Tricyclic and monoamine oxidase-inhibitor antidepressants, in *Handbook of Psychopharmacology,* Vol. 14: *Affective Disorder: Drug Actions in Animal and Man* (L. L. Iverson, S. D. Iverson, and S. Snyder, eds.). Plenum, New York, 1978, pp. 199-232.

34. A. Nies and D. Robinson, Monoamine oxidase inhibitors, in *Handbook of Affective Disorders* (E. Paykel, ed.). Churchill Livingstone, Edinburgh, 1980.

35. M. Steiner, R. F. Haskett, and B. J. Carroll, Premenstrual tension syndrome: The development of research diagnostic criteria and new rating scales. *Acta Psychiatr. Scand.* 62:177-190 (1980).

36. C. W. Serif, A psychosocial perspective on the menstrual cycle, in *The Psychobiology of Sex Differences and Roles* (S. I. Parson, ed.). Hemisphere Publ. Co., New York, 1980, pp. 245-268.

13 Estrogens and Central Nervous System Function: Electroencephalography, Cognition, and Depression

EDWARD L. KLAIBER   The Worcester Foundation for Experimental Biology, Shrewsbury, Massachusetts

DONALD M.BROVERMAN, WILLIAM VOGEL, and JAMES A. KENNEDY
Worcester State Hospital, Worcester, Massachusetts

CONRAD J. L. NADEAU   University of Massachusetts Medical Center, Worcester, Massachusetts

The possibility that estrogens have psychotropic properties has long been of historic interest (Sevringhaus, 1933; Wiesbader and Kurzrok, 1938; Ripley et al., 1940). Recently, this possibility has been the subject of increased investigation by both basic and clinical researchers. A systematic approach to this problem requires several levels of inquiry.

First, there is a need to establish rational physiological mechanisms by which estrogens might exert an influence on central nervous system neural functioning. Second, techniques must be established which permit objective measurements of the postulated effects of estrogens on central nervous system functioning. Third, if estrogens do affect central nervous system functioning, and if estrogens are to be considered psychotropic agents, behavioral manifestations of these influences should exist in cognitive activity and/or emotional states.

This chapter is organized around these three problem areas and will present the theoretical viewpoint that estrogens do act to enhance or facilitate adrenergic functioning in the central nervous system through a number of physiological mechanisms.

The requirement of an objective index of estrogens' effects on brain function is dealt with by describing studies of the influence of estrogens on electroencephalographic (EEG) responses to photic stimulation, an index known to be sensitive to adrenergic stimulants and depressants.

The psychotropic effects of estrogens are demonstrated by two studies: one examines changes in cognitive task performances across the menstrual cycle; the second investigates the use of estrogen in the treatment of depression in women. Estrogen's effect in both instances is believed to be achieved through stimulation of the adrenergic portion of the central nervous system.

I. Mechanisms of Action of Estrogens on Central Nervous System Adrenergic Functioning

Estrogens have been reported to affect several different physiological mechanisms which could influence central nervous system adrenergic functioning. These mechanisms include: (1) stimulation by estrogens of the synthesis of adrenergic neurotransmitters; (2) an estrogen-induced inhibition of the degradation of adrenergic neurotransmitters; and (3) blocking by estrogens of the synaptic reuptake of norepinephrine with a consequent potentiation of the neurotransmitters synaptic activity.

II. Effects of Estrogens on the Synthesis of Adrenergic Neurotransmitters

The administration of ethinyl estradiol to mice pretreated with monoamine oxidase (MAO) inhibitors resulted in an increased norepinephrine content in various portions of the brain (Greengrass and Tonge, 1974). A similar significant norepinephrine increase was found in the hypothalamus of the anestrous ewe following estradiol treatment (Kendall and Narayana, 1978). However, since there was no pretreatment with an MAO inhibitor, the increase in norepinephrine could have been due to an inhibitory effect of estrogen on MAO activity.

Tyrosine hydroxylase is the rate-limiting enzyme in the synthesis of norepinephrine. An increase in the activity of this enzyme should result in an increase in the synthesis of norepinephrine. Beattie et al. (1973) found that estrogen administration produced a rise in hypothalamic tyrosine hydroxylase activity in the ovariectomized rat. However, Luine et al. (1977), using a different experimental design, failed to find this effect.

III. Effects of Estrogens on Neurotransmitter Degradation

Estrogens may also decrease the rate of degradation of adrenergic neurotransmitters. Estradiol has been reported to inhibit MAO in rat hypothalamus (Kobayashi et al., 1966); in rat amygdala and hypothalamus (Luine et al., 1975); and in mouse pituitary (Srivastava et al., 1978). MAO is the principle enzyme involved in the intraneuronal metabolism of adrenergic neurotransmitters. Estrogens have also been reported to inhibit MAO activity in human plasma (Klaiber et al., 1971; Klaiber et al., 1972); and plasma estradiol levels have been found to be negatively correlated with plasma MAO activity (Briggs and Briggs, 1972).

Estradiol treatment has also been found to sustain levels of norepinephrine in the lateral septum of ovariectomized rats that were treated with a norepinephrine synthesis blocking agent (Crowley et al., 1978), suggesting that estradiol inhibited the destruction of norepinephrine by MAO.

Finally, catechol estrogens, metabolites of estradiol, have been demonstrated to inhibit competitively the enzymatic methylation and biologic inactivation of circulating norepinephrine by catechol-o-methyltransferase with a concommitant potentiation of norepinephrine pressor effects (Ball et al., 1972).

IV. Effects of Estrogens on Neurotransmitter Uptake

Estrogens may block the neuronal reuptake of adrenergic neurotransmitters at the synapse, potentiating their synaptic action. Estradiol has been reported to inhibit the uptake of norepinephrine by synaptosomes (Janowsky and Daris, 1970); and synaptosomal membrane fragments from rat brain bound significantly less norepinephrine in the presence of estradiol (Inaba and Kamata, 1979).

V. Interactions of Estrogen with Progesterone and Testosterone

While estrogens may significantly influence certain neural mechanisms in the adrenergic portion of the central nervous system, other gonadal hormones, such as progesterone and testosterone, may block or oppose the actions of estrogens. For instance, whereas estradiol has been reported to increase tyrosine hydroxylase activity, progesterone apparently decreases the activity of this enzyme (Beattie et al., 1973). Progesterone also blocked estrogen's action in sustaining brain norepinephrine levels in ovariectomized rats treated with a norepinephrine synthesis blocking agent (Crowley et al., 1978); and the administration of medroxyprogesterone has been reported to reverse the estrogen-induced inhibition of plasma monoamine oxidase activity in women (Klaiber et al., 1971).

While estradiol administration lowered MAO activity, testosterone administration increases MAO activity in female rat tissue (Wurtman and Axelrod, 1963). Further, testosterone blocked estradiol's inhibition of the binding of norepinephrine by the synaptosomal membrane fragments (Inaba and Kamata, 1979).

The actions of progesterone and testosterone in blocking or opposing estrogen's effects on adrenergic mechanisms should be considered when attempting to assess estrogen's influence on central nervous system adrenergic functioning.

An abundance of evidence supports the possibility that physiological mechanisms exist which could enable estrogens to facilitate or enhance central nervous system adrenergic functioning. Section VI deals with objective studies demonstrating such an effect of estrogens.

VI. Effects of Estrogen and Progesterone on the EEG Photic Driving Index

EEG rhythms tend to synchronize with the frequency of a bright flashing light, and this is termed an EEG photic driving response. Previous research has shown that the frequency of EEG photic driving responses is sensitive to drugs which either stimulate or block adrenergic functions. Adrenergic stimulants such as noradrenaline, amphetamine, nicotine (cigarette smoking), and MAO inhibitors have been reported to diminish the frequency of EEG photic driving responses (Floru et al., 1962; Shetty, 1971; Vogel et al., 1974; Vogel et al., 1977). On the other hand, substances which block central adrenergic functioning, such as the phenothiazines, tend to increase the frequency of EEG photic driving responses (Jorgensen and Wulff, 1958; Wilson and Glotfelthy, 1958; Misurec and Nahanek, 1964; Killam et al., 1967). The frequency of EEG photic driving responses would, therefore, seem a useful index of central adrenergic nervous system functioning.

VII. Cyclic Changes of EEG Photic Driving Responses Across the Menstrual Cycle

Since cyclic changes in estrogen and progesterone production occur across the menstrual cycle, and since we hypothesize that these hormones influence central adrenergic functioning, it can be predicted that corresponding cyclic changes in the frequency of EEG photic driving responses would also occur across the menstrual cycle.

The specific hormonal events of interest in the menstrual cycle are the sharp rise and fall of blood estradiol levels just before ovulation; and the secondary rise of blood estradiol with the accompanying rise of blood progesterone after ovulation (Fig. 1). As stated earlier, the rise in progesterone is important since progesterone in some instances opposes the neurophysiological effects of estradiol (Klaiber et al., 1971); Rodier, 1971; Beattie et al., 1973; Crowley et al., 1978).

The basal body temperature reflects the changes in blood levels of estradiol and progesterone across the menstrual cycle. The lowest point of the basal body temperature, the thermal nadir, coincides with the peak blood estradiol level just before ovulation. After ovulation, a sustained rise in basal body temperature occurs as progesterone blood levels increase. Peak temperatures coincide with the highest progesterone levels (De Allende, 1956).

In the preovulatory phase of the cycle, when estrogen levels are rising and when progesterone levels are at their lowest point, central adrenergic states should be enhanced and the frequency of EEG photic driving responses should be reduced. On the other hand, in the postovulatory phase of the cycle when levels of both estrogen and progesterone are high, the opposition of progesterone to estrogen should result in a diminished central adrenergic state, and, consequently, the frequency of EEG photic driving responses should be greater.

This predicted cyclicity in EEG photic driving responses was observed across two menstrual cycles in 14 healthy young women who had basal body temperature records suggestive of ovulation in both cycles (Fig. 2) (Vogel et al., 1971).

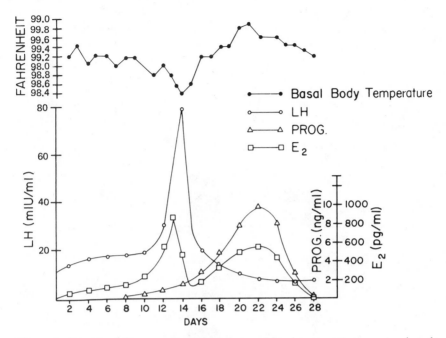

Figure 1 Basal body temperature and hormonal levels across the menstrual cycle. LH = luteinizing hormone, PROG = progesterone, E_2 = estradiol. (From Broverman et al., Copyright 1981 by the American Psychological Association. Reprinted/adapted by permission of the publisher and author.)

VIII. Manipulations of EEG Photic Driving Responses in Amenorrheic and Depressed Women by the Administration of Estrogens

Women with secondary amenorrhea do not have the cyclic changes of estrogen and progesterone observed in regularly menstruating women. Interestingly, the mean level of EEG photic driving responses in a group of six women with secondary amenorrhea was found to be significantly elevated compared with that found in both the pre- and postovulatory phases of the menstrual cycles of regularly menstruating women (Fig. 3).

The administration of oral conjugated estrogens to amenorrheic women resulted in a significant decrease in the frequency of EEG photic driving responses, while the administration of a progestin (medroxyprogesterone) in conjunction with the estrogen resulted in an increase in the frequency of EEG photic driving responses to a level significantly greater than that observed with estrogen alone (Fig. 3) (Vogel et al., 1971). A similar suppressive effect of oral conjugated estro-

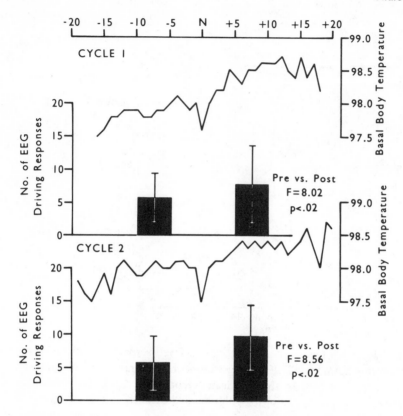

Figure 2 EEG driving responses pre- and postovulation in 14 regularly menstruating women. (From E. L. Klaiber, D. M. Broverman, W. Vogel, and Y. Kobayashi, Rhythms in plasma MAO activity, EEG, and behavior during the menstrual cycle, *Biorhythms and Human Reproduction,* M. Ferin, F. Halberg, R. M. Richart, and R. L. Vande Wiele, eds. John Wiley and Sons, New York, 1974.)

gen administration on EEG photic driving responses in a group of outpatient depressed women was reported by Klaiber et al. (1972).

   Both correlative and manipulative data, therefore, support the hypothesis that estrogen and progesterone affect EEG photic driving responses. The variations in the frequency of EEG photic driving responses induced by the gonadal steroid hormones reflect, we believe, corresponding variations in central nervous system adrenergic functioning. The EEG results also suggest that central nervous system adrenergic functioning is enhanced in the preovulatory phase of the menstrual cycle compared with the postovulatory phase of the cycle.

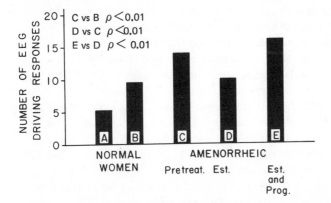

Figure 3   EEG driving responses in six amenorrheic women before and after treatment with estrogens and estrogens and a progestin. (From E. L. Klaiber, D. M. Broverman, W. Vogel, and Y. Kobayashi. Rhythms in plasma MAO activity, EEG, and behavior during the menstrual cycle, *Biorhythms and Human Reproduction,* M. Ferin, F. Halberg, R. M. Richart, and R. L. Vande Wiele, eds. John Wiley and Sons, New York, 1974).

IX. Estrogens and Cognitive Task Performances

The EEG studies described above support the hypothesis that estrogens augment central nervous system adrenergic functioning. Estrogens might be expected to affect human behavior similarly to adrenergic stimulants. Adrenergic stimulants and depressants are known to affect two categories of behaviors differentially: "automatized" behaviors and "perceptual-restructuring" behaviors.

Automatized behaviors refer to those behaviors that so highly practiced and overlearned that minimums of conscious attention are required for their effective execution (Ach, 1905). Automatization ability is measured by such tasks as speed of reading, color naming, naming objects, etc. (Broverman, 1964).

Perceptual-restructuring tasks are tasks in which the initial "automatized" perceptual responses to obvious stimulus attributes must be inhibited or set aside in favor of responses to less obvious, hidden or embedded stimulus attributes, e.g., the Embedded Figures test (Witkin, 1950).

A cluster of perceptual-restructuring tasks has been identified by factor analytic studies (Broverman, 1964; Goodenough and Karp, 1961; Podell and Phillips, 1959; Thurstone, 1944). Besides the Witkin Embedded Figures Tasks, this cluster includes such other well-known tasks as the Thurstone Gottschaldt (Thurstone, 1944), the Wechsler (Kohs) Block Design subtest (Wechsler, 1955), and the Porteus Mazes (Porteus, 1950).

Adrenergic stimulants such as amphetamine and caffeine enhance performances of such automatized tasks as color naming (Callaway and Stone, 1960), speed of reading (Florey and Gilbert, 1943), and typing (Hollingworth, 1912). On the other hand, a recent unpublished study in our laboratory indicates that caffeine, an adrenergic stimulant, impairs performance of the Embedded Figures Task (Witkin, 1950), a perceptual-restructuring task.

The adrenergic depressant, chlorpromazine, has been reported to impair performances of automatized tasks, such as tapping speed (Lehmann and Csank, 1957), Digit Symbol subtest (Kornetsky et al., 1957), and a repetitive task requiring perceptual alertness (Primac et al., 1957). On the other hand, chlorpromazine facilitated performances of such perceptual-restructuring tasks as the Porteus Maze test (Helper et al., 1963), and speed of counting backwards, which requires inhibition of the automatized tendency to count forwards (Shatin et al., 1956). Similar effects of these drugs have been reported on performances of analogous tasks by animals (Broverman, et al., 1968).

Considerable evidence supports the hypothesis that adrenergic stimulants enhance the performances of "automatized" tasks and impair the performances of "perceptual-restructuring" tasks. This pattern of change in cognitive functioning should occur with estrogen administration if estrogen acts as an adrenergic stimulant. Ideally, this hypothesis should be tested in a manipulative study which involves cognitive testing before and after estrogen administration. Unfortunately, no such study has been carried out.

Another approach to testing the hypothesis is a correlative examination of cognitive performances across situations in which estrogen levels are known to vary, e.g., the menstrual cycle.

Our theory predicts that, in women who ovulate, the peaking of estrogen blood levels just before ovulation should enhance performances of automatized tasks and impair performances of perceptual-restructuring tasks. In contrast, since progesterone appears to block some of the physiologic actions of estrogen, the rising levels of progesterone after ovulation should act to impair performances of automatization tasks and enhance performances of perceptual-restructuring tasks (Fig. 4).

This hypothesis was supported in a study of 87 regularly menstruating women (Broverman et al., 1981). However, the extent of the predicted changes in performances of the two categories of tasks was a function of how close the testing sessions were to the preovulatory estradiol peak; and to the postovulatory progesterone peak, as inferred from basal body temperature records. The greater the temporal distance from the peaks, the less evident were the predicted effects.

The predicted effects were also not evident in 21 women whose basal body temperature records suggested that ovulation did not occur in the observed cycles. The usual rise and fall of estradiol and progesterone does not occur in anovulatory cycles. In any sample of regularly menstruating women, approximately 25% of their cycles are anovulatory (De Allende, 1956).

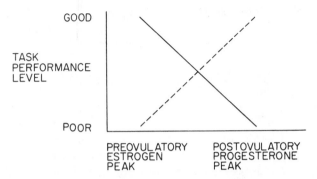

Figure 4   Theoretically predicted performance levels of automatization (solid line) and perceptual-restructuring (broken line) task at different phases of the menstrual cycle. (From Broverman et al., Copyright 1981 by the American Psychological Association. Reprinted/adapted by permission of the publisher and author.)

Failure to exclude anovulatory cycles, and failure to take into account the precise time of the testing periods relative to the presumed hormonal peaks may account for the many studies reporting a noncyclicity of cognitive performances across the menstrual cycle (Wickham, 1958; Sommer, 1972; Messent, 1976; Munchel, 1979).

As noted above, the effects of the gonadal hormones on cognitive performances differ as a function of type of cognitive task employed. Other tasks, which are neither automatized nor perceptual-restructuring in nature, may show no hormonal effects at all. Task selection is therefore also a critical factor in demonstrating the effects of gonadal hormones on behavior.

The adaptive values of the two categories of cognitive behaviors sensitive to menstrual cycle hormonal changes, automatization and perceptual-restructuring behaviors have been noted in the literature. For instance, the ability to automatize tasks is considered essential for the release of attention from performances of learned aspects of behavior so that attention may be focused on mastery of novel tasks (Ford, 1929). Conversely, an inability to automatize effectively would preclude proficiency in such critical "automatized" behaviors as speech (Humphrey, 1951) and reading (Bryan and Harter, 1899). Empirically, poor automatization ability has been found in dyslexic children (Drake and Schnall, 1966; Eakin and Douglas, 1971; Vogel et al., 1976). Men with superior automatization ability were found to have higher socioeconomic status occupations and greater income compated with men of comparable age and intelligence but with lesser automatization ability (Broverman, 1964).

The ability to perform perceptual-restructuring tasks, on the other hand, has been linked to developmental status and adult creativity (Witkin et al., 1962);

and to superior ability in the physical sciences (Macfarlane Smith, 1964). Both categories of behavior appear to have adaptive value.

Whether or not cognitive abilities vary systematically across the menstrual cycle is a legitimate concern of feminists. Their concern is that if cognition were shown to vary with the menstrual cycle, this would be used as evidence against the suitability of women for various types of employment. It should therefore be noted that our study was not designed to assess the functional significance of the observed changes in performances, and the results should not be taken as evidence of a functionally significant impairment or enhancement of abilities at different stages of the cycle. Moreover, cyclicity in cognitive performance is not unique to women. Comparable changes in the performances of these same tasks were observed in men from morning to afternoon, which is when significant diurnal changes in testosterone production are known to exist (Mackenberg et al., 1974). The present study was designed to test the theoretical hypothesis that menstrual-cycle-related changes of gonadal hormones affect cognitive functions in adult women in predictable ways. Our results are therefore primarily of theoretical importance.

X. Estrogens and Mental Depression

We have hypothesized that estrogens enhance central nervous system adrenergic functioning. Schildkraut (1965) has hypothesized that depression involves a deficiency of norepinephrine in the adrenergic portion of the central nervous system. If both hypotheses are correct, it would be reasonable to expect that estrogens might act as antidepressants.

This hypothesis was confirmed in a double-blind study (Klaiber et al., 1979). Forty pre- and postmenopausal inpatients with primary, recurrent, unipolar, incapacitating, endogenous, major depressive disorders were studied. These patients had failed to respond to conventional therapies. After a month of placebo medication, large doses (15 to 25 mg/day) of oral conjugated estrogens were administered for 3 months to 23 of the women, while placebos were continued over 3 months in the remaining 17. The decision to employ high doses of estrogens was based on preliminary empiric observations made during a pilot study. In this study, it was observed that alleviation of symptoms in severe depressed states required high doses of estrogen. The estrogen administration was cyclic with the addition of a progestin (medroxyprogesterone) in the last 5 days of estrogen administration. Weekly ratings of depression were obtained throughout the study period using the Hamilton rating scale (Hamilton, 1960). The posttreatment Hamilton ratings of depression were significantly reduced in the estrogen-treated group, but not in the placebo group.

Table 1 shows that the estrogen and placebo treatment groups had very similar mean Hamilton pretreatment scores (31.2 and 30.6, respectively). However,

Table 1 Mean Hamilton Depression Ratings Before and After 3 Months of Estrogen or Placebo Treatment

		Pretreatment	Posttreatment	Posttreatment minus Pretreatment
Estrogen-treated patients (n = 23)	Mean	31.2	22.0	9.2
	SD	5.3	8.2	8.2
Placebo-treated patients (n = 17)	Mean	30.6	30.5	0.1
	SD	7.2	9.2	5.1
t test				4.01
				P <0.0005

Source: E. L. Klaiber, D. M. Broverman, W. Vogel, and Y. Kobayashi, Estrogen therapy for severe persistent depressions in women, *Arch. Gen. Psychiatry* 36:550-554. Copyright 1979, American Medical Association.

the score for the estrogen treatment group declined an average of 9.2 points (from 31.2 to 22.0), whereas the score for the placebo treatment group declined only 0.1 point. This difference was statistically significant ($t = 4.01; P < 0.0005$, df = 38).

Although a statistically significant improvement was observed in the 23 estrogen-treated patients, their average Hamilton level after 3 months of treatment was still quite high (22.0). However, for these severely depressed subjects, the average 9.2 point improvement seemed to trained observers to be clinically as well as statistically significant. Moreover, as shown in Table 2, considerable variability existed in the Hamilton ratings after 3 months of treatment. For example, six of the estrogen-treated patients showed improvements of more than 15 points and had a posttreatment mean Hamilton rating of 13.8. For some of the patients, therefore, the response to estrogen therapy was very marked. However, two patients became worse on estrogen treatment. In comparison, none of the patients in the placebo group showed 10 or more points of improvement, and the condition of eight patients worsened.

In view of the wide range of response to the estrogen therapy, we attempted to ascertain what factors, if any, were associated with improvement in response to estrogen treatment.

Neither menopausal status nor age were significantly related to amount of improvement. Length of previous illness was the only variable found to be significantly related to degree of improvement.

Table 2 Amounts of Improvement in Hamilton Ratings of Depression Before and After 3 Months of Estrogen or Placebo Treatment

Amount of improvement	Estrogen treatment			Placebo treatment		
	Number of patients	Mean pretreatment	Mean posttreatment	Number of patients	Mean pretreatment	Mean posttreatment
15 or more points	6	33.1 ± 4.9	13.8 ± 6.5	0	—	—
10 to 14 points	5	33.0 ± 4.1	21.2 ± 3.4	0	—	—
5 to 9 points	4	29.7 ± 6.1	22.2 ± 5.6	3	29.4 ± 10.2	22.5 ± 9.5
0 to 4 points	6	29.9 ± 6.6	26.7 ± 7.5	6	29.7 ± 6.5	26.8 ± 6.6
Became worse	2	27.8 ± 2.8	34.1 ± 3.9	8	31.6 ± 7.4	36.2 ± 7.9

Source E. L. Klaiber, D. M. Broverman, W. Vogel, and Y. Kobayashi, Estrogen therapy for severe persistent depressions in women, *Arch. Gen. Psychiatry* 36:550–554. Copyright 1979, American Medical Association.

The results of this study support the hypothesis that estrogens have antidepressant properties. Other studies have also reported that estrogens act to improve mood and psychological status of both elderly institutionalized and noninstitutionalized women (Kantor et al., 1978; Kantor et al, 1973; Kerr, 1968). However, these subjects were not severely depressed, and dosage levels of estrogens were conventional, e.g., 0.3 mg Premarin daily. Schiff et al. (1979) also reported tha nondepressed menopausal women treated with oral conjugated estrogen (0.625 mg daily) showed an improvement in psychological functioning and sleep activity.

XI. Adverse Effects of High Dose Estrogen Therapy

A major issue in the use of high doses of estrogens as antidepressants is the possible adverse effects of therapy. This issue may be addressed by weighing the possible risks of the therapy against the risks associated with the patient's illness. The women we treated were chronically and severely depressed. All had failed to respond to conventional antidepressant treatment. The risk of suicide in such a population is high. Twenty-five of the 40 patients (62.5%) had made serious suicide attempts before entering this program. All of the patients expressed suicidal thoughts ranging from mild to severe, and a number of suicides were attempted during the study period. In addition to the suicide risk, these women faced an extremely high risk of life-long debilitation from their severe chronic depressive state.

Several other studies (Smith et al., 1975; Mack et al., 1976) have reported an increased risk of endometrial cancer in postmenopausal women who received estrogen therapy as treatment for menopausal symptoms. It has been known for many years that sustained estrogen treatment can induce endometrial hyperplasia (Lipsett, 1974). An advanced stage of endometrial hyperplasia, adenomatous hyperplasia, has been shown to be a precursor of endometrial carcinoma in some cases (Gusberg, 1947). The risk of endometrial hyperplasia can be reduced if estrogens are administered cyclically with a progestin added near the end of the cycle (Kistner, 1971; Campbell et al., 1978; Paterson et al., 1980). All of our patients were treated in this manner. Recent reports (Gambrell et al., 1979; Hammond et al., 1979) indicate that the use of a progestin in conjunction with estrogen treatment significantly reduces the risk of endometrial carcinoma compared with estrogen treatment alone. In fact, in one study (Gambrell et al., 1979) fewer cancers were observed in the estrogen-progestin-treated group than in an untreated group, although this was not a statistically significant difference. Obviously, further time and study are required to determine if progestin truly protests against endometrial cancer. In the meantime, all women receiving high dose estrogen treatment for depression must be carefully monitored.

Our patients receiving high doses of estrogen have been followed with periodic endometrial biopsies to assess the status of the endometrium. Endometrial hyperplasias have been detected in 12% of our patients. When hyperplasia is detected, the progestin dosage is increased in an attempt to reverse the hyperplasia. If hyperplasia persists, estrogen treatment is discontinued. It is our opinion that this regime decreases the risk of endometrial carcinoma.

At present, however, because of the carcinoma risk factor, we are using high dose estrogen treatment only in severely depressed women who have a history of resistance to conventional therapy. In such instances, estrogen may be life-saving because of the high incidence of suicidal attempts in these women when their depressive states cannot be relieved.

Other adverse effects of estrogen include breast tenderness, nausea, and vomiting. We observed few such problems and they tended to disappear after a month of treatment. Reports exist of increased risk of thrombophlebitis with oral contraceptives (Inman et al., 1970; Boston Collaborative Drug Surveillance Program, 1973). However, no documented reports of thrombosis or embolism attributable to conjugated estrogens exist (Boston Collaborative Drug Surveillance Program, 1974), and we did not observe these problems in our patients treated with high doses of estrogens.

XII. Hormonal Characteristics of Depressed Women

The fact that estrogens act as antidepressant agents in depressed women raises questions regarding the hormonal status of these women compared with nondepressed women. As noted earlier, neither menopausal status nor age were significant factors in the therapeutic response to estrogens, i.e., estrogen administration was effective in both elderly menopausal women and younger women with regular menstrual cycles. The effectiveness of exogenous estrogens in the latter group is particularly puzzling since, presumably, these women already had adequate endogenous estrogens as evidenced by their regular menstrual cycles. The antidepressant response to estrogen of these young women could, conceivably, be a pharmacologic effect induced by the massive doses of administered estrogens, or the result of an abnormality involving estrogen metabolism in the depressed patients. The study described below was an attempt to explore this possibility (Vogel et al., 1978).

Testosterone metabolism in depressed women was also studied because testosterone may, in some instances, oppose the action of estrogens (Inaba and Kamata, 1979). The studies involved blood concentrations of estradiol and testosterone as well as metabolic clearance and production rates of these hormones.

Plasma estradiol and testosterone concentrations were studied across the menstrual cycle in 22 ovulatory depressed women and in 10 ovulatory nondepressed women who served as control subjects. The two groups were of equivalent mean age.

The results indicated that the mean plasma estradiol levels of the depressed women were significantly higher than those found in the nondepressed women in the week before ovulation and in the week after ovulation, but not during ovulation itself. Significant positive correlations were observed between the weekly estradiol levels of the depressed patients and their Hamilton ratings of depression for the same period; the greater the blood estradiol concentration, the higher the Hamilton rating of depression.

Plasma testosterone concentrations were also found to be significantly elevated in the depressed women compared with the nondepressed women.

Blood metabolic clearance and blood production rates of estradiol and testosterone were determined in 11 depressed ovulatory women and 10 nondepressed ovulatory women. Both groups were matched for age and body weight. Baird et al. (1969) have published a full discussion of these techniques.

The ovulating depressed women had significantly lower mean metabolic clearance rates of estradiol, but not significantly different production rates of estradiol compared with the nondepressed women. Thus, the depressed women were producing estradiol at a normal rate, but were clearing it from the blood at a significantly reduced rate which may account for the elevated plasma estradiol levels noted in depressed women earlier.

The depressed women also had significantly higher production rates of testosterone than did nondepressed women.

In summary, depressed women compared with nondepressed women, have significant elevations in (1) plasma estradiol levels, (2) plasma testosterone levels, and (3) blood production rates of testosterone. However, depressed women have significantly lower metabolic clearance rates of estradiol. No significant difference exists between the blood estradiol production rates of depressed and nondepressed women.

These results do not, in themselves, provide a definitive understanding of the role of gonadal hormones in depression. They do, however, raise many questions and suggest several possibilities.

We have previously reported that the administration of large doses of estrogens to depressed women tended to alleviate depressive symptoms. However, our data indicate that depressed women tend to have normal production rates of estradiol and high levels of circulating estradiol. Apparently, the adequate amounts of estradiol produced and circulating in depressed women are unable to achieve the antidepressant effects accomplished by additional exogenous estrogens. Therefore, in the depressed women an unknown factor may be producing a resistance to estrogen by preventing the adequate endogenous supplies of estradiol from carrying out their physiological function on brain tissue.

A physiological resistance to estrogen could occur in several ways. For example, an excessive binding of estradiol by a specific binding protein in the plasma would make less unbound circulating estradiol available for action at tissue receptor sites. Large amounts of administered estrogen might be capable of saturating the plasma binding capacity, thereby increasing the level of unbound estradiol available to tissue receptors. If excess binding of estradiol in the plasma exists in depressed women, thereby producing a retention and elevation of estradiol in the plasma, and if estrogen is an antidepressant, a positive correlation might be expected between plasma estradiol and the degree of depression, as we reported above.

Other mechanisms that could produce an estorgen resistance would be (1) a deficiency of estradiol tissue receptor sites, or (2) an abnormally low affinity for estradiol of the estradiol tissue receptors. High doses of estrogen might overcome either problem by stimulating the producition of estradiol receptors or by overcoming a low affinity by mass action. Again, these possibilities would not account for the elevated plasma estradiol levels nor their positive correlation with the degree of depression.

The increased testosterone production found in depressed women may influence estrogens actions on the brain since testosterone blocks or opposes some estrogen activity.

Finally, the high doses of estrogen required to alleviate depressive symptoms may be required, not to overcome an estrogen resistance factor, but rather to exert a pharmacologic antidepressant effect of unknown nature.

XIII. Conclusion

Our review supports the hypothesis that estrogens act to enhance adrenergic functioning in the central nervous system. Several physiological mechanisms that might produce this effect have now been reported.

Our data on changes in EEG photic driving across the menstrual cycle and before and after estrogen administration (Vogel et al., 1971) provide objective evidence that both endogenous and administered estrogens significantly affect brain function in a manner that would be expected if estrogens act as adrenergic stimulants.

Similarly, the changes in performances of cognitive tasks across the menstrual cycle (Broverman et al., 1981) are the changes expected if estrogesn act as adrenergic stimulants.

Finally, large doses of estrogens administered to clinically depressed women significantly ameliorated depressive symptoms (Klaiber et al., 1979). Again, this would follow from the perspective of Schildkraut's (1965) catecholamine deficiency hypothesis of depression, if estrogens enhance central nervous system adrenergic functioning.

Our review, however, also revealed a number of complicating factors that may have acted to obscure or prevent earlier demonstrations of an adrenergic effect of estrogen. These include (1) the capacities of other steroid hormones, primarily progesterone, but also testosterone, to oppose the physiological and behavioral effects of estrogen; (2) the need to align closely behavioral measures across the menstrual cycle with the relatively brief midcycle peak of estradiol and the postovulatory peak of progesterone; and (3) endocrine abnormalities that may exist in depressed persons which may result in a need for higher than usual doses of estrogen to produce desired or expected effects.

Finally, we must recognize the many claims of serious side effects associated with estrogen administration. Some of these concerns appear to be inappropriate generalizations from birth control preparations and other synthetic estrogens that do not apply to conjugated estrogens. However, the most serious warning is the possibility that oral conjugated estrogen administration increases the risk of endometrial carcinoma. The methodology, significance, and shortcomings of the studies involved have been discussed at length (Weiss, 1975; Gordan and Greenberg, 1976; Horowitz and Feinstein, 1978). There is a growing feeling among many physicians that the original warnings were overstated.

Perhaps the most important recent development in this area of concern is the appearance of several new studies indicating that the cyclic administration of estrogen with progestins reduces the risk of endometrial cancer (Gambrell et al., 1979; Hammond et al., 1979). Nevertheless, close monitoring of patients and periodic endometrial biopsies continue to be appropriate when administering estrogens.

The apparent and potential benefits of estrogens suggest that intensive research must be continued in this area of the effects and clinical uses of estrogen.

Acknowledgment

These studies were supported, in part, by USPHS grants MH-18757, MH-11291, MH-26424, and a grant-in-aid from Ayerst Laboratories.

References

Ach, N. (1905). Uber die Willenstaetigkeit und das Denken. Goettingen, Vandenhoeck und Ruprecht. Translated in *Organization and Pathology of Thought* (D. Rapaport, ed.). Columbia University Press, New York, 1951.

Baird, D. T., R. Horton, C. Longcope, and J. F. Tait (1969). Steroid dynamics under steady-state conditions. In *Recent Progress in Hormone Research*, vol. 25 (E. B. Astwood, ed.). Academic, New York, pp. 611-664.

Ball, P., R. Knuppen, M. Haupt, and H. Breuer (1972). Interactions between estrogens and catechol amines. III. Studies on the methylation of catechol estrogens, catechol amines and other catechols by the catechol-o-methyltransferase of human liver. *J. Clin. Endocrinol.* 34:736-746.

Beattie, C. W., C. H. Rodgers, and L. F. Soyka (1973). Influence of ovariectomy and ovarian steroids on hypothalamic tyrosine hydroxylase activity in the rat. *Endocrinology* 91:276-286.

Boston Collaborative Drug Surveillance Program (1973). Oral contraceptives and venous thromboembolic disease, surgically confirmed gallbladder disease, and breast tumours. *Lancet* 1:1399-1404.

Boston Collaborative Drug Surveillance Program (1974). Surgically confirmed gallbladder disease, venous thromboembolism, and breast tumors in relation to postmenopausal estrogen therapy. *N. Engl. J. Med.* 290:15-19.

Briggs, M., and M. Briggs (1972). Relationship between monoamine oxidase activity and sex hormone concentration in human blood plasma. *J. Reprod. Fertil.* 29:447-450.

Broverman, D. M. (1964). Generality and behavioral correlates of cognitive styles. *J. Consult. Psychol.* 28:487-500.

Broverman, D. M., E. L. Klaiber, Y. Kobayashi, and W. Vogel (1968). Roles of activation and inhibition in sex differences in cognitive abilities. *Psychol. Rev.* 75:23-50.

Broverman, D. M., D. Majcher, D. Shea, V. Paul, E. L. Klaiber, and W. Vogel (1981). Changes in cognitive task performance across the menstrual cycle. *J. Comp. Physiol. Psychol.* 95:646-654.

Bryan, W. L., and N. Harter (1899). Studies on the telegraphic language: the acquisition of a hierarchy of habits. *Psychol. Rev.* 4:345-375.

Callaway, E. III, and G. Stone (1960). Re-evaluating focus of attention, in *Drug and Behavior* (L. Uhr and J. G. Miller, eds.). John Wiley, New York, pp. 393-398.

Campbell, S., J. McQueen, J. Minardi, and M. I. Whitehead (1978). The role of progesterone in peri- and post menopausal hormone replacement therapy. *Postgrad. Med. J.* 54:1-100.

Crowley, W. R., T. L. O'Donohue, H. Wachslight, and D. M. Jacobowitz (1978). Effect of estrogens and progesterone on plasma gonadotrophins and on catecholamine levels and turnover in discrete brain regions of ovariectomized rats. *Brain Res.* 154:345-357.

De Allende, I. L. C. (1956). Anovulatory cycles in women. *Am. J. Anat.* 98: 293-305.

Drake, C., and M. Schnall (1966). Decoding problems in reading. *Pathways Child Guidance* 3:1-12.

Eakin, S., and V. I. Douglas (1971). Automatization and oral reading problems in children. *J. Learning Disabil.* 4:31-33.

Florey, C. D., and J. Gilbert (1943). The effects of benzedrine sulfate and caffeine citrate on the efficiency of college students. *J. Appl. Psychol.* 27:121-134.

Floru, R., A. Costin, V. Nestianu, and M. Sterescu-Volanschi (1962). Researches concerning the effect of noradrenaline upon the electrical activity of the central nervous system and upon the evoked rhythm of intermittent photic stimulation in cats with chronic electrodes. *Electroencephalogr. Clin. Neuriphysiol.* 14:566.

Ford, A. (1929). Attention-automatization: the transitional nature of mind. *Am. J. Psychol.* 41:1-32.

Gambrell, R. D., F. M. Massey, T. A. Castaneda, A. J. Ugenas, and C. A. Ricci (1979). Reduced incidence of endometrial cancer among women treated with progestogens. *J. Am. Geriatr. Soc.* 27:389-394.

Goodenough, D. R., and S. A. Karp (1961). Field dependence and intellectual functioning. *J. Abnorm. Soc. Psychol.* 63:241-246.

Gordan, G. S., and S. G. Greenberg. (1976). Exogenous estrogens and endometrial cancer. *Postgrad. Med.* 59:66.

Greengrass, P. M., and S. R. Tonge (1974). The accumulation of noradrenaline and 5-hydroxytryptamine in three regions of mouse brain after tetrabenazine and iproniazid: effects of ethinyloestradiol and progesterone. *Psychopharmacologia* 39:187-191.

Gusberg, S. B. (1947). Precursors of corpus carcinoma estrogens and adenomatous hyperplasia. *Am. J. Obstet. Gynecol.* 54:905.

Hamilton, M. (1960). A rating scale for depression. *J. Neurol. Neurosurg. Psychiatry* 23:56-62.

Hammond, L. B., F. R. Jelovsek, K. L. Lee, W. T. Creasman, and R. T. Parker (1979). The effects of long-term estrogen replacement therapy. II. Neoplasia. *Am. J. Obstet. Gynecol.* 133:537-547.

Helper, M. M., R. C. Wilcott, and S. L. Garfield (1963). Effects of chlorpromazine on learning and related processes in emotionally disturbed children. *J. Consult. Psychol.* 27:1-9.

Hollingworth, H. L. (1912). The influence of caffeine on mental and motor efficiency. *J. Arch. Psychol.* 3:1-166.

Horowitz, R. I., and A. R. Feinstein (1978). Alternative analytic methods for case-control studies of estrogen and endometrial cancer. *N. Engl. J. Med.* 299:1089-1094.

Humphrey, G. (1951). *Thinking.* John Wiley, New York.

Inaba, M., and K. Kamata (1979). Effect of estradiol-17 beta and other steroids on noradrenaline and dopamine binding to synaptic membrane fragments of rat brain. *J. Steroid Biochem.* 11:1491-1497.

Inman, W. H. W., M. P. Vessey, B. Westerholm, and A. Engelund (1970). Thromboembolic disease and the steroidal content of oral contraceptives: a report to the Committee on Safety of Drugs. *Br. Med. J.* 2:203-209.

Janowsky, D. S., and J. M. Daris (1970). Progesterone-estrogen effects on uptake and release of norepinephrine by synaptosomes. *Life Sci.* 9:525-531.

Jorgensen, R. S., and M. H. Wulff (1958). The effect of orally administered chlorpromazine on the electroencephalogram of man. *Electroencephalogr. Clin. Neurophysiol.* 10:325.

Kantor, H. I., C. Michael, and H. Shore (1973). Estrogen for older women. *Am. J. Obstet. Gynecol.* 116:115.

Kanton, H. I., L. J. Milton, and M. L. Ernst (1978). Comparative psychological effects of estrogen administration on institutional and non-institutional elderly women. *J. Am. Geriatr. Soc.* 26:9-16.

Kendall, D. A., and K. Narayana (1978). Effects of oestradiol-17 beta on mono-amine concentrations in the hypothalamus of anoestrous ewe. *J. Physiol.* 282:44-45.

Kerr, M. D. (1968). Psychohormonal approach to the menopause. *Mod. Treat.* 5:587.

Killam, K. F., E. K. Killam, and R. Naquet (1967). An animal model of light sensitive epilepsy. *Electroencephalogr. Clin. Neurophysiol.* 22:497-513.

Kistner, R. W. (1971). *Gynecology Principles and Practice.* Year Book Med. Publ., Inc., Chicago.

Klaiber, E. L., D. M. Broverman, W. Vogel, Y. Kobayashi, and D. Moriarty (1972). Effects of estrogen therapy on plasma MAO activity and EEG driving responses of depressed women. *Am. J. Psychiatry* 128:1492-1498.

Klaiber, E. L., D. M. Broverman, W. Vogel, and Y. Kobayashi (1979). Estrogen therapy for severe persistent depression in women. *Arch. Gen. Psychiatry* 36:550-554.

Klaiber, E. L., Y. Kobayashi, D. M. Broverman, and F. Hall (1971). Plasma monoamine oxidase activity in regularly menstruating women and in amenor-rheic women receiving cyclic treatment with estrogens and a progestin. *J. Clin. Endocrinol. Metab.* 33:630-638.

Kobayashi, T., T. Kobayashi, J. Kato, and H. Minaguchi (1966). Cholinergic and adrenergic mechanisms in the female rat hypothalmus with special reference to feedback of ovarian steroid hormones, in *Steroid Dynamics* (G. Pincus, T. Nakao, and J. Tait, eds.). Academic Press, New York and London, pp. 305-307.

Kornetsky, C., O. Humphries, and E. V. Evarts (1957). Comparison of psycho-logical effects of certain centrally acting drugs in man. *Arch. Neurol. Psychiatry* 77:318-324.

Lehmann, H. E., and J. Csank (1957). Differential screening of phrenotropic agents in men: Psychophysiologic test data. *J. Clin. Exp. Psychopathol.* 18:222-235.

Lipsett, M. B. (1974). Endocrine responsive cancers of man, in *Textbook of Endocrinology,* 5th ed. (R. H. Williams, ed.). Saunders, Philadelphia, pp. 1071-1083.

Luine, V. N., R. I. Khylchevskaya, and B. S. McEwen (1975). Effects of gonadal steroids on activities of monoamine oxidase and choline acetylase in rat brain. *Brain Res.* 86:293-306.

Luine, V. N., B. S. McEwen, and I. B. Black (1977). Effect of 17-β estradiol on hypothalamic tyrosine hydroxylase activity. *Brain Res.* 120:188-192.

Macfarlane Smith, I. (1964). *Spatial Ability.* Robert R. Knapp, San Diego, California.

Mack, T. M., M. C. Pike, B. E. Henderson, R. I. Pfeffer, V. R. Gerkinds, M. Arthur, and S. E. Brown (1976). Estrogens and endometrial cancer in a retirement community. *N. Engl. J. Med.* 294:1262-1267.

Mackenberg, E. J., D. M. Broverman, W. Vogel, and E. L. Klaiber (1974). Morning-to-afternoon changes in cognitive performances and in the electroencephalogram. *J. Educ. Psychol.* 66:238-246.

Messent, P. R. (1976). Female hormones and behavior, in *Exploring Sex Differences* (B. Lloyd and J. Archer, eds.). Academic Press, London.

Misurec, J., and K. Nahanek (1964). Changes in photo-metrazol (photo-myoclonic) threshold in treatment with some psychopharmacological drugs. *Electroencephalogr. Clin. Neurophysiol.* 17:607.

Munchel, M. E. (1979). The effects of symptom expectations and response styles on cognitive and perceptual-motor performance during the premenstrual phase. Indiana University. *Dissert. Abstr. Int.* 39:3531-3532.

Paterson, M. E., T. Wade-Evans, D. W. Sturdee, M. H. Thom, and J. W. W. Studd (1980). Endometrial disease after treatment with oestrogens and progestagens in the climacteric. *Br. Med. J.* 280:822-824.

Podell, J. E., and L. Phillips (1959). A developmental analysis of cognition as observed in dimensions of Rorschach and objective test performance. *J. Pers.* 27:439-463.

Porteus, S. D. (1950). *The Porteus Maze Test and Intelligence.* Pacific Books, Palo Alto, California.

Primac, D. W., A. F. Mirsky, and H. E. Rosvold (1957). Effects of centrally acting drugs on two tests of brain damage. *Arch. Neurol. Psychiatry* 77:328-332.

Ripley, H. S., E. Shorr, and G. N. Papanicolaou (1940). The effect of treatment of depression in the menopause with estrogenic hormone. *Am. J. Psychiatry* 96:905-915.

Rodier, W. I., III. (1971). Progesterone-estrogen interactions in the control of activity-wheel running in the female rat. *J. Comp. Physiol. Psychol.* 74:365-373.

Schiff, I., Q. Regestein, D. Tulchinsky, and K. J. Ryan (1979). Effects of estrogens on sleep and psychological state of hypogonadal women. *JAMA* 242:2405.

Schidlkraut, J. J. (1965). The catecholamine hypothesis of affective disorders: a review of supporting evidence. *Am. J. Psychiatry* 122:509-522.

Sevringhaus, E. L. (1933). The use of folliculin in involutional states. *Am. J. Obstet. Gynecol.* 25:361-365.

Shatin, L., L. Rockmore, and I. C. Funk (1956). Response of psychiatric patients to massive doses of thorazine. II. Psychological test performance and comparative drug evaluation. *Psychiatr. Q.* 30:402-416.

Shetty, T. (1971). Photic responses in hyperkinesis of childhood. *Science* 174: 1356-1357.

Smith, D. C., R. Prentice, D. J. Thompson, and W. L. Herrmann (1975). Association of exogenous estrogen and endometrial carcinoma. *N. Engl. J. Med.* 293: 1164-1167.

Sommer, B. (1972). Menstrual cycle changes and intellectual performance. *Psychosom. Med.* 34:263-269.

Srivastava, K., P. K. DasGupta, and P. K. Mehrotra (1978). Monoamine oxidase activity in the pituitary of mice after estrogen, progesterone and centchroman treatment. *Indian J. Physiol. Pharmacol.* 22:310.

Thurstone, L. L. (1944). *A Factorial Study of Perception.* Psychometric Monograph 4. University of Chicago Press, Chicago.

Vogel, W., D. M. Broverman, and E. L. Klaiber (1971). EEG responses in regularly menstruating women and in amenorrheic women treated with ovarian hormones. *Science* 172:388-391.

Vogel, W., D. M. Broverman, and E. L. Klaiber (1977). EEG responses to photic stimulation in habitual smokers and nonsmokers. *J. Comp. Physiol. Psychol.* 91:418-422.

Vogel, W., D. M. Broverman, E. L. Klaiber, and Y. Kobayashi (1974). EEG driving responses as a function of monoamine oxidase. *Electroencephalogr. Clin. Neurophysiol.* 36:205-207.

Vogel, W., D. M. Broverman, E. L. Klaiber, Y. Kobayashi, and F. Clarkson (1976). A model for the integration of hormonal, behavioral, EEG, and pharmacological data in psychopathology, in *Psychotropic Action of Hormones* (T. M. Itil, G. Laudahn, and W. M. Herrmann, eds.). Spectrum Publ., New York, pp. 121-134.

Vogel, W., E. L. Klaiber, and D. M. Broverman (1978). Roles of the gonadal steroid hormones in psychiatric depression in men and women. *Prog. Neuropsychopharmacol.* 2:487-503.

Wechsler, D. (1955). *Wechsler Adult Intelligence Scale.* Psychological Corp., New York.

Weiss, N. S. (1975). Risks and benefits of estrogen use. *N. Engl. J. Med.* 293: 1200-1202.

Wickham, M. (1958). The effects of the menstrual cycle on test performance. *Br. J. Psychol.* 49:34-41.

Wiesbader, H., and R. Kurzrok (1938). The menopause: a consideration of the symptoms, etiology, and treatment by means of estrogens. *Endocrinology* 23:32-38.

Wilson, W. P., and J. S. Glotfelthy (1958). Effect of intravenous promazine on arousal responses in man. *Dis. Nerv. Syst.* 19:307-309.

Witkin, H. A. (1950). Individual differences in ease of perception of embedded figures. *J. Pers.* 19:1-15.

Witkin, H. A., R. B. Dyk, H. F. Faterson, D. R. Goodenough, and S. A. Karp (1962). *Psychological Differentiation.* John Wiley, New York.

Wurtman, R. J., and J. Axelrod (1963). Sex steroids, cardiac ^{3}H-norepineph-rine, and tissue monoamine oxidase levels in the rat. *Biochem. Pharmacol.* 12:1417-1419.

14 The Menstrual Cycle in Anorexia Nervosa

KATHERINE A. HALMI   The New York Hospital-Cornell Medical Center, Westchester Division, White Plains, New York

Since amenorrhea is a major diagnostic symptom of anorexia nervosa, extensive studies have been conducted on the hypothalamic-pituitary-ovarian axis in patients with this disorder. Anorexia nervosa, which occurs predominantly in pubertal and young women, is characterized by behavior directed towards losing weight, peculiar patterns of handling foods, weight loss, intense fear of gaining weight, disturbance of body image, and, in women, amenorrhea. Hypotheses explaining the cause of amenorrhea in anorexia nervosa have ranged from psychological to physiological explanations. Is the amenorrhea in anorexia nervosa a result of an emotional or nutritional disturbance or is it secondary to a substantial weight loss?

It is known that menstruating obese women may become amenorrheic when they are on low-calorie diets [1]. A severe reduction in caloric intake may trigger the amenorrhea before substantial weight loss occurs in anorexia nervosa.

There is evidence that amenorrhea occurs in many patients with anorexia nervosa before weight loss has occurred [2,3]. Early onset amenorrhea would favor the hypothesis that psychological factors cause the amenorrhea in anorexia nervosa.

It is known that amenorrhea is present in chronically undernourished women who cannot obtain enough food [4]. Late onset amenorrhea would support the idea that weight loss causes the amenorrhea in anorexia nervosa.

Another theory is that the amenorrhea is caused by a primary distrubance of hypothalamic function and that the full expression of this disturbance is brought about with psychological stress [5]. Russell [6] has suggested that the malnutrition of anorexia nervosa perpetuates the amenorrhea but is not primarily responsible for the endocrine disorder which could be attributed partly to psychological disturbance and partly to unknown causes.

After treatment, the return of normal menstrual cycles lags behind the return to a normal body weight [7]. A normal body weight is essential for the return of menstruation but does not guarantee that return. Crisp postulates that a normal dietary pattern including adequate carbohydrate ingestion is necessary for the return of menstrual function [8]. Resumption of menses in anorexia nervosa is also associated with marked psychological improvement [7].

With the refinement of bioassay techniques, it has been possible to examine some of these hypotheses by careful endocrine evaluations of anorexia nervosa patients. Early investigations showed that urinary excretion of estrogen was diminished in emaciated anorectics [9]. It was then necessary to determine whether these patients had a primary failure of ovarian function. If the latter were true one would expect high levels of urinary gonadotropins. Later studies showed that both the urinary excretion and plasma levels of gonadotrophins are decreased, indicating that the ovarian failure is secondary to a disturbance in hypothalamic-pituitary function [10,11].

One strategy in assessing the hypothalamic-pituitary regulation of ovarian activity is to examine the effect of estrogen administration on serum lutinizing hormone (LH) levels. In healthy women exogenous estrogen will decrease LH levels during the follicular phase of the menstrual cycle (negative feedback effect of estrogen). Several days after the exogenous estrogen is given there is an acute release of LH (positive feedback effect). In one study negative feedback effects of estrogen were present in patients with detectable levels of LH [12]. None of the 19 patients tested showed a positive feedback release of LH to the estrogen stimulus. With weight restoration, 11 out of 12 patients showed the negative feedback effects of estrogen but the positive release of LH was present in only three patients. Two of those three patients resumed regular menstruation within 6 months of reaching normal weight. The authors suggested a sequence in the return of normal hypothalamic-pituitary-ovarian activity. The recovery of the hypothalamus to respond normally to the negative feedback effects of estrogen followed by the return of the positive feedback response eventually leads to the return of menstruation. In those patients of normal weight who failed to menstruate, continuing impairment of the hypothalamus to respond normally to the feedback effects of estrogen on gonadotrophin release is suggested.

Another way of assessing the hypothalamic-pituitary-ovarian axis is by measuring the effect of chlomiphene, an antiestrogen, on LH levels. Chlomiphene is reported to compete with estrogen at hypothalamic receptor sites and thus prevent the negative feedback effect of estrogen. Chlomiphene thus increases the secretion of releasing factors from the hypothalamus which in turn cause secretion of the pituitary LH. One study showed that malnourished anorectics had a deficient LH response to chlomiphene. Both the first and second LH peaks were absent and subsequent menstrual bleeding did not occur. After weight gain the patients showed the initial rise in LH after clomiphene but the second LH peak was not present. Of the six patients who maintained a normal body weight for at least six months after chlomiphene, only three resumed normal menstruation. This suggests a hypothalamic defect and that the defect is not related to the patient's nutritional status [13].

A common cause of secondary amenorrhea in young women is hyperprolactinemia [14]. Several studies have shown serum prolactin levels to be within normal range in anorectic patients before and after weight gain [15,16].

It is now necessary to evaluate whether there is an impairment in the hypothalamic gonadotrophin-releasing hormone (GnRH) and/or an impairment in the pituitary response of GnRH. Synthetic GnRH has been used to evaluate the capacity of the pituitary gland to release LH and follicle stimulating hormone (FSH). Studies with synthetic GnRH have shown an impaired gonadotrophin response in emaciated anorectic patients [17-19]. The FSH response was normal and LH response diminished resulting in a reversed FSH-LH ratio [20,21]. The observation of an FSH response to GnRH greater than the LH response is similar to a pattern reported in prepubertal girls [22]. The LH response to GnRH returned to normal with weight gain. These studies indicate that the anorectics' malnourished state interferes with the pituitary synthesis and release of gonadotrophins. However, the explanation is not so simple. It was noted that in normal women LH response to GnRH is increased with repeated doses of GnRH [23]. It was then demonstrated that follicular maturation and ovulation could be induced in underweight amenorrheic women with anorexia nervosa by injections of 500 μg of GnRH every 8 h over a 4 week period [24]. When human chorionic gonadotrophin was given with the GnRH, ovulation and normal corpus luteum function occurred. One woman became pregnant while receiving this treatment. Constant administration of GnRH normalized basal LH and FSH secretion and induced a cyclic gonadotrophin secretory pattern with differential changes of the LH and FSH responses to GnRH [25]. Thus persistent exposure of the pituitary to GnRH produced the same changes in FSH and LH response to GnRH that occurred with restoration of weight.

The most compelling evidence that amenorrhea in anorexia nervosa is secondary to disturbed hypothalamic regulation of gonadal function is the finding of an "immature" pattern of release of gonadotrophins from the pituitary over a 24 h period. In normal adult women LH is released in bursts throughout the day and night [26]. Boyar et al. have shown that prepubertal children have smaller bursts of LH secretion during both day and night and very low levels of LH [26]. In early puberty the bursts of LH increase in magnitude during sleep. In late puberty, the bursts of LH during the day increase in magnitude but the night bursts are still greater.

In a study of nine women with anorexia nervosa, Boyar et al. [27] found that eight showed patterns of LH secretion resembling those found in prepubertal and pubertal children. In a later study of women with anorexia nervosa who had regained their weight, those patients who continued to have abnormal eating patterns also continued to have an immature LH secretory pattern [28]. Those women who showed both weight gain and normalization of the LH pattern were also improved psychologically. In this same study, the return of menses did not show a simple relation to weight or maturity of the LH secretory pattern [28].

These findings were confirmed by another group of investigators from the Max Planck Institute [29]. They found that 14 of 16 patients had a prepubertal LH secretory pattern. An adult secretory LH pattern was seen in their patients only with a body weight greater than 80% of the ideal body weight.

Recent studies of estrogen metabolism in anorexia nervosa complicate the tidy formulation of hypothalamic malfunction as the cause of amenorrhea in anorexia nervosa. In seven patients with anorexia nervosa, estradiol metabolism was studied by following an injection of a tracer dose of estradiol [30]. The same study was done in eight control women and four obese women. In the anorectic patients, there was a shift of estradiol metabolism from 16 alpha-hydroxylation to 2-hydroxylation and consequently a disproportionate increase in catecholestrogens. Estrone can be 16-hydroxylated to 16-hydroxyestrone which is rapidly oxidized to estriol [31]. An alternate metabolic route is to the catecholestrogen, 2-hydroxyestrone. The age matched obese women in the above study [30] showed a marked increase in the transformation of estradiol to estriol and a decrease in 2-hydroxyestrone formation. This study indicates that a change in body weight can cause significant alterations in the metabolism of biologically active estrogen.

In an excellent review article on neuroendocrine regulation of the menstrual cycle Yen discusses catecholestrogens. He points out that they have both a catechol phase and an estrogen phase and thus have the potential of interacting with both the catecholamine-mediated and the estrogen-mediated systems in the central nervous system (CNS) and pituitary [32]. Through its catechol structure the molecule may inhibit dopamine and norepinephrine biosynthesis by blocking the rate-limiting enzyme tyrosine hydroxylase or decrease o-methylation of nor-epinephrine by competing with catechol-o-methyltransferase, which degrades norepinephrine in the synapse. Through the estrogen structure, it may act as an antiestrogen, blocking estrogen receptors in the hypothalamus or pituitary.

It is now possible to postulate that the change in estrogen metabolism associated with weight loss has an effect through the formation of catecholestrogens in the brain on catecholamine and dopamine metabolism in the brain. This in turn may influence the development of some of the behavioral signs and symptoms of anorexia nervosa.

Summary

The documented disturbances in the hypothalamic-pituitary-ovarian system in anorexia nervosa patients are: (1) a decrease in estrogen secretion, (2) a decrease in pituitary secretion of LH, (3) "immature" pattern of LH secretion, (4) a decrease in LH response to estrogen stimulation, and (5) a shift of estradiol metabolism towards a disproportionate increase in catecholestrogens. There is evidence that weight loss and psychological disturbances can be associated with amenorrhea [33,34]. Since amenorrhea occurs in one-fifth to one-third of anorexia nervosa patients before weight loss has occurred [35] and since restoration to a normal weight does not insure the resumption of normal menstruation, it seems reasonable to propose that a "vulnerable" hypothalamus in response to environmental stress develops an impairment in the regulation of a secretion of gonadotrophin-releasing hormone. Subsequent weight loss further sustains the amenorrhea by other mechanisms.

References

1. G. F. M. Russell and C. J. Beardwood, Amenorrhea in the feeding disorders: anorexia nervosa and obesity. *Psychother. Psychosom.* 18:358-364 (1970).

2. P. Dally, *Anorexia Nervosa.* Heinemann, London, 1969.

3. S. Theander, Anorexia nervosa. *Acta Psychiatr. Scand. [Suppl.]* 214:77-78 (1970).

4. S. Zubiran, F. Gomez-Mont, and J. Laguna, Endocrine disturbances and their dietetic background in undernourished in Mexico. *Ann. Intern. Med.* 42:1259-1269 (1955).

5. G. F. M. Russell, Metabolic, endocrine and psychiatric aspects of anorexia nervosa. *The Scientific Basis of Medicine, Annual Reviews,* London, pp. 236-255 (1969).

6. G. F. M. Russell, Premenstrual tension and "psychogenic" amenorrhea: psychophysical interactions. *J. Psychosom. Res.* 16:279-287 (1972).

7. H. G. Morgan and G. F. M. Russell, *Psychol. Med.* 5:355-371 (1975).

8. A. H. Crisp and E. Stonehill, Relation between aspects of nutritional disturbance and menstrual activity in primary anorexia nervosa. *Br. Med. J.* 3:149-151 (1971).

9. E. P. McCullagh and W. R. Tupper, Anorexia nervosa. *Ann. Intern. Med.* 14:817-838 (1940).

10. J. C. Marshall and T. R. Fraser, Amenorrhea in anorexia nervosa: assessment and treatment with chlomiphene citrate. *Br. Med. J.* 4:590-592 (1971).

11. G. F. M. Russell, J. A. Loraine, E. T. Bell, and R. A. Harkness, Gonado-

trophin and estrogen excretion in patients with anorexia nervosa. *J. Psychosom. Res.* 9:79-85 (1965).

12. A. Wakeling, V. A. DeSouza, and C. J. Beardwood, Assessment of the negative and positive feedback affects of administered estrogen on gonadotrophin release in patients with anorexia nervosa. *Psychol. Med.* 7:397-405 (1977).

13. A. Wakeling, J. C. Marshall, C. J. Beardwood, V. F. A. DeSouza, and G. F. M. Russell, The effects of chlomiphene citrate on the hypothalamic pituitary gonadol axis in anorexia nervosa. *Psychol. Med.* 6:371-388 (1976).

14. H. G. Bohnet, H. G. Dahlen, and W. Wuttke, Hyperprolactinemic and ovulatory syndrome, *J. Clin. Endocrinol. Metab.* 42:132-143 (1976).

15. A. Wakeling, V. F. A. DeSouza, M. B. R. Gore, M. Sabur, D. Kingstone, and A. M. B. Boss, Amenorrhea, body weight and serum hormone concentrations, with particular reference to prolactin and thyroid hormones in anorexia nervosa. *Psychol. Med.* 9:265-272 (1979).

16. K. A. Halmi and B. M. Sherman, Prediction of treatment response in anorexia nervosa. *Biol. Psychiat. Today.* Elsevier-North-Holland Biomedical Press, pp. 609-614 (1979).

17. R. A. Vigersky, D. L. Loriaux, A. E. Anderson, R. S. Mecklenburg, and J. L. Vaitukaitais, Delayed pituitary hormone response to LRF and TRF in patients with anorexia nervosa and with secondary amenorrhea associated with simple weight loss. *J. Clin. Endocrinol. Metab.* 43:893-900 (1976).

18. P. Travaglini, P. Beck-Peccoz, C. Ferrari, B. Ambrosi, A. Paracchi, A. Severgnini, A. Spada, and G. Faglia, Some aspects of hypothalamic-pituitary function in patients with anorexia nervosa. *Acta Endocrinol.* 81:252-262 (1976).

19. B. M. Sherman, K. A. Halmi, and R. Zamudio, LH and FSH response to gonadotrophin releasing hormone in anorexia nervosa: effect of nutrition of rehabilitation. *J. Clin. Endocrinol. Metab.* 41:135-142 (1975).

20. K. A. Halmi and B. M. Sherman, Gonadotrophin response to LH-RH in anorexia nervosa. *Arch. Gen. Psychiatry* 132:875-885 (1975).

21. M. P. Warren, R. Jewelewicz, I. Dyrenfurth, R. Ans, S. Khalaf, and R. L. Vandewiele, The significance of weight loss in the evaluation of pituitary response to LH-RH in women with secondary amenorrhea. *J. Clin. Endocrinol. Metab.* 40:601-611 (1975).

22. J. C. Job, P. E. Garnier, J. L. Chaussain, and G. Milhaud, Response of FSH and LH to GnRH in young women. *J. Clin. Endocrinol. Metab.* 35:473-475 (1972).

23. J. D. Hoff, B. L. Lasley, C. F. Wang, and S. S. C. Yen, The two pools of pituitary gonadotrophin: regulation during the menstrual cycle. *J. Clin. Endocrinol. Metab.* 44:302-312 (1977).

24. S. J. Nillius and L. Wide, Gonadotrophin-releasing hormone treatment for induction of follicular maturation and ovulation in amenorrheic women with anorexia nervosa. *Br. Med. J.* 16:405-408 (1975).

25. S. J. Nillius and L. Wide, Affects of prolonged lutinizing hormone-releasing hormone therapy on follicular maturation, ovulation and corpus luteum function in amenorrheic women with anorexia nervosa, *Upsala J. Med. Sci.* 84:21-35 (1979).

26. R. Boyar, J. Finkelstein, H. Roffwarg, S. Kapen, E. Weitzman, and L. Hellman, Synchronization of augmented luteinizing hormone secretion with sleep during puberty. *N. Engl. J. Med.* 287:582-586 (1972).

27. R. M. Boyar, J. Katz, J. W. Finkelstein, S. Kapen, H. Weiner, E. L. Weitzman, and L. Hellman, Anorexia nervosa, immaturity of the 24-hour luteinizing hormone secretory pattern. *N. Engl. J. Med.* 291:861-865 (1974).

28. J. L. Katz, R. M. Boyar, and H. Roffwarg, LH-RH responsiveness in anorexia nervosa: intactness despite prepubertal circadian LH patterns. *Psychosom. Med.* 39:241-251 (1977).

29. K. M. Pirke, M. M. Fichter, R. Lund, and P. Doerr, 24-hour sleep-wake pattern of plasma LH in patients with anorexia nervosa. *Acta Endocrinol.* 92:193-204 (1979).

30. J. Fishman, R. M. Boyar, and L. Hellman, Influence of body weight on estradiol metabolism in young women. *J. Clin. Endocrinol. Metab.* 41:989-991 (1975).

31. R. M. Boyar, Endocrine changes in anorexia nervosa. *Med. Clin. North Am.* 62:297-303 (1978).

32. S. Yen, Neuroendocrine regulation of the menstrual cycle. *Hosp. Pract.* 14:83-97 (1979).

33. J. S. Rakoff, L. A. Rigg, and S. C. Yen, The impairment of progesterone induced pituitary release of prolactin and gonadotrophin in patients with hypothalamic chronic and ovulation. *Am. J. Obstet. Gynecol.* 130:807-812 (1978).

34. R. J. Santen, J. N. Friend, and D. Trojanowski, Prolonged negative feedback suppression after estradiol administration: proposed mechanism of eugonadal secondary amenorrhea. *J. Clin. Endocrinol. Metab.* 47:1220-1229 (1978).

35. A. Borghi, G. Forte, S. Fusi, C. Vigiani, E. Calabresi, and G. Cattani, Disorders of the hypothalamic-pituitary-ovarian axis in anorexia nervosa, in *The Endocrine Function of the Human Ovary*. Academic, London, 1976, pp. 291-304.

15 Psychopathology and the Menstrual Cycle

STEPHEN W. HURT, RICHARD C. FRIEDMAN, JOHN CLARKIN,
RUTH CORN, and MICHAEL S. ARONOFF The New York Hospital-
Cornell Medical Center, Westchester Division, White Plains, New York

In 1931, Frank described a syndrome of premenstrual tension (PMT) occurring 7 to 10 days preceding menstruation and relieved by menstrual flow [1]. Shortly thereafter, Benedek and Rubenstein carried out their classic investigation of the relationship between the mental functioning of patients in psychoanalysis and the menstrual cycle [2]. It is difficult to overestimate the influence of these two investigations on the form and content of subsequent research. Recently, a number of reviews have integrated modern developments in psychobiology and psychopathology with other work carried out since the 1930s [3-9]. Rather than restating concepts already previously emphasized and extensively reviewed in this volume, we will discuss important areas for understanding psychopathology that have previously not been the focus of attention in the literature.

The term "premenstrual syndrome" connotes the time bound nature of a group of symptoms that regularly covary together. The term suggests that a group of symptoms have been described and that their temporal course has been well established. As Abplanalp et al. have noted in a recent review [9], this appears not to be the case. They observed that the time course of symptoms within cycles has not yet been definitely described. The number and combination of symptoms making up the syndrome and reported to be associated with the premenstrual phase also tend to differ across studies [9]. In Frank's original description of 15 women, irritability, extreme tension, decreased impulse control, and decreased judgment were all emphasized as important parts of the clinical picture. In general, subsequent clinical research has tended to validate that these

299

behaviors do tend to covary together premenstrually in certain subtypes of
patients.

Ambiguity about the role of depression in the syndrome, however, illustrates
that the critical point of view advanced by Abplanalp et al. is well taken. Two
women in Frank's original series manifested suicidal depression and another became "despondent" premenstrually. Studies of women who are not psychiatric
patients have demonstrated that depressed mood does appear to occur frequently
premenstrually [5]. Premenstrual depression was also frequently reported in
Benedek and Rubenstein's psychoanalytic patients [2]. Severity of depression
has been shown to be related to suicide as is evident in the incidence of depressive symptoms in suicidal samples and in the relationship between severity of depression and degree of suicidal intent in suicide attemptors [10,11]. Moreover,
menstrual cycle phase appears to influence the timing of suicidal behavior. Calls
to suicide prevention centers, suicide attempts, and successful suicides all tend
to occur more frequently in the luteal or menstrual phases of the cycle than can
be expected by chance [12,13]. Moderate or marked degrees of a "premenstrual
affective syndrome" have been found to be associated with seeking treatment for
affective disorders [14], the presence of clinically significant episodes of depression [15], and a slightly increased incidence of depressive illness among first-
degree relatives [16]. Using a validated instrument to measure suicidal intent,
Pallis and Holding have found that women with extremely high degrees of suicidal intent were more likely to make suicide attempts during the premenstrual
period [17].

This research suggests that depression might indeed constitute part of a "premenstrual affective syndrome" (PAS). However, Haskett et al. [18] recently
described a subgroup of women who manifested premenstrual irritability, lability
of mood, tension, and restlessness, but who were without major psychopathology
intermenstrually. These investigators found that depression was not characteristically exacerbated premenstrually unless the patient already experienced various
types of psychopathology. These investigators argued, therefore, that depression
is not an essential factor of the premenstrual affective syndrome [18]. A recent
study by Endicott et al [20] suggests that whether significant depression occurs
premenstrually might depend on the presence or absence of a lifetime diagnosis
of affective disorder. In this investigation, only women who met Research Diagnostic Criteria [20] for a lifetime diagnosis of affective disorder developed significant premenstrual depression. We believe that the role of depression in a premenstrual affective syndrome has not been clearly established. The literature to
date suggests that premenstrual affective syndrome is not a single entity. Criteria
for describing each of the many possible syndromes remain to be more explicitly
defined. (For further discussion of this topic, the reader is referred to Chapter
12, by Endicott and Halbreich.) It would appear, however, that depression is a
recurrent symptom for one subgroup of women. Whether these women have current psychopathology, as Haskett et al. have suggested [18] or lifetime histories

of affective disorder, as Endicott et al. have suggested [19], or both, has yet to be clearly demonstrated.

The role of depression in PAS illustrates another source of confusion in the literature. Some clinicians and investigators have argued that a qualitative distinction should be made between patients who experience PMT but who are otherwise normal intermenstrually (as in the Haskett, et al. study), and patients who suffer from a diagnosed psychiatric illness and also experience regular symptoms associated with the menstrual cycle. This approach is attractive because it allows for the detailed study of a well-characterized subgroup of patients. Based on the limited data available to date, however, it would appear that patients with a variety of types of psychiatric illnesses could experience the same recurrent premenstrual symptoms as women who are psychiatrically normal intermenstrually. Admittedly, women with preexisting illnesses could also experience exacerbation of the symptoms of their illness in addition to the group of symptoms that "normally" occur premenstrually, thus producing a confounded picture. Therefore, we feel that the wisest approach to open nosologic problems is to assess premenstrual symptoms using explicit criteria and simply to note whether conditions of major psychopathology (according to DSM-III criteria) are present.

The lack of clarity in conceptualizing relationships between psychopathology and the menstrual cycle has also been due to the evolution of psychodiagnostic nomenclature during the last half century. It was not until 1952, well after Frank's and Benedek and Rubenstein's investigations, that the first standardized edition of the *Diagnostic and Statistical Manual of the American Psychiatric Association* (DSM-I) appeared. This was modified in a second edition (DSM-II) in 1968. These editions provided quite general guidelines for diagnosis, and it was subsequently found that methods of making psychiatric diagnoses varied greatly in response to theoretic orientation, local preferences, and other non-standardized factors. More recent efforts have been directed at standardizing criteria for the identification of homogenous groups of patients and have tended to focus on phenomenology rather than underlying, common psychodynamics. Growing out of the efforts of a group at Washington University during the 1970s, the current version of the *Diagnostic and Statistical Manual of the American Psychiatric Association* (DSM-III) was published in 1980 [21]. Each of its clinical syndromes is described in terms of its essential and associated features and specifies both inclusionary and exclusionary criteria.

Use of DSM-III greatly increased the likelihood that investigators throughout the world, regardless of theoretic orientation (or bias), would agree on the category of behaviors represented by a diagnostic term. There is currently no specific diagnostic term with a unique code number in DSM-III to connote premenstrual tension syndrome (PTS) or premenstrual affective syndrome (PAS). With ever-increasing research in this area, however, such a diagnosis might be possible in a subsequent edition of the DSM.

Regardless of how ways of conceptualizing psychiatric illness have changed with time, basic psychodynamic concepts of unconscious conflict, defense, neurotic symptom formation, and, more recently, object relations theory have proved extremely helpful in understanding psychopathology. These concepts have also been useful in exploring relationships between psychopathology and the menstrual cycle. Unfortunately, much early work in this field was carried out within a broad cultural context of social discrimination against women and a basically phallocentric clinical-behavioral context. Freud's view of the psychosexual development of women must, in our opinion, be distinguished from more useful aspects of psychodynamic theory that still retain power to explain aspects of psychopathology. Freud suggested that women have feelings of inferiority because of the absence of a penis rather than normatively developing positive self-regard as a result of possessing uniquely female attributes. Freud also suggested that women might be less adequate than men in more global ways than those restricted to the development of body ego and self esteem [22]. The phallocentric aspects of Freud's view of psychosexual development had great influence until relatively recently. These concepts were criticized by Horney [23-25] and by Thompson [26-29]. However, not until Kinsey's studies [30,31] in the 1940s and 1950s and the work of Masters and Johnson [32] and Sherfey [33] in the 1960s was the power of this model of sex differences in behavior seriously diluted. The phallocentric view, in our opinion, is not an essential aspect of psychodynamic theory, despite its historic impact.

The importance of psychodynamic constructs in understanding psychopathology and menstrual cycle relationships can be seen in the classic psychoanalytic investigation of Benedek and Rubenstein [2]. The limitations of this ambitious investigation are well-known and need not be reviewed here. Nevertheless, it is the only study we are aware of in which a serious attempt was made to understand the behavior of the whole patient over time. The investigators reported systematic fluctuations in mental activity closely associated with menstrual cycle phase. Affects fluctuated along a pleasure/displeasure continuum and certain specific types of negative affects, namely irritability, anxiety, and depression, constituted dysphoria when present. Sexual feelings also fluctuated in intensity and the fantasies associated with sexual desire were different during different phases of the cycle. The luteal phase appeared to be associated with procreational fantasies in contrast with the stimulatory erotic fantasies of the follicular phase. Benedek and Rubenstein were the first investigators to note this association between menstrual cycle phase and the content of these women's fantasies. Adams et al. [34] recently studied a small sample of normal college-aged women to determine the link between menstrual cycle phase and sexual activity. Unlike previous investigators who focused solely on heterosexual activity (coitus), Adams et al. also studied autosexual activity and distinguished between male-initiated, female-initiated, and mutually initiated heterosexual activity. They found an increase in the incidence of female-initiated and mutually initiated sexual activity at the midpoint of the cycle. Autosexual activity was also elevated. Male-initiated sexual activity showed no change at midcycle. Importantly, Adams et al. reported that these midcycle elevations in certain types of sexual activity were restricted to women not taking oral contraceptives.

Taken in conjunction, the data of Adams et al. and the observations of Benedek and Rubenstein illustrate the complex synchronization of physiological, psychological, and behavioral events with menstrual cycle phase. In the neurotic patients of Benedek and Rubenstein, a second observation of clinical relevance was made. They underscored the importance of these patients' unconscious sexual conflicts by noting many instances in which sexual feelings and fantasies were associated with affects stemming from these unconscious sexual conflicts. On the strength of these data, it would seem reasonable to assume that women with other psychopathologic conditions might also manifest affective changes that could be traced to unresolved, unconscious sexual conflicts brought into focus by the reproductive issues of the menstrual cycle. This psychodynamic orientation of Benedek and Rubenstein provides a model for understanding the relationship between the physiological changes of the menstrual cycle and the concommitant psychological changes in affects and fantasies linked to unconscious sexual conflicts. Furthermore, the specific behavioral manifestations of these relationships would need to be considered in the context of the psychobiographic, psychosocial, and psychodynamic variables unique to each.

Benedek and Rubenstein paid particular attention to psychodynamic factors. They pointed out that the strength of ego defenses appeared to fluctuate with the cycle. They observed that ego defenses were weakest during the late luteal phase of the cycle. In psychodynamic theroy, any weakening of the ego's defenses increases the possibility that impulses will achieve direct behavioral expression. When this is considered in light of their model linking menstrual cycle phases with affects and conflicts, it suggests clearly that psychopathologic behaviors are most likely to occur during the latter half of the cycle. These behaviors would presumably be characteristic of the style with which individuals coped with conflict and would be expressed according to the degree to which ego defenses were weakened. Benedek and Rubenstein's model is therefore compatible with the large body of clinical studies relating pathologic acts of various types to phases of the menstrual cycle. O'Conner et al. have recently reviewed multiple studies of many hundreds of women and involving psychiatric hospitalization, attempts at suicide, calls to suicide prevention centers, arrests and convictions, disturbances of a disorderly nature in women's prisons, sickness in industry, and accidents [5]. The maximum incidence of such activity occurs during the premenstrual or menstrual phases of the cycle, and another peak occurs at the projected time of ovulation. As Parlee has noted [4], these correlations say nothing about the probability of normal women committing pathologic acts as a consequence of cyclicity of psychohormonal functioning. This clinical literature, taken in total, says nothing about what "women in general" may be like premenstrually. The samples studied are aberrant and probably represent psychopathologic subgroups. This is an important distinction in view of the evidence that the performance of normal women, at a variety of tasks, has not been shown to fluctuate with the cycle. Data from deviant subgroups can be used in a biased and prejudicial fashion if applied inappropriately. Given this reservation, however, there seems little doubt that, within the universe of those prone to commit pathologic acts, such acts occur at a relatively high frequency during the paramenstrual period.

Parlee [4] has also appropriately emphasized that no comparable studies correlate cycle phase with unusually positive behaviors such as acts of heroism or great creativity. Data about behavioral events and cycle phase may reflect a bias since investigators in this area have tended to be interested in psychopathology per se. This possible bias should not obscure the fact that data on behavioral abnormality and cycle phase has, in our view, added a helpful perspective in understanding psychopathology.

Our own work in psychopathology and the menstrual cycle has involved the premenstrual affective syndrome, as manifested by specific criteria, in women with independent psychopathologic syndromes. One diagnostic category thought to have particular relevance for psychopathology associated with the menstrual cycle is that of the (DSM-III) borderline personality disorder. These patients, more likely to be women than men, fluctuate widely in the effectiveness and maturity of their characterologic defenses. They appear to have well-integrated personality structures at some times, and at other times appear to function at an extremely primitive level. They characteristically experience transient affective dysphoria, identity diffusion, perceptual distortions, and manifest a loss of reality testing for brief periods [21]. We believed that borderline patients might most clearly manifest premenstrual exacerbations of dysphoric symptoms because of the propensity for ego disorganization characteristic of the borderline disorder.

To investigate this hypothesis, we collected data on the menstrual cycle symptoms of a hospitalized group of borderline pateints with and without a superimposed major depressive syndrome and compared our findings with groups of patients diagnosed as experiencing major depression only and schizophrenia. Briefly, we found that the prevalence of a PAS was greatest in women who met DSM-III criteria for borderline personality disorder and major depression concurrently. It was interesting that borderline pathology without concurrent affective pathology did not appear to predispose towards PAS.

Our study involved psychiatric inpatients between 14 and 45 years of age who were neither pregnant nor taking oral contraceptives and were diagnosed on admission to the hospital as having major affective disorder, borderline personality disorder, or schizophrenia. All patients were interviewed on a single occasion by a research nurse who obtained informed consent and completed a menstrual history form to determine the physical characteristics of the menstrual cycle. A structured interview was then administered to determine the presence of PAS according to the (slightly modified) criteria of Kashiwagi et al. [15] (Table 1).

Table 1 Criteria for Premenstrual Affective Syndrome (PAS)

Criteria of Kashiwagi et al. [15]	Current criteria
At least one of the following behavioral symptoms:	At least one of the following behavioral symptoms:
Sad, blue, depressed	Sad, blue, depressed
Tense or nervous	Tense, on edge, irritable
Cry easily	Nervous, agitated, pacing
Decreased energy	Tired, listless, decreased energy
Increased mood or energy	Increased mood, felt more positive or better
	Worried, fearful, panicky
	Hostile, quarrelsome, assaultive
At least one of the following somatic symptoms:	At least one of the following somatic symptoms:
Swelling of legs	Swelling of legs or ankles
Swelling of abdomen	Swelling of abdomen
Tenderness of breasts	Swelling or tenderness of breasts
Weight gain	Weight gain
Subjective rating of symptoms (moderate or severe)	Subjective rating of symptoms (moderate or severe)
Objective recognition	Objective recognition

Patients were asked about the premenstrual and menstrual phases of their last three cycles. For probable PAS, a behavioral symptom indicating dysphoric mood of at least moderate severity, and at least one somatic symptom during the premenstrual week were required. In addition, patients either had to rate the overall severity of symptomatic impairment as moderate or severe, or believe that any behavioral or somatic change would be severe enough to allow someone else to recognize when they were about to menstruate. For definite PAS, both of these latter criteria had to be met.

A questionnaire on attitudes towards menstruation was then administered [35]. This contains 33 statements representing beliefs about the physiologic concomitants of menstruation, styles of dealing with menstruation, the effect of menstruation on performance, and general evaluation of menstruation. Each item is rated on a seven-point agreement scale with the midpoint (4) defined as "neither agree nor disagree." Each statement was read to the patient to be sure it was understood. Previous work with the questionnaire [35] has identified five dimensions reflecting attitudes towards menstruation: as a debilitating event (e.g., "I am more easily upset during my premenstrual or menstrual periods than at other times of the month"); as a predictable event (e.g., "I have learned to anticipate my menstrual period by the mood changes which precede it"); as a bothersome event (e.g., "Menstruation is something I just have to put up with"); as a positive event (e.g., "Menstruation is a recurring affirmation of womanhood"); and denial of effect (e.g., "Women who complain of menstrual distress are just using that as an excuse"). Scores on each dimension were calculated by dividing the sum of all items in a dimension by the number of items.

A chart review to establish definitively each patient's diagnosis was conducted by judges unaware of the menstrual data. Patients were given a DSM-III diagnosis if they unequivocally met DSM-III criteria for a specified condition. In equivocal cases, a second independent chart review was done. If these two independent reviewers agreed on a diagnosis, the patient was given that diagnosis. In rare cases of disagreement, a third reviewer reviewed the chart independently. The diagnosis chosen by two of three reviewers was used. If all three disagreed, the patient was dropped from the study (N = 3). We report on a total of 45 patients in four diagnostic groups: borderline personality disorder (without Axis I diagnosis [N = 9] ; mean age = 21.2 years), schizophrenia (N = 13; mean age = 23.2), major depressive episode (N = 11; mean age = 26.1), and major depressive episode with borderline personality disorder (N = 12; mean age = 22.5).

Our data on the general characteristics of these patients' menstrual cycles revealed that two-thirds (N = 30) of our total sample of psychiatric inpatients (N = 45) reported regular cycles of 25 to 35 days in the year preceding their hospitalization. Table 2 illustrates how our slightly modified criteria for PAS were related to the diagnoses of these patients. In analyzing this relationship, we noted a trend across the diagnostic groups. Patients with DSM-III, axis II pathology only (borderline personality disorder) reported the lowest prevalence of PAS. Those patients with DSM-III, axis I pathology only (schizophrenia or major depression) reported a higher prevalence of PAS. Finally, those patients with concurrent diagnoses of borderline personality disorder and major depression reported the highest prevalence of PAS.

Although these differences in prevalence are not statistically significant, they do provide some support for the model we propose. In the presence of pronounced affective dysphoria and severe character pathology, the prevalence of PAS is greatest. We also found confirming evidence in the specific association of these symptoms with the premenstrual phase of the cycle (Table 3). Those patients reporting PAS also reported a significant decrease in the overall severity of dysphoric symptoms during the menstrual phase of the cycle compared with their premenstrual levels ($t = 4.87; P < 0.001$). There was no significant change

Table 2 Premenstrual Affective Syndrome Criteria and Psychiatric Diagnosis (%)

	Axis I			
	Borderline	Depression	Schizophrenia	Borderline with depression
A. Three or more behavioral symptoms	11[a]	64	62	83
B. Two or more somatic symptoms	33	45	62	75
C. Moderate or severe interference	44	73	69	92
D. Recognizable by others	33	55	38	58
E. Probable or definite PAS (A+B+C or D)	33	64	62	83
Mean age (yrs)	21.2	26.1	23.3	22.8

[a] $\chi^2 = 7.79$, $P < 0.01$ compared with remaining three diagnostic groups combined.

Table 3 Comparison of Total Behavioral Symptom Scores by PAS Status and Menstrual Cycle Phase

	Menstrual cycle phase			
PAS Status	Premenstrual	Menstrual	t	$P<$
PAS Probable or Definite n = 28	18.39 ± 4.16[a]	13.96 ± 3.81	4.87	0.001
No PAS n = 17	11.05 ± 3.87	8.71 ± 3.85	1.80	not significant
t	5.76	4.36		
$P<$	0.001	0.001		

[a]Mean total behavioral symptom score calculated by sum of severity scores for all seven behavioral symptoms (range 7 to 28) ± standard deviation.

in dysphoric symptoms between cycle phases among those patients who failed to meet criteria for the PAS ($t = 1.80; P > 0.05$).

Of major importance is the prevalence of the dysphoric (behavioral) symptoms of the PAS. If dysphoric symptoms are considered separately, significant differences emerge between diagnostic groups. We found a significant difference in the prevalence of three or more premenstrual dysphoric symptoms between patients with borderline personality disorder alone and patients in the three other diagnostic groups combined ($\chi^2 = 7.79; P < 0.01$). Only 11% of the patients with Axis II pathology alone (borderline personality disorder) reported three or more psychological symptoms of premenstrual dysphoria. Sixty-four percent of the depressive and 62% of the schizophrenic patients reported three or more psychological symptoms of premenstrual dysphoria while, again at the extreme end of the range, 83% of the patients with both borderline personality disorder and major depression reported three or more psychological symptoms of premenstrual dysphoria. These data clearly indicate that major psychopathology (DSM-III, axis I), particularly affective psychopathology if coexistent with severe character pathology (borderline personality disorder with major depression), is related to the increased prevalence of PAS.

As the study sample included both young adult and adolescent patients, we considered that these data might be confounded by an age effect. PAS has generally been reported to reach its peak prevalence between the ages of 25 and 40 [36]. Our data revealed no significant age effects on either the prevalence or severity of PAS and showed no confounding influence of age and diagnosis. Our results suggest that PAS, as manifested by specific criteria, is as common among adolescent psychiatric inpatients as it is among adults and is not, therefore age-dependent. Moreover, symptoms which regularly fluctuate with the cycle are associated with significant distress in both adolescent and adult inpatient samples and are of clinical significance.

These data could be interpreted merely as indicating that the overall severity of psychiatric disturbance is associated with PAS. Thus, the presence of personality disorders alone (Borderline personality disorder) is associated with the lowest prevalence of the PAS. Intermediate levels of PAS are associated with the more severe forms of psychopathology denoted by DSM-III, axis I conditions (major depression and schizophrenia). Finally, the joint occurrence of DSM-III, axis I, and axis II conditions (major depression and borderline personality disorder) is associated with the highest prevalence of PAS. To test this hypothesis, the data from the study of Kashiwagi et al. [15], involving outpatients with less severe forms of psychiatric illnesses, were compared with our data.

Table 4 shows this comparison. Our major finding was a difference in the prevalence of moderate or severe levels of interference in functioning due to the PAS between our combined inpatient groups and Kashiwagi et al.'s combined outpatient groups with diagnosable psychiatric illness ($\chi^2 = 10.85; P < 0.001$). A significant difference in moderate or severe levels of interference was also found between our borderline personality disorder alone group and Kashiwagi et al.'s "other psychiatric illness" group ($\chi^2 = 6.94; P < 0.01$). Otherwise, the two groups closely resembled one another. Interestingly, Kashiwagi et al. also reported that their sample included 15 patients with hysterical character pathology, 12 of whom concurrently met diagnostic criteria for depression. Among these 12 patients, 11 reported definite or probable PAS while none of the three remaining patients with hysterical character pathology but without depression met positive PAS criteria.

Taken together with the outpatient data of Kashiwagi, et al. [15], our findings do not support the proposition that severe character pathology is, in itself, associated with an increased prevalence of PAS. However, when severe character pathology is present in conjunction with major depression, there is a marked prevalence of PAS.

Table 5 shows the data from the Menstrual Attitudes Questionnaire (MAQ) in our sample and the control data of Brooks et al. [35]. Two-way analysis of variance comparisons of diagnosis by PAS status for the mean item values for the five dimensions yielded no significant differences between diagnostic groups nor between PAS status. The positive PAS patients tended to agree more often (mean item score > 4.00) that menstruation was bothersome ($\chi^2 = 3.09; P < 0.10$).

When compared with the control data of Brooks et al. [35], these MAQ data indicate that the positive PAS patients, regardless of age, believed that menstruation was somewhat more debilitating, bothersome, and predictable. Patients who did not meet criteria for positive PAS also believed menstruation to be

Table 4 Premenstrual Affective Syndrome Criteria in Inpatient and Outpatient Psychiatric Samples (%)

Symptoms	Current sample				Kashiwagi et al. [10]		
	Borderline N=9	Depressed n=11	Schizophrenic n=13	Borderline with Depression n=12	Affective n=43	Other n=14	None n=24
A. One or more behavioral symptoms	78	82	77	92	100	100	92
Two or more behavioral symptoms	44	64	69	83	72	21	41
Three or more behavioral symptoms	11	64	62	83	-	-	-
B. One or more somatic symptoms	56	82	69	92	77	79	59
Two or more somatic symptoms	33	45	62	75	-	-	-
C. Moderate or severe interference	56	73	69	92	51	0	25
D. Recognizable by others	33	55	38	58	67	14	13
Probable or definite PAS (A+B+C or D)	33	64	62	83	65	14	21

Table 5 Menstrual Attitude Questionnaire

Factors	PAS	No PAS	Controls[a]
Debilitating			
Mean item value	4.02[b]	3.80[b]	3.39
% agree	(50)	(35)	(32)
Bothersome			
Mean item value	4.65[b]	4.24	4.18
% agree	(82)	(53)	(59)
Positive			
Mean item value	4.86	4.58	4.64
% agree	(82)	(82)	(77)
Predictable			
Mean item value	4.97[b]	4.54[b]	3.79
% agree	(89)	(76)	(54)
Denial			
Mean item value	2.70	2.91	2.73
% agree	(4)	(18)	(12)
Mean age	22.8	24.5	19.3

[a]Figures for 191 college women reported by Brooks et al. [11].
[b]$P < 0.05$ compared with controls.

somewhat more debilitating and predictable when compared with the Brooks et al. controls. Negative PAS patients did not report menstruation to be more bothersome.

These data are consistent with the general relationships noted above between psychiatric illness and PAS. The attitude of our sample toward menstruation indicates a significant and generally negative impact of the menstrual cycle on their behavior. Their view of menstruation as both debilitating and predictable suggests the hypothesis that, in women predisposed to adaptive failure, the menstrual period of the cycle is predictably associated with behavioral changes. This association is strongest in those inpatients meeting criteria for probable or definite PAS.

Our interpretation of these data, as suggested by our general model, is that the repetitive dysphoria experienced by these women during the premenstrual interval produces recognizable changes in their psychological state associated with the approaching onset of menstruation. Their menstrual attitudes are clearly consistent with their retrospective accounts of recent menstrual experience which demonstrate a significant premenstrual increase in dysphoric affect relieved by the onset of menstruation. This finding is only in the positive PAS group.

The findings presented thus far suggest that the relationship between psychiatric illness and PAS is complex. Severe character pathology, as exemplified by the presence of the borderline syndrome in our study, contributes slightly to an increase in the prevalence of PAS over that found among Kashiwagi et al.'s [15] control group. Of greater importance, however, is the presence of a major psychiatric illness such as major depression or schizophrenia. When one of these illnesses (major depression) appears in conjunction with severe character pathology, the prevalence of PAS is further increased. The prevalence of PAS among our schizophrenic patients suggests that level of ego integration does contribute to an individual's susceptibility to premenstrual exacerbation of dysphoric symptoms.

Our findings are at variance with some recent studies appearing in the psychiatric literature. Coppen reported that dysphoric menstrual symptoms were less prevalent among schizophrenic than among control patients. He also reported more severe dysphoric menstrual symptoms in neurotic than in control patients while, except for depression, his affective disorder sample was indistinguishable from the control sample [37]. Diamond et al. [38] also reported no significant increase in premenstrual or menstrual dysphoria among their patients with affective disorder compared with controls. Differences between their samples and ours may account for the differences between the results of the studies. Both Coppen's and Diamond et al.'s samples were older (mean ages 39.3 and 35.7 years, respectively). Coppen's sample also consisted of both inpatients and outpatients while Diamond et al.'s sample differed from ours in being less acutely ill and composed mainly of patients with bipolar disorder.

In reviewing the charts of these 45 patients, we were also interested in common clinical factors which might be associated with the development of PAS. In particular, in keeping with the generalized model of a relationship between sexual conflicts and the menstrual cycle, we attended to the psychosexual histories of these 45 patients. All of the data reported below were taken from a review of these patients' charts and was unknown to us before the chart review. Moreover, in reviewing the charts, we intentionally remained blind to the PAS status of the patient.

We found that 57% of the patients who satisfied criteria for probable or definite PAS had grossly abnormal sexual histories. The details are summarized in Table 6. Of the remaining patients who failed to satisfy criteria for positive PAS, only 5% had an abnormal sexual history. This difference in proportion of patients with abnormal sexual histories in the two groups is statistically and clinically significant.

Among the positive PAS patients, the abnormal sexual histories included rape (n = 6) and childhood molestation or incest (n = 4). These events were emotion-

Table 6 Sexual Histories

Patient	Diagnosis	Present age	Sexual history
1	Depression	41	Raped at age 30.
2	Depression	34	Unplanned pregnancy at age 18. While pregnant she developed multiple sclerosis. As a result, the father of the child left her 1 month before delivery. Baby was then given up for adoption.
3	Schizophrenia	22	Raped at age 16.
4	Schizophrenia	22	Sexually molested by an adult at age 5.
5	Schizophrenia	18	Raped at age 16.
6	Borderline	19	Juvenile onset gender identity disorder.
7	Borderline	15	Repeated sexual contact with stepfather from age 12. Prostitution, onset age 12.
8	Borderline plus Depression	18	Raped at age 16.
9	Borderline plus Depression	22	Reported sexual contact with a friend of father's, when she was age 8. Oral sex with two older brothers, early adolescence. Abortions at ages 15, 19, and 20.
10	Borderline plus Depression	41	Raped twice at age 21. Incest with older brother and sex with older brother's friends, onset age 7.
11	Borderline plus Depression	37	Totally inhibited sexual desire following gyn surgery at age 25.
12	Borderline plus Depression	17	Ego dystonic homosexuality, onset age 11.
13	Borderline plus Depression	18	Juvenile onset gender identity disorder.
14	Borderline plus Depression	25	Raped at age 14.
15	Borderline plus Depression	15	Ego dystonic homosexuality, onset age 13.

(continued)

Table 6   (continued)

Patient	Diagnosis	Present age	Sexual history
16	Borderline plus Depression	21	Ego dystonic homosexuality, onset age 19.
17[a]	Schizophrenia	21	Child out of wedlock at age 17. Family "right to life" Catholic and had several "unwed mothers" boarding with them during patient's early adolescence. She is described as a "rebel" and although her parents were angry about her pregnancy, had no choice but to allow her to bear child.

[a]Patient denies history of PAS.

ally painful for patients to recall and their involvement was a source of consciously perceived conflict. Three additional patients met DSM-III criteria for ego dystonic homosexuality and two for gender identity disorder. In one case, gynecologic surgery that had no effect on menstruation was followed by inhibited sexual excitement, and in another, an out-of-wedlock pregnancy and abandonment by the child's father coincided with the onset of multiple sclerosis. Finally, two patients also gave histories of medical abortions. In this series of patients, all those who gave histories of childhood molestation or incest, rape, ego dystonic homosexuality, or other sexual pathology or abortions were confined to the positive PAS group. Of the two patients who had had marital pregnancies, and subsequent adoption of the child, one was included in the positive and one in the negative PAS group.

Felice et al. [39] stated that PAS might be one type of psychosomatic difficulty resulting from such trauma as rape. We believe that other abnormal sexual events such as those described above and occurring predominantly among our positive PAS patients might have similar consequences.

In conceptualizing relationships between psychodynamics, psychopathology, and biologic rhythms associated with the menstrual cycle, we have applied the initial observations and hypotheses of Benedek and Rubenstein [2] to a wider psychopathologic domain than the neuroses. Our clinical research suggests that level of ego organization and severity of affective disturbance both appear to play an important, but unequal, role in the prevalence of a premenstrual affective syndrome in various psychiatric groups. The prevalence of the premenstrual affective syndrome is somewhat greater in those groups characterized by both a low level of ego integration and the concurrent presence of severe affective disturbance. We have also presented data indicating that, particularly for these patients, unresolved sexual conflicts, as induced by severe, early sexual trauma, might be of etiologic significance. We would speculate that abnormal sexual experience during early (prepubertal) development creates a specific sense of sexual vulnerability in many women. This vulnerability is evident in the cyclic strain associated with the menstrual cycle and its highlighting of sexual and reproductive conflicts after puberty. The association of an increased prevalence of premenstrual affective syndrome with psychopathologic conditions characterized by the concurrent presence of dysphoric symptoms and poor ego integration is compatible with this model.

The complexities of the interrelationship of biologic and psychodynamic factors are not to be minimized. We can postulate that, in many cases, the interactions of physiology, psychosocial stress, and intrapsychic conflict may lead to PAS. We must also consider that developmental psychodynamics and biologic frames of reference are not mutually exclusive. Therefore, it is a multifaceted view of the menstrual cycle and its relation to psychopathology that presents us with this intriguing and interesting area of study.

Acknowledgment

The author gratefully acknowledge the most helpful assistance of Ms. Pat Cobb in the preparation of this chapter.

References

1. R. T. Frank, *Arch. Neurol. Psychiatry* 26:1053 (1931).
2. T. Benedek and B. B. Rubenstein, *Psychosom. Med.* 1:245, 461 (1939).
3. S. L. Smith, in *Topics in Psychoendocrinology* (E. J. Sachar, ed.). Grune & Stratton, New York, 1975.
4. M. B. Parlee, *Psychol. Bull.* 80:454 (1973).
5. J. F. O'Conner, E. M. Shelly, and L. O. Stern, in *Biorhythms and Human Reproduction* (M. Ferin, G. Halberg, R. M. Richart, and R. L. Vande Wiele, eds.). John Wiley, New York, 1974.
6. M. Steiner and B. J. Carroll, *Psychoneuroendocrinology* 2:321 (1977).
7. R. H. Moos, *The Menstrual Distress Questionnaire Manual.* Stanford University, Stanford, 1977.
8. B. Sommer, *Psychosom. Med.* 35:515 (1973).
9. J. Abplanalp, R. F. Haskett, and R. M. Rose, *Psychiatr. Clin. North Am.* 3:327 (1980).
10. K. Minkoff, E. Bergman, A. T. Beck, and R. Beck, *Am. J. Psychiatry* 130:455 (1973).
11. M. A. Silver, M. Bohnert, A. T. Beck, and D. Marcus, *Arch. Gen. Psychiatry* 25:573 (1971).

12.   A. J. Mandell and M. P. Mandell, *JAMA* 200:132 (1967).
13.   R. D. Wetzel and J. N. McClure, *Comp. Psychiatry* 13:369 (1972).
14.   R. D. Wetzel, T. Reich, J. N. McClure, and J. A. Wald, *Br. J. Psychiatry* 127:219 (1975).
15.   T. Kashiwagi, J. N. McClure, and R. B. Wetzel, *Dis. Nerv. Syst.* 37:116 (1976).
16.   M. A. Schuckit, V. Daly, G. Herrman, and S. Hineman, *Dis. Nerv. Syst.* 36:516 (1975).
17.   D. J. Pallis and T. A. Holding, *J. Biosoc. Sci.* 8:27 (1976).
18.   R. F. Haskett, M. Steiner, J. N. Osmun, and B. J. Carroll, *Biol. Psychiatry* 15:121 (1980).
19.   J. Endicott, U. Halbreich, and S. Schacht, *Psychosom. Med.* 43:88 (1981).
20.   R. L. Spitzer, J. Endicott, and E. Robins, *Arch. Gen. Psychiatry* 35:773 (1978).
21.   *Diagnostic and Statistical Manual of Mental Disorders,* Third Edition. American Psychiatric Association, Washington, D.C., 1980.
22.   S. Freud, *The Complete Introductory Lectures on Psychoanalysis.* W. W. Norton & Co., Inc., New York, 1966, p. 576.
23.   K. Horney, *New Ways in Psychoanalysis.* W. W. Norton & Company, Inc., New York, 1939.
24.   K. Horney, *The Collected Works of Karen Horney,* Vol. I. W. W. Norton & Co., Inc., New York, 1937-1945.
25.   K. Horney, *Feminine Psychology.* W. W. Norton & Co., Inc., New York, 1967.
26.   C. Thompson, *Psychiatry* 4:1 (1941).
27.   C. Thompson, *Psychiatry* 6:123 (1943).
28.   C. Thompson, *Psychoanalysis: Evaluation and Development.* Hermitage House, New York, 1950.
29.   C. Thompson, in *Psychoanalysis and Female Sexuality* (H. M. Ruitenbeek, ed.). College & University Press, New Haven, 1966.
30.   A. C. Kinsey, W. B. Pomeroy, C. E. Martin, and P. H. Gebhard, *Sexual Behavior in the Human Male.* Saunders, Philadelphia, 1948.
31.   A. C. Kinsey, W. Pomeroy, C. Martin, and P. H. Gebhard, *Sexual Behavior in the Human Female.* Saunders, Philadelphia, 1953.
32.   W. H. Masters and V. E. Johnson, *Human Sexual Response.* Little, Brown Boston, 1966.
33.   M. J. Sherfey, *J. Am. Psychoanal. Assoc.* 14:28 (1966).
34.   D. B. Adams, A. R. Gold, and A. D. Brut, *N. Engl. J. Med.* 299:1145 (1978).
35.   J. Brooks, D. Ruble, and A. Clark, *Psychosom. Med.* 39:288 (1977).
36.   J. L. Kramp, *Acta Psychiatr. Scand. [Suppl.]* 203:261 (1968).
37.   A. Coppen, *Br. J. Psychiatry* 111:155 (1965).
38.   S. B. Diamond, A. A. Rubinstein, D. L. Dunner, and R. R. Fieve, *Compr. Psychiatr.* 17:541 (1976).
39.   M. Felice, J. Grant, B. Reynolds, S. Gold, M. Wyatt, and F. P. Heald, *Clin. Pediatr.* 17:311 (1978).

16 Premenstrual Tension in Borderline and Related Disorders

MICHAEL H. STONE   University of Connecticut Health Center, Farmington, Connecticut

Recently, borderline syndromes have received considerable attention in the psychiatric literature. A number of investigators have also noted an uneven sex distribution among "borderline" cases, however defined, within and across cultures. The female preponderance is in the range of 2:1 (Spitzer et al., 1979; Stone and Oestberg, 1979; Stone, 1980). Given such an uneven distribution, it would not seem inappropriate to search for explanations involving phenomena specific to females. Psychological trauma stemming from sexual molestation (including incest) might constitute one contributory factor, as has been suggested by Brooks (1980), since this is trauma to which girls are considerably more vulnerable than boys. Trauma of this sort may have been experienced by 5% of all women in our culture, and probably by a higher percentage of those who will later be labeled "borderline." Moderate to severe psychological symptoms recurring at some point in the menstrual cycle (usually premenstrually, but in many instances menstrually or in the preovulative phase): (O'Connor et al., 1973) affect an even higher percentage of women: one-sixth to one-half, depending on how severity is defined (cf. Haskett et al., 1980). Possible connections between these "premenstrual" syndromes and borderline or related disorders have nonetheless remained unexplored. Clinicians who work primarily with borderline patients are often struck by the severity of menstrual-cycle-related symptoms in their female patients (or in certain ostensibly neurotic women, whose symptom picture is aggravated premenstrually to reach the borderline level of pathology).

This chapter will explore this hitherto neglected area. This exploration, it should be noted, is undertaken with a certain measure of presumptuousness, since, as Parlee (1973) has pointed out in her careful review, psychological studies have "... not as yet established the existence of a class of behaviors and moods, *measurable in more than one way,* which can be shown to fluctuate throughout the course of the menstrual cycle" (p. 463). Here we shall assume that it *is* nevertheless meaningful to speak of a "premenstrual syndrome," despite its possessing, by the most exacting scientific standards, no more than "face validity" (Parlee, 1973). [Emphasis added]

I. Historical Note

That many women experience emotional and physical discomfort around the time of their menses has been known for millenia and has been commented upon by the earliest medical writers, from the time of Hippocrates. Simon (1978) cites a relevant passage from Hippocrates' *Diseases of Women,* where hysterical diseases were ascribed, at times, to retained menstrual blood, and characterized by women "gnashing their teeth" or "doing all sorts of unheard-of things" (pp. 242-243). Retained menses were viewed as capable of provoking delusory thinking as well, or raving madness or suicidal thoughts.

The ancients were also much concerned with possible influences of the sun and the moon upon body or soul; it did not seem fantastic to them, as it often does to modern physicians, that the moon could cause thythmic variations in temperament, enough to justify allusion to a "lunar" cycle, analogous to the more familiar menstrual cycle. Men were seen as vulnerable to these lunar effects as much as were women. These positions were argued, for example, by the renowned 17th century English physician, Richard Mead, whose treatise on lunar and solar influences is the more known to us for its having been plagiarized a century later by Mesmer (Pattie, 1956). Mead (1748) citing one of his predecessors, mentions a case supposedly exemplifying the effects of the full moon:

Carolus Piso . . . related [the case] of a girl, who, about each full moon of the Spring season, was seized with such obstinate hysterical symptoms, that they continued the whole third quarter. The first day she was convulsed, then she was seized with a loss of speech, and fell into a deep sleep, which lasted two days; and the remaining four days she spent in doing insignificant things, crying out for help; or . . . in a slight delirium, without a wink of sleep.

Pinel's awareness of menses-related symptoms, that could on occasion be extremely florid, is reflected in the following passage from his 1799 *Nosographie:*

A young girl of dark complexion and of strong and healthy constitution fell into a state of "mania" at the age of seventeen, without any apparent cause. The mania consisted in a series of extravagant acts: talking to herself, leaping about, ripping off her clothes and throwing them into the fire. This went on for some five months . . . and was followed by her first menstrual period. After three cycles in which there was no flow, she then manifested hysterical crises at each successive period. At first there would be a disinclination for her customary activities, frequent crying for no obvious reason, a gloomy and taciturn demeanor, and soon thereafter—loss of speech, flushed facies, spasmodic tightening in the neck and a sense of being choked. These symptoms would last three or four days . . . following which all her functions would return to normal.

Clinicians in Pinel's day could have no understanding of the specific hormones connected with the menstrual cycle, nor of their normal cyclic variations. Yet Pinel was aware that pregnancy, by eliminating the menses for the better part of a year, eliminated the premenstrual turbulence to which certain women were prone. Hence he recommended early marriage and frequent pregnancies as a palliative, however unwieldy, for this condition. Similar advice was tendered by Esquirol's pupil, Voisin (1826) in the case of a young woman who experienced premenstrual nymphomania, Hippocrates, however, had recommended the same remedies two millenia earlier (Simon, 1978, p. 243). In our own time Coppen and Kessel (1963) observed that the tendency to severe premenstrual symptoms seemed to diminish with increasing parity.

Spurzheim (1818), the celebrated advocate of Gall's phrenology, would have cautioned against pregnancy in these cases, since it may be accompanied by emotional disorders as severe as the premenstrual condition it was to remedy:

At puberty, many girls of delicate constitution, with precocious disposition and overactive imagination, become melancholic, inactive and indifferent to things which once interested them—for example, the cleanliness of body and habits, displays of friendship, etc. All too often they end up succumbing to a general apathy or dementia. Besides, the menstrual flow, pregnancy, delivery and nursing are frequent causes of madness in women.*

Something closer to the modern description of the premenstrual syndrome is to be found in the famous textbook of Prichard (1835):

Some females, at the period of the catamenia, undergo a considerable degree of nervous excitement: morbid dispositions of mind are displayed by them at these times, a wayward and capricious temper, excitability in the feelings, moroseness in disposition, a proneness to quarrel with their dearest relatives, and sometimes a dejection of mind approaching to melancholia."

---

*To which, in a momentary lapse of chivalry, Spurzheim added, "one can therefore understand why the number of severely disturbed females is so great."

The elements of tension, depression, and irritability, highlighted in the landmark (for our century) paper of Frank (1931), are clearly adumbrated in Prichard's remarks.

Other commentators of the day who were cognizant of the tendency, in premenstrual afflictions, to *dysphoric* symptoms include Esquirol and another of his pupils, A. Brierre de Boismont. In the first volume of Esquirol's text (1838) we find: "Young women who haven't menstruated or those who have menstrual difficulties are prone to depression and suicide, as Hippocrates had once remarked."

In his monograph on suicide, Brierre de Boismont (1856) had the following observations:

Difficulties with menstruation, the return of the cycle to its critical point, often induce in women a boredom with life and a desire to put it to an end. It is not rare, especially among the mentally ill and the epileptic, to see women who, during the menstrual flow, search for every imaginable means of destroying themselves, and who forget all about such wishes throughout the rest of the month.

II. Definition of Borderline Syndromes

The term *borderline* derived from attempts to classify certain patients referred for psychoanalytic treatment whose psychopathology was later discovered to be greater than could be handled effectively by that method (Stern, 1938). Borderline demarcated a region between psychosis and classic "analyzable" neurosis. Other definitions were formulated where the emphasis was on the proximity of the proposed "borderline" case to core schizophrenia (Knight, 1953). A variety of competing terms not embodying "borderline" as an adjective, which were briefly popular, describe cases resembling those already being grouped within the borderline terminology. These terms are numerous and include *ambulatory schizophrenia* (Zilboorg, 1941), *as-if personality* (Deutsch, 1942), *latent psychosis* (Bychowski, 1953), and *pseudoneurotic schizophrenia* (Hoch and Polatin, 1949). The nearness of some cases to schizophrenia was suggested by Ekstein's "borderline schizophrenia" (1955) and by Rado's "schizotypal" (1956); in other cases the similarity to manic depression is suggested "cyclothymic depression" (Jacobson, 1953). Frosch (1964) emphasized in his descriptions of the *psychotic character* that brief psychotic episodes might occur sporadically and take the form of either ordinary schizophrenia or manic-depressive illness.

Some of the prominent symptoms displayed by these borderline patients included narcissism, inordinate hypersensitivity to rejection or criticism, a poor capacity to tolerate stress, a strong tendency to externalize (close, at times, to paranoia), and mild difficulties (short of delusion) with reality testing, especially in the realm of interpersonal relationships (Stern, 1938). Deutsch's "as-if" patients displayed a masking of aggressive tendencies and an inner emptiness.

Knight, although concerned with differentiating *borderline* from unequivocal schizophrenia, tended to use the term as a separate. The chief features were weakening of such ego functions as secondary process thought and realistic planning, along with a general primitive level of defense mechanisms (with domination of denial and projection, instead of healthier defenses such as rationalization and intellectualization).

After this time, borderline is used almost exclusively to denote clinical entities considered by their promulgators as distinct from other diagnostic entities. This is true of the definitions proposed by Grinker et al. (1968); Kernberg, (1967, 1977), and Gunderson and Singer (1975). More recently others (Stone, 1977, 1980; Akiskal et al., 1977; Carroll et al., 1980) have been impressed by the degree to which many cases subsumed under the borderline label closely resemble, or later evolve directly into, primary affective disorder.

The Grinker criteria, although influenced by the position on borderline conditions taken by the Chicago Psychoanalytic institute, emphasized phenomenologic rather than strictly psychoanalytic impressions. The most common characteristics were (1) anger is the main or only affect, (2) there is a defect in affectional relationships, (3) the sense of identity is weak and inconsistent; and (4) depression characterizes life. Grinker's group believed that their patients could be classified into four subdivisions. Details of these subgroups have been summarized elsewhere (Perry and Klerman, 1978; Stone, 1980, p. 29). For our purposes, it is important to note that affective, chiefly depressive, symptoms are prominent in three; the other subgroup resembles Deutsch's as-if personality. Grinker's Type IV, for example, showed anaclitic depression and anxiety, as well as narcissistic characterologic features.

One of the difficulties with the Grinker schema is the absence of readily objectifiable criteria analyzable by computer, which hampers the development of a common language between Grinker's group and psychiatrists at other centers. Several contemporary investigators have sought to rectify this.

Kernberg's formulations (1967, 1977) are the result of his ambitious attempt to bring objectification and a standardized approach within the context of a psychoanalytic system. There are two basic criteria: (1) the patient must preserve the capacity to test reality even in the interpersonal realm and (2) the sense of identity or "ego-integration" is enfeebled. The first rules out psychosis; the latter neurosis (in the sense of a classically analyzable condition). Nonspecific criteria include: (1) a lowered capacity to tolerate stress, (2) impulsivity, and (3) poor functioning in the realms of school, avocations, or work. Finally, primitive defenses predominate: denial, projective identification, splitting (where sharply contradictory views of the self and of others exist side by side in the mind without being seriously questioned). Core schizophrenia and even schizotypal but nondelusional conditions are almost always excluded by the first item mentioned above: patients with these more serious disorders usually cling to their distorted views of themselves and others, even in the face of persuasive confrontation. Although Kernberg did not have the primary affective disorders in mind when he established his criteria, many patients who emerge as borderline in his schema happen to exhibit, or go on to exhibit at follow-up, many of the signs of manic-depressive illness (depressive more than bipolar); their close relatives also exhibit various affective disorders in an unexpectedly high proportion (Stone 1977; Stone et al., 1980). A sizeable subgroup of Kernberg borderline patients (two-thirds of whom are female) are affectively ill. Their relative youth (their average age in most samples will be in the 20s) means they have not passed through much of the age of risk for the classic psychoses (schizophrenia and manic-depression). However, unipolar depressive criteria are fulfilled, or nearly so, in a fair percentage of cases, especially if followed for several years.

One of the chief values of the Kernberg system is that it defines an overall *level of function,* more than a restrictive syndrome. The breadth of applicability and its utility are closely related to this fact.

Midway between the psychoanalytic and the phenomenologic, the borderline schema elaborated by Gunderson (Gunderson and Singer, 1975; Gunderson and Kolb, 1978) selects a patient sample that is smaller, but located almost entirely within, Kernberg's borderline *level* of personality organization. The Gunderson definition adheres more closely to the usual definition of a *syndrome,* and has as its chief characteristics: (1) lowered achievement (this distinguished "borderline" from "neurotic"), (2) impulsivity, (3) manipulative suicide threats, (4) mild or brief psychotic episodes, (5) good superficial socialization (whereas core schizophrenics tend to show *poor* socialization), and (6) disturbances in close relationships. The latter consists either of general ragefulness or a tendency to be depressive; and vulnerable, should a love relationship become threatened, to suicide gestures or angry outbursts. The "borderline personality disorder," as the Gunderson syndrome is usually called, may also be further subdivided into a (smaller) schizotypal variety and a (larger) affectively ill group, many cases of which can, as with comparable cases in the Kernberg schema, be seen as formes frustres of major depressive (or, at times, bipolar-II: see Dunner et al., 1976) disorder.

Gunderson and his co-workers have devised a 119 item questionnaire, the Diagnostic Interview for Borderlines (DIB) to objectify the diagnostic entity they have proposed.

The contribution of Spitzer and his group toward resolving some of the confusion that besets this borderline realm of diagnosis is their attempt (Spitzer et al., 1979) to determine, through a survey of American psychiatrists and psychoanalysts, what signs and symptoms cropped up most frequently among cases labeled "borderline." An effort was also made to factor-analyze their results, to see if certain diagnostically cohesive variants emerged. Although only a minority of borderline patients could be viewed as pure-types, two factors did appear to merit separate standing: the *schizotypal* and the "unstable." The unstable items will outnumber the schizotypal in a sample of borderline patients (Stone and Oestberg, 1979); many would be recognized as related to, if not a part of, the primary *affective* disorders: unstable interpersonal relationships, intense anger, self-damaging acts, affective instability, impulsivity, and feeling frantic when alone.

Even more tilted toward the affective pole of disorders is the *hysteroid dysphoria* syndrome elaborated by Klein and Shader (1975). Although the term borderline is not part of this label, the majority of hysteroid dysphoric patients happen to fall within the borderline region, as defined by Kernberg (Stone, 1979). These rejection-sensitive patients, almost all of whom are female, experience frequent bouts of depression, often in conjunction with romantic disappointments, and tend to abuse alcohol or other drugs, make suicide threats, and show marked lowering of self-esteem.

III. Psychiatric Syndromes Related to the Menstrual Cycle

Women may experience a variety of psychological symptoms connected with the menstrual cycle, including dysmenorrhea and "premenstrual tension" (PMT). The combination of anxiety, headache, mood lability, fatiguability, breast swelling, and insomnia, mentioned by Perr (1958) or the collection of factors (pain, changes in ability to concentrate, social avoidance, autonomic reactions, water retention, negative affect, notably irritability and tense depression, etc.) outlined by Moos (1968) are the basic ingredients of the premenstrual tension syndrome. Although these symptoms were reported in Frank's original and oft-quoted article (1931) as occurring 10 to 7 days before the menses, several authors have pointed out that (1) not every affected woman shows all of these symptoms during any or each cycle, and (2) the timing is not always confined to the premenstruum per se, but may occur during the menses (Beaumont, et al., 1975) or (usually in a milder form) just before ovulation (Greene and Dalton, 1953; May, 1976; O'Connor et al., 1973). Alterations in sexual behavior, including nymphomania, are noted in some women, as part of the PMT syndrome (Gray, 1941). Coppen and Kessel (1963) and Cullberg (1972) believed that PMT symptoms were exacerbations of preexisting neurotic personality traits; in a sample of women with dysmenorrhea, on the other hand, symptoms occurred only *during* the time of menstrual flow; the women who experienced painful menses, furthermore, did not score higher than other women on a scale of neuroticism.

There are few women who do not experience some cycle-related symptoms during their reproductive life. Smith (1975), citing Torghele (1957), mentions that 216 of 272 women (79%) in a state hospital reported varying degrees of premenstrual discomfort. Similar findings were noted in cross-cultural studies. "Periodic psychosis" in Japanese women, for example, usually occurred in the luteal phase (Smith, 1975). Likewise, 42% of acute psychiatric admissions in a Danish hospital took place in the premenstrual part of the patient's cycle (Kramp, 1968); similar findings were also reported by Glass (1971). Perhaps 30 to 60% of women experience at least mild to moderate premenstrual symptoms; the more severe

forms, necessitating restriction of daily activities or bed rest, are experienced by
a smaller percentage (7% in Coppen and Kessel's 1963 estimate; 5% "severe" and
16% "moderate," in an earlier study cited by Tonks, 1975).

In agreement with the authors mentioned above, who believed that the PMT
syndrome resulted from an interaction of biologic factors with preexisting "neuroticism," are the observations of Tonks (1975): women with known psychiatric
disorders had a much higher incidence of *severe* (32% as against 5%) or *moderate*
(30% instead of 16%) symptoms than women in the general population.

The irritability, tension, depression, etc. that comprise the PMT syndrome are
not the sole emotional disorders to which women are vulnerable at critical points
in the cycle (premenstrual, menstrual, and preovulatory, in descending order of
risk). Crimes committed by women may occur predominantly during the premenstruum (Perr, 1958). Besides the increase in general psychiatric emergencies at this
time, noted by Glass et al. (1971) and Dalton (1959), suicide threats and calls to
suicide-prevention centers are also more frequent (Wetzel et al., 1971a, 1971b;
Wetzel and McClure, 1972). Williams and Weekes (1952), in an anecdotal study,
mentioned how often acute psychoses (schizophrenia, mania, etc.) occurred premenstrually, although (as Haskett et al., 1980, also noted), *not* always accompanied by the typical PMT symptoms.

Of considerable interest here, because of its location at the interface of the
two entities under consideration, is the "wrist cutting" alluded to by Graff and
Mallin (1967) and Grunebaum and Klerman (1967). Both sets of authors describe
a series of young women who cut their wrists or otherwise mutilate themselves as
pathologic means of easing "indescribable tension." Exploitation of this action for
emotional gain was a common feature, since it was often done in the hospital, when
the doctors and nurses most familiar with them had gone home for the evening or
when the patient had hoped to coerce a staff member into providing some attention
or favor. Other characteristic elements of these patients were their chaotic interpersonal relationships, sexual disorders (including episodic promiscuity), history
of childhood incestuous or other sexual trauma, and tendency to abuse alcohol
or other substances. Grunebaum and Klerman believed these patients ". . . belong
to a syndrome in the borderline group, with specific assets and liabilities in ego
development" (p. 532), but none of these authors mentions the menstrual cycle
as a possible contributing factor. However, one can hardly read the case descriptions without speculating that the self-mutilation episodes were an expression of
(pre)menstrual tension. Five years later, Rosenthal et al. (1972), in similarly
psychodynamically oriented article, nevertheless paid close attention to menstrual
phenomena: "most striking was the high correlation between the act of cutting
and the point in the patient's menstrual cycle. More than 60% of the cutting
gestures were not all "premenstrual," but were evenly divided between the premenstruum and menstruation.

These patients do not represent the only intersection of the borderline and
the premenstrual syndromes. Others have suggested that women with primary

affective disorders are at a greater risk for severe PMT. Schuckit et al. (1975), for example, noted a trens: 11% of women with severe PMT also satisfied Feighner et al.'s (1972) criteria for recurrent unipolar depression (as opposed to 5% of a control group). A family history of depressive illness was greater in the PMT sample as well. McClure et al. (1971), describing several women with bipolar symptoms in the premenstrual phase, who also had a family history of mania, believed that women with primary affective disorders were particularly likely to report premenstrual depression.

These observations have led to speculation that the PMT syndrome may be a variant or atypical expression of primary affective disorder (manic-depressive illness (Coppen, 1965; Kashiwagi et al., 1976). A logical extension of this argument would be, recognizing that isogenic conditions need not always be isophenic (Cancro, 1975), that severe PMT and recurrent affective disorders are different phenotypic expressions of common genetic source. A more conservative, and probably more accurate, view would be that the PMT syndrome and primary affective disorder are usually etiologically separate, but overlap in their occurrence, interacting in such a way that a predisposition to one aggravates any tendency to the other. Diamond et al. (1976) attribute many of the PMT syndrome symptoms to premenstrual hormonal changes that affect electrolyte and fluid balances in the body. These electrolyte shifts (e.g., increase in residual sodium) might contribute to depression and hence *worsen* the affective state. If, as seems likely, PMT syndrome is etiologically heterogeneous, we would not expect one remedy to suffice for all cases. Sletten and Gershon (1966), for example, reported promising results with lithium in eight women with severe premenstrual irritability who also had significant degrees of water retention. This might lend support to the hypothesis that severe PMT is close to bipolar affective disorders. But in a more recent and more controlled study, Singer et al. (1974) found that lithium was only slightly more effective than placebo in 19 Chinese women with PMT syndrome. In a similar vein, Steiner et al. (1980), after administering lithium to 15 women selected for the severity of their premenstrual symptoms, found only three who responded favorably. These three also met diagnostic criteria for cyclothymic disorder (i.e., subclinical form of primary affective disorder: Akiskal et al., 1977). Two of the three had a family history of affective disorder.

To the extent that suicide may be an expression of genetic loading for affective disorder, the heightened incidence of completed suicide in the *luteal* phase (MacKinnon and MacKinnon, 1956; MacKinnon et al., 1959) might be the other side of the same coin: PMT and suicide as two of the many faces of manic-depression. The menstrual-cycle-related suicide threats of which Wetzel and his collaborators had written, and the manipulative suicidal gestures such as wrist cutting, could be seen as less extreme examples of the same phenomenon. Here again, one must resist the appeal of a theory whose simplicity would probably prove more attractive than accurate (that the PMT syndrome is a variant of manic-depression).

Smith (1975) underlined certain differences between the PMT syndrome and at least those forms of primary affective disorder that satisfy the most exacting diagnostic criteria: women exhibiting premenstrual dysphoria have fewer "vegetative" signs than are encountered in clear-cut unipolar disease; early morning sleep disturbances are not encountered with any regularity in women with premenstrual disturbances. Haskett et al. (1980) noted that women with high scores on a menstrual distress questionnaire (MDQ) in the estrogen-dominated *follicular* phase, rather than in the expected luteal phase, often had high scores on scales for neurotic-depression in general. Their MDQ scores did not increase markedly as they entered the premenstrual week. These data, again, point more in the direction of *interaction* between, rather than *identity* between, the PMT syndrome and manic-depression.

A number of biochemical studies have sought to clarify relationships between cycle phases and the symptoms peculiar to these phases. Investigators impressed by the correlation between premenstrual water retention and premenstrual irritability have sought cyclic variations in electrolyte concentration that might account for both the water retention and the symptoms. Coppen and Shaw (1963) found an increase in intracellular and in some bone sodium ("residual Na") in states of *depression*. Similar findings were reported by Sletten and Gershon (1966) in women experiencing severe PMT (where depression was a prominent part of the clinical picture). Cortisol, whose excretion is increased in many instances of depression, causes heightened levels of intracellular sodium (Coppen and Shaw, 1963), making this hormone a possible beginning point in any theory of PMT syndrome. More recently, however, the primacy of water-retention in the PMT syndrome has been questioned. Some women with severe PMT symptoms report little gain in weight premenstrually; others experience weight gain before ovulation, but no symptoms at that time (Greene and Dalton, 1953).

Other investigators have focused on the role of estrogens and progesterones. Rees (1953), for example, believed that as progesterone levels diminished in the late luteal phase, still circulating estrogens were suddenly "unopposed," leading to water retention and premenstrual swelling and tension.

Possible interactions between female sex hormones and the factors underlying manic-depression have been suggested by the work of Gordon et al. (1980): estrogen appears to exert antidopaminergic effects which could then aggravate a depression. Gordon's study was prompted by the observation that postmenopausal women were especially at risk for tardive dyskinesia secondary, perhaps, to the waning of ovarian estrogen production. Paige (1971), studying the effects of oral contraceptives on paramenstrual "negative affect" (hostility, anxiety, depression), noted that some women taking these compounds showed no cyclic variations in affect. He ascribed this flattening of the normal curve in part to a drug-related diminution in menstrual flow, in part to altered monoamine oxidase (MAO) activity. The PMT syndrome, Paige speculated, may stem from heightened MAO activity, secondary to increased progesterone levels (cf. Grant and Pryse-Davis,

1968); estrogen, by inhibiting MAO activity might be conducive to the maintenance of normal mood. Despite these intriguing correlations between the catecholamine hypothesis of depression and changes in monoamine activity provoked by female hormones, no substantial evidence unifies primary affective disorder and the paramenstrual mood disorders. Paige cautions that there is ". . .
no empirical evidence to justify the assumption that specific affective changes
in the cycle occur in direct response to specific biochemical changes" (p. 516).

Invoking a somewhat different biochemical model relevant to depression,
Smith (1975) speculated that, in certain women with a history of depressive disorder, estrogen may lead to exacerbation of symptoms through its interference
with tryptophan metabolism (leading to a lowered central nervous system serotonin level). Some cases of PMT syndrome may therefore reflect estrogens excess (cf. Frank, 1931), but, as Smith stresses, not all. Perhaps in only a minority
of women are hormonal changes of primary importance in their paramenstrual
symptoms.

For a more detailed discussion of late-luteal rise in endometrial MAO, the
role of progesterone, and the possible relationship to premenstrual depression,
the paper of Grant and Pryse-Davies (1968) should be consulted. The implication
for *treatment* resulting from the often-conflicting results among investigators are
discussed at length by Paige (1971) and Sampson (1979). The latter's double-
blind cross-over study of progesterone therapy for PMT syndrome failed to
demonstrate more benefit than placebo.

IV. Psychodynamic Considerations

Both borderline and premenstrual tension syndromes seem to be heterogeneous
and multifactorial in origin. Psychogenic factors would appear to play an important role: as "necessary" in neither; but "sufficient" in some borderline cases.
In the latter, overwhelmingly stressful early environments alone can, on occasion,
lead, by themselves, to the rigidification of personality and primitivity of defenses
that make up the criteria for most of the various "borderline" labels (Stone, 1980,
pp. 308-310).

To the extent that the PMT syndrome results in most instances from interaction between biologic and psychological forces,* it is important to note whether
certain types of psychological trauma are particularly conducive to the manifestation of this syndrome, and if so, whether they would tend to exert their pathogenic influence at particular points in the menstrual cycle.

A number of psychoanalysts have addressed themselves to these questions.
Daly (1935) believed that both men and women harbored unconscious fantasies

---

*The biologic forces are sufficient only for a minority (Friedman et al., 1980). In Cullberg's
opinion (1972): "Some women may suffer painful moods at certain points in the cycle and
not suffer from additional global forms of psychopathology."

in which menstruation was experienced as a castrative punishment for infantile sexual strivings. Rodrigue (1955) described a 26-year-old woman (who may have been manic-depressive functioning at the borderline level) in whom recurrent bouts of depression, dysmenorrhea, and ego boundary loss occurred in the paramenstrual part of her cycle. Dreams during that phase depicted bodily mutilation: she would seem to swallow her own flesh, or to see a hole in the center of her face. Her father was violent; in the course of her analysis, it was revealed that menstruation, for her, was seen as a sadistic form of sex. A comparable viewpoint was expressed by Helene Deutsch (1965). Writing on the narcissistic component of reactions to loss, she mentioned that menstrual depressions could be reactions to loss, either in the sense of (fantasied) castration, or as fantasied loss of a possible (incestuously conceived) pregnancy.

Several investigators have searched for links between mental content and menstrual phase in normal women. Using 5 min random tape-recorded conversations (analyzed for anxiety and hostility), Gottschalk et al. (1961) noted transient decreases in the levels of anxiety and hostility against the self at ovulation. These authors stressed the importance of studying more than one cycle, to negate the effects of random, but possibly pathogenic, interpersonal events. Women may tend to rationalize an upset as being due to some "cause" in their interpersonal environment (husband forgot anniversary; boyfriend showed up half-an-hour late, etc.). But if the "causes" sre such that most women take them in stride, and if they occur only at specific times in one cycle after another, the suspicion is heightened that, in cases of PMT syndrome, the provocative factors are more within the patient's biology.

Ivey and Bardwick (1968) used a similar approach to that of Gottschalk and studied normal college students. Premenstrual anxiety levels were found to be increased significantly over those observed at ovulation. Conversational themes in the premenstrual phase centered around hostility, depression, self-depreciation, death, sexuality (including incest), and general failure to cope. In the opinion of the authors, the endocrine changes influenced psychological behavior even in normal women, such that their spontaneous verbalizations changed character in lock-step with changes in the phase of the menstrual cycle.

The most thorough attempt to correlate psychodynamic contents with specific phases of the cycle was actually the first: that of Benedek and Rubinstein in 1939. This study comes closest to answering Parlee's criticism of the absence of reports using more than one technique or frame of reference for issues concerning the PMT syndrome. While Benedek was recording sequential material from women in analytic treatment, Rubinstein was carrying out sequential measures of their hormone levels. Their findings were briefly: the *estrogenic* phase is characterized by active heterosexual libido, stimulating, in normal women, wishes for sexual gratification. In neurotic women, jealousy may be stirred up and lead to aggressive feelings toward a (male) sexual partner. The few days immediately *before ovulation,* when estrogen levels suddenly diminish, are accompanied by increased narcissistic concerns, heterosexual hostility, and fears relating to the mother. These tendencies give way in the succeeding *ovulative* phase to attitudes of passive dependency, relaxation, pleasure, and heightened identification with the child role (with being her mother's child). At the time of peak progesterone levels in midluteal phase, the dominant feelings are associated with being or becoming a mother; impregnation wishes become more conscious, as does the wish to nurse a baby. There is a longing for closeness at this time. Finally, in the *premenstrual* phase, aggressive tendencies assert themselves to an even greater degree than during the preovulative phase. The woman's preexisting state is apparently important: Benedek reported that in those women whose unconscious relationship to their mothers was predominantly *hostile,* the "oral" material becomes aggressively tinged and tensions develop. These destroy the otherwise pleasant passive-dependent and narcissistic feelings of the postovulative phases and may prompt a severe *depressive* reaction.

To summarize, the available information suggests that even *normal* women are "lived" by their biochemical changes, to the extent that certain psychosexual preoccupations and feelings will surface at particular points in the menstrual cycle. Negative emotions (rage, hostility, sadness) are particularly likely, if they occur at all, to manifest themselves in the two paramenstrual phases and, to a lesser extent, in the preovulative phase. In women who are neurotic, or who, episodically or continually, function at the borderline level, these tendencies are often exaggerated, sometimes flagrantly. In these more severely affected women, anamnestic exploration will usually reveal pronounced and still unresolved conflicts concerning gender identity and reproductive life. The borderline wristcutters of Rosenthal et al. (1972), for example, often felt ". . . more like their fathers than their mothers" (p. 1365). Although promiscuity and sexual perversions were not manifested by many of these patients, the wrist cutters studied by Graff and Mallin (1967) did exhibit sexual disorders of this type. Negative reactions to the menarche were also typical in the (borderline) wrist cutting group, but were not typical of the normal controls (Rosenthal et al., p. 1364). Self-mutilative acts were never noted before the menarche. During their childhood years, the wrist-cutting patients had often been the passive victims of an unusually frightening experience (illness or surgery). Similarly, the borderline patients in a sample studied at the New York Hospital-Westchester Division, were often the victims of sadistic incestuous experiences with their fathers (Brooks and Stone, 1980). Impulse control and tolerance for interpersonal stress are low, by definition, in borderline women. These capacities are especially vulnerable paramenstrually (Friedman et al., 1980), and may account for many of the flamboyant suicide gestures of borderline women in this part of the cycle, and for many other unusual behaviors, such as trichotillomania (cf. Stone, 1980, case #16).

V. Case Histories

Neither borderline nor premenstrual tension syndrome is a unitary entity, nor
are there universally accepted diagnostic criteria. Haskett et al. (1980) have proposed a set for the PMT syndrome. Borderline does not figure among the diagnostic criterion sets of Feighner et al. (1972) nor the research diagnostic criteria
(RDC) of Spitzer et al. (1975). Kernberg and Gunderson's borderline schemes
generate similar patient samples, but are not coextensive. The Spitzer checklist
has now been incorporated into the DSM-III (1980), but, again, does not constitute the single, nor even the most popular, method of categorizing a patient as
borderline. Diagnosticians, for whom patients are considered "undiagnosible"
(Welner et al., 1973), or essentially free of psychopathology (unless they happen
to satisfy some accepted set of criteria), will tend to overlook certain clinical
pictures apparent to those with a different perspective. Perhaps some of Steiner
and Haskett's (1980) patients who, apart from their PMT syndrome, were believed
to be "without" psychopathology, may have functioned at the borderline level
(according to Kernberg), even while failing to meet criteria for unipolar depression, etc.

When borderline is used as a level of personality organization (Kernberg, 1977),
or level of function, consistency over time is implied. If a course of intensive psychotherapy is long enough and successful enough, the level, admittedly, may as-
cend to the higher neurotic level. Usually a patient diagnosed as borderline at one
time will, untreated, continue to warrant this label at any other time. But there
are exceptions. Many of these exceptional cases are precisely the ones are of special interest here: women with severe paramenstrual episodes, who would be diagnosed borderline (by almost any criteria) at the height of the symptom-outbreak,
but who, if evaluated during the rest of the cycle, would be seen as "neurotic."
Some women, in whom the premenstrual build-up of irritability, tension, hostility,
mood lability, or impulsivity may last 7 to 10 days, where the personality changes
do not revert to normal for another day or two after onset of menses, appear
borderline for *nearly half their reproductive life.* Are they to be considered
fundamentally borderline, but with some asymptomatic interludes? Or fundamentally neurotic with recurring decline in functional level and personality organization? These questions are not trivial, because the clinician treating such a
woman is necessarily prejudiced one way or the other, depending upon which
diagnosis seems more "real." Women with pronounced and recurrent fluctuations of this sort are often particularly puzzling to their therapists, for the very
reason that neither party has paid attention to the importance of the menstrual
factor. The rage attacks which figure so prominently in the Gunderson criteria,
for example, will often, if one takes the trouble to notice, be seen to occur not
only cyclically but paramenstrually. To ignore that juxtaposition would force a
therapist to give excessive importance to psychodynamic factors, and agree too
readily with the patient about some minor life event as "provoking" the outburst.

The case histories that follow, taken both from practice and hospital supervisory experience, will show something of the variety of clinical situations at the intersection of the premenstrual and the borderline (or borderlinelike) syndromes. They are presented in descending order of psychopathology, from the most ill (when first seen) to the least.

I. Miss A., a 23-year old art student, had been admitted to the emergency unit of a psychiatric hospital following serious suicide attempt. She had taken a large overdose of sleeping pills after an argument with her boyfriend. Having told no one of her suicidal intentions, she was discovered by a roommate who had returned to their apartment unexpectedly. The patient was transferred to a long-term facility, where she was noted to be sullen, depressed, almost uncommunicative, still preoccupied with thoughts of suicide, and tense. Her speech was coherent and she showed no "productive" signs of psychosis. Symptoms were predominantly affective (depressed, in this instance); personality organization was borderline. Guarded closely by the staff (who had placed her on "suicidal" precautions), she awoke on the second day after admission chipper and cheerful, as though nothing had happened, and went about the ward making encouraging comments to the other patients and asking if she could help out in the kitchen with mealtime chores. This transformation was noted by someone to coincide with the onset of her menses. This calm and considerate mood persisted for the next 3 weeks when, suddenly, she experienced extreme despair (ostensibly over the failure of her therapist to grant a minor request), and in the middle of the night, eluding her guard, ran into the shower where she tried to hang herself with a belt. Had not an orderly making rounds prevented her, she would have died. Her period came later that morning, however, and again her mood brightened instantly. The day before her next period, she tried to cut her wrists with broken glass.

The cyclic, and premenstrual, nature of her mood changes now having become obvious to the staff, a course of Lithium was prescribed. This had no beneficial effect, but Elavil (300 mg/day) did reduce the premenstrual tension so that she made either no, or only a mild, suicide threat. Gynecologic consultation revealed an ovarian cyst, removal of which contributed to amelioration of symptoms. She spent 16 months in the hospital. Upon discharge, she was able to work, and resumed her relationship with her boyfriend, with less tendency to arguments and suicide gestures during the premenstruum. Intensive psychotherapy focused on her hostile-dependent relationship with her mother, who had twice received electroconvulsive therapy for unipolar depression, and an unresolved longing for closeness with a schizoid and emotionally unavailable father.

The steepness and suddenness of functional decline premenstrually (and before treatment), in this woman exceeded that of any other patient with severe PMT syndrome known to this writer.

II. Mrs. B. had begun psychotherapy at age 26. Her marriage was deteriorating and divorce was imminent. She had become depressed, anxious, tearful, and less able to perform her usual duties at work. At times she strongly considered suicide. Several weeks after she and her husband separated, she panicked, abused alcohol, and drove recklessly on the highway, half intending to kill herself in an accident. The panic attack came two days before her period and she was subsequently hospitalized. Premenstrual symptom aggravation was noted by the hospital staff over the course of her next three periods. The most prominent symptoms were crying, paranoid feelings, hostility, anxiety of near-panic proportions, and preoccupation with suicide. Her personality organization was considered borderline. Prominent affective symptoms made tricyclic antidepressants seem a useful therapeutic adjunct. She responded to these with euphoria, giddiness, and pressured speech: a hypomanic attack, provoked by tricyclics in someone who could best be viewed, diagnostically, as bipolar-II, at the borderline level. She responded fairly well to Lithium: the premenstrual attacks were largely ameliorated. Severe forms of unipolar and bipolar depression had been present in several close maternal and paternal relatives. Her mother and a sister also experienced marked premenstrual tension.

After 2 years of intensive psychotherapy, supplemented with Lithium and sometimes an anxiolytic drug for the week preceding her period, she had become more stable. In addition, the sharply contradictory feelings toward self and others, the hallmark of the borderline ego integration defect in Kernberg's metapsychology, had been largely resolved. Her personality organization was now at the neurotic level. She still experienced occasional depressive episodes, only some of which occurred in the premenstrual phase.

Psychodynamic factors included a seductive father (although overt incestuous behavior had not occurred) and an extremely hostile, rejecting mother. The patient had three sisters and a brother, but, of the daughters, was the only one who adopted conventionally feminine values and attire. Her sisters also had frequent episodes of premenstrual tension: one exhibited, at this phase of the cycle, outbursts of rage and trichotillomania; another, promiscuity and depression.

III. Mrs. C. sought psychiatric consultation because of marital conflict and depressive episodes. She was 43 and had three grown children. "Every so often," she related, she and her husband would get into a heated argument (each blaming the other) that generally culminated in verbal and physical violence, and, on her part, abuse of alcohol, a crying spell, and a suicide gesture. This pattern repeated itself during the course of her therapy, and was seen to coincide invariably with the 3 or 4 days before her period. Following each outburst of hostility and depression came an "aftermath," during which she would feel puzzled at her previous irascibility, contrite toward her husband, and discouraged about her ever becoming stable enough to pursue postgraduate studies she had hoped to complete.

In the anamnesis it was revealed that her father had been a bipolar manic-depressive, severely alcoholic, and a compulsive gambler. One of her daughters had, in her 20s, begun to experience recurrent bouts of severe depression and had twice made serious suicide attempts.

Treatment consisted of regular visits to Alcoholics Anonymous, Elavil (and at times Thorazine) the 10 days before an anticipated period, and psychotherapy directed at her marital conflict. This succeeded in stabilizing her life, as desired, along with considerable easing of her premenstrual irritability and depression. As with many women with this condition, neither she nor her husband, despite years of sudden "inexplicable" mood shifts, had connected the dysphoric episodes and the particular phase of the menstrual cycle in which they occurred. Before her recovery, she fluctuated between borderline and neurotic, depending on the time of the month.

IV. Miss D. was in her late 30s when she began psychotherapy, having led a nomadic and eccentric existence for the 15 years since her graduation from college. She had never been regularly employed, but was supported by a generous trust from a grandparent. Two first-degree relatives had been hospitalized: her mother with "psychotic depression," a sibling, with paranoid schizophrenia. Ordinarily affable although socially withdrawn, circumstantial, good-hearted, and preoccupied with mysticism, astrology, and superstitions, premenstrually she became a "different person." For 2 or 3 days before her period, she was alternately irascible and tearful, self-depreciatory and paranoid, suicidal, hostile, loud, and abusive (slamming doors, phones, etc.). A succession of medications, including tricyclics, phenothiazines, Lithium, diuretics, and minor tranquilizers, had no appreciable benefit. She was very careful, however, to note on a calendar when her "bad days" were likely to come. She was impressed by medical fads and popular cure-alls and found a book that advised the addition of manganese to her diet as a sure means of curbing her depressive tendency. I expressed disapproval for unfounded remedies for serious conditions, but she began a manganese-rich diet and has been relatively asymptomatic before her periods ever since. Whether this was a placebo effect or a new cure for PMT was not determined.

She has remained relatively unresponsive to psychotherapy, however, and although now able to work, continues to lead an unfulfilled, schizoid existence. She was diagnostic puzzle for some time, but was eventually placeable (along a continuum from schizophrenia to manic-depression) as a predominantly affective schizoaffective patient, functioning at the borderline level.

V. Miss E., a single employed woman aged 32, was the eldest of three children, raised in poor circumstances by grandparents following the death of their mother (of cancer) when the patient was seven. Her father became alcoholic, as had been two of his brothers and a grandfather. Two aunts had received electroconvulsive therapy (ECT) for depression. Her grandmother was rejecting and strict to the point of cruelty. Each of the patient's male relatives in three generations tried to force her into sexual acts from the time she was 9. To some she acquiesced, after which she experienced strong guilt feelings, despite having been a victim with no advocate. Those feelings seemed to underlie her incapacity to experience orgasm until she had explored her sexual problems for many years in psychotherapy. She experienced recurrent episodes of depression, headache, tearfulness, self-denigration, and mild irritability, usually confined to the premenstruum but sometimes lasting 1 or 2 days after onset of menstruation. Tricyclic antidepressants were tried, partly because of the family history of major depressive disease. Her response was favorable and premenstrual symptoms were reduced to quite tolerable levels. Diagnostically, her personality organization has been neurotic, although at the height of a premenstrual episode she would momentarily appear borderline because of her (temporary) incapacity to view herself or those close to her realistically.

VI. Miss F. was a 35-year-old orchestral musician who had been in psychotherapy for many years becasue of difficulties in romantic relationships and with her fellow musicians. She had always been markedly eccentric, made almost no friends among women, but was successful at striking up acquaintances with men, with whom, however, she usually had only brief relationships. The emphasis of psychotherapy was on how to make a relationship last, in the face of her habit of finding minor faults in her boyfriends, whom she would then "scrap" in favor of some new potentially "better" partner. This patient was moderately irritable almost all the time, tended to be snappish with her colleagues in the orchestra, was extremely self-centered, and would often complain of "depression." The latter was seldom composed of sadness, tearfulness, or the more customary depressive symptoms, but was a heightening of her "baseline" irritability. Suicidal ruminations would sometimes accompany these spells, but never led to self-destructive gestures. These symptoms were markedly intensified the week before her period; her awareness of this tendency led her to plan vacations and other special occasions at times least likely to include a menstrual period.

Diagnostically, she fulfilled criteria for "schizotypal borderline" (Spitzer et al., 1979; DSM-III). In dimensional terms, she exhibited enough affective symptoms, as outlined above, with premenstrual worsening to justify a diagnosis of "predominantly schizotypal schizoaffective disorder with borderline function."

Her mother was hospitalized on many occasions for paranoid schizophrenia; her father, who eventually committed suicide, experienced recurrent depressions.

VII. Mrs. G., married and the mother of two, was referred for chemotherapy management by her therapist who had noticed the marked lability of her moods and believed a diagnosis of cyclothymic personality might be justified. The therapist wondered if a trial of Lithium might not be warranted.

Mrs. G. entered therapy becasue of marital discord, an important element of which was her episodic outbursts of hostility toward her husband, for which the provocation seemed, even in her own judgment, minimal. Her mother and her sister experienced recurrent depressions; both had an "irritable" temperament (Kraepelin, 1921; Stone, 1980). Functionally, she was at the neurotic level, although there would have been some question about a borderline diagnosis if she had been evaluated during a crisis. Her outbursts of anger always occurred 7 or 8 days before her period and were accompanied by headaches, mild nausea, bad dreams, jitteriness, and tearfulness. As she described it: "Just before my period, everything is blown out of context; I react to everything out of proportion, get angry at everything . . . everybody seemed to be in the wrong except me. The day of my period, or even the day before, it all subsides."

The PMT syndrome of this patient (diagnosed as bipolar-II, with cyclothymic personality, and neurotic personality organization) has been much less severe on a regimen of Lithium and tricyclic antidepressants.

VIII. Mrs. H. was referred for psychotherapy at the age of 28 because of irritability and abusiveness toward her two young children. There were strong undercurrents of hostility toward the older child (a boy of six) particularly: labor and delivery had been unusually prolonged and painful; as a baby he had been colicky, and now was "willful" and difficult. Relations with her husband had always been strained: he made disparaging comments about her intelligence, although she was very bright; sexually, she was unresponsive. She regarded her husband as crude and bullyish. Prone to tearfulness and depression, she became either panicky or aggressive hostile (violent toward her children) premenstrually. This rhythmic fluctuation in mood had existed for years, without her being aware of the correlation between cycle and symptoms. Her mother had similarly severe premenstrual tension and had received ECT for depression at the time of menopause. An older sister was extremely irritable, promiscuous, depressive, and abused alcohol. The patient, an "oedipal winner," had been much favored by the father; her mother resented that closeness and behaved more rejectingly toward Mrs. H. than toward her other two children.

During the remainder of her cycle, Mrs. H. was more relaxed, less petulant, had a certain joie de vivre and charm, and was more consistently loving toward her dhildren.

When first evaluated, Mrs. H. had sharply contradictory attitudes about herself and the members of her immediate and original families. She was intensely guilt-ridden about the two episodes of premarital sex with her husband, the month before their marriage. Her self-esteem was severely impaired and blamed her problems on her sexual "indiscretion" 10 years previously. Her level of function was initially borderline. She exhibited the features of "hysteroid dysphoira" (Klein, 1977) or subclinical affective disorder (cf. Akiskal et al., 1977).

On a regimen of 100 mg/day Elavil during the first year of her therapy and small amounts of Thorazine when panicky, her premenstrual tension was well-controlled. This facilitated concentration on her sexual and interpersonal conflicts. She largely overcame the neurotic guilt toward her mother for being her father's favorite, began to see femaleness as no longer an inferior condition, the way her mother and sisters apparently regarded it, and grew less resentful of her mother's indifference. By the time she left therapy 3 years later when the family moved to another city, she was functioning at the neurotic level. At follow-up

12 years later, she had divorced, completed graduate studies, made a second marriage that was much more gratifying than the first, taught school, and was asymptomatic (including premenstrually).

VI. Discussion

The borderline syndromes are of special interest to clinicians concerned with menstrual-cycle-related emotional disorders. Although methodic epidemiologic studies at the meeting of these entities have not yet been carried out, it would appear that women considered borderline by any of the currently popular diagnostic schemata are at high risk for paramenstrual aggravation of symptoms. Similarly, women who first come to a physician's attention because of a severe premenstrual disorder will, in many instances, also be found to satisfy criteria for one or several of the borderline syndromes. Women with primary affective illness, whether bipolar or unipolar, and whether clear-cut (satisfying research diagnostic criteria) or "subclinical" (cf. Akiskal et al., 1977), appear over-represented among borderline patients, or those with severe PMT syndromes (Stone, 1980). AS we have seen, available evidence lends more weight to the idea that primary affective disorders and severe PMT stem from different sets of factors rather than that both are merely different expressions of genetic loading for manic-depression.

It is not surprising that many women with severe PMT are considered borderline in function, at least if evaluated at the height of their distress, because many of the signs and symptoms of PMT (impulsivity, dysphoria, inability to tolerate stressful situations, irrationality or unreasonableness that, however pronounced, falls short of delusion) are said to characterize *borderline personality organization* (Kernberg, 1977) or (adding rageful affect, manipulative suicide gestures and substance abuse to the list) *borderline personality disorder* (Gunderson and Singer, 1975).

For similar reasons, women with severer forms of PMT are said either to be at risk for affective disorder (especially of the depressive type) or to exhibit a variant form of a primary affective disorder (cf. Kashiwagi, 1976). Again, the items by which these conditions are ordinarily diagnosed include many elements in common. Whereas affinities between borderline and primary affective disorder have been suggested by the surplus of close relatives with the latter among borderline probands (Stone, 1977; Stone et al., 1980), comparable studies beginning with PMT probands have not, to my knowledge, been completed.

Attenuated forms of schizophrenia, as exemplified by the "schizotypal borderline" (Spitzer et al., 1979), may, according to a number of clinicians, be associated with a lower incidence of PMT syndrome than would be found in association with primary affective disorder (cf. Coppen, 1965). Borderline schizophrenic women are not, however, immune to premenstrual turbulence, as shown by Patient VI. In the report of Torghele (1957) the PMT syndrome was noted in a high proportion of hospitalized schizophrenic women. My impression is that

Table 1 Premenstrual Tension in Borderline Office Patients

	Severity of PMT syndrome	
Diagnostic subtype	None to mild	Moderate to severe
Affective (N = 10)	5	5
Schizotypal (N = 8)	7	1

schizotypal women are more vulnerable to PMT than normal/neurotic women but less so than women with affective illness. This derives in part from clinical experience with 35 borderline patients in private practice over the past 14 years. Of these, 25 were women. Eight were distinctly schizotypal; 10 were distinctly affective in their symptoms. Defining *severe* PMT as involving gross impairment of function with minipsychotic episodes and *moderate* PMT as involving considerable discomfort, destabilization of interpersonal (especially, sexual) relationships, but no work impairment, the two women with severe PMT were confined to the affective-disordered group. Moderate degrees of PMT were noted in *four,* of whom only *one* was schizotypal. These data are summarized in Table 1, where a cut-off is made between mild and moderate.

Clearly, the sample is too small to permit statistical support of an assumption about heightened vulnerability in the affective group. But if a similar proportionality were to emerge in a larger series, a significant trend might be established.

Because there have been so few methodic surveys of PMT in borderline patients, we are left with intuitive impressions whose validity, as with that of the assumption about schizotypal patients, awaits careful testing. It may be useful at this point to set forth in some systematic fashion the impressions thus far generated, since this may help in the design of the future research protocols by which our assumptions will be assayed. Table 2 summarized my estimation of the *likelihood,* given one of the conditions listed on the left side of the Table, that a woman would also exhibit one of the other conditions on which we have been focusing our attention.

To the extent that these assumptions were to be corroborated in future studies, we could claim that the highest degrees of correlation and predictability were noted in the intersection of *borderline* × *PMT* and of *primary affective disorder* × *PMT*; i.e., that the presence of either *borderline* or *primary affective disorder* predicted a moderate to severe case of PMT. Many women with primary affective disorder function predominantly on the neurotic level; this condition predicts borderline function only to a mild (in some samples to a moderate) degree. Those women who show signs of both primary affective disorder and a borderline syndrome are probably at very high risk for severe PMT. Of more interest to both clinician and geneticist would be the degree to which *severe PMT,* whether or not coupled with a *borderline* condition, predicted a primary affective disorder (and, *a fortiori,* close relatives with unipolar or bipolar affective ill-

Table 2 Possible Predictability Among Borderline, Premenstrual, Primary
Affective, and Schizotypal Disorders

	Borderline syndrome	PMT syndrome	Primary affective disorder	Schizotypal disorder
Borderline syndrome	—	high	moderate	low
PMT syndrome[a]	moderate	—	moderate	low
Primary affective disorder	low	high	—	0
Schizotypal disorder	moderate[b]	low	0	—

"high" = > 50%; "moderate" = 25 to 50%; "low" = < 25%.

[a]moderate to severe, as defined in the text.

[b]"moderate," especially with respect to Gunderson borderline system; "low" with respect
to the Kernberg system.

ness). The Bayesian algebra required to estimate the probability depends on percentages only a few of which (viz., the percentage of women in the general population with severe PMT) are known with any reliability. Even if severe PMT were merely *strongly correlated* with affective disorder, this would be of great interest to clinicians in making decisions about whether to use psychopharmacologic agents and, if so, which ones. If women presenting with moderate to severe PMT also had a superabundance of close relatives with unipolar and bipolar illness, (or later developed such disorders themselves), one might begin to search for biologic markers common to the two conditions. Granting the probable heterogeneity of the PMT syndrome, is there a subset in which the symptoms are largely an expression of genetic loading for primary affective disorder?

Even if it were confirmed that women with severe PMT had a strikingly high incidence of primary affective disorders *and* similarly affected close relatives, this should not be interpreted as proof that PMT was one particular manifestation of genetic loading for affective illness. It would probably be nearer the truth to suppose that PMT and affective illness in their severe forms are so often found in conjunction as to appear unitary in their essence and origin. In this group, personality function is so often at the borderline level as to make the Venn diagram for borderline, severe PMT, and primary affective illness (especially depressive) nearly perfectly overlapping. But if one chose to examine only those women with mild degrees of the PMT syndrome, only a small fraction, perhaps 10% or less, would be borderline and a still smaller fraction manic-depressive. We might expect the proportions for borderline or primary affective disorder to be slightly higher than in the general population of women. If we begin with *mild* PMT, the concepts of borderline, primary affective disorder, and PMT itself are easily separable. But if we concentrate on *severe* PMT, the three entities begin to merge. I find tenable the hypothesis that factors strongly predisposing to PMT interact with the genetic factors predisposing to manic-depression to bring more instances of the latter to the surface, clinically, and thus contribute importantly to the over-representation of females with borderline syndromes.

Affective disordered women might also be more vulnerable to PMT than their schizophrenic counterparts. The PMT syndrome, from the psychological standpoint, is primarily a disorder of mood and affect. Presumably the harboring of risk genes for manic-depression could intensify the mood-disrupting potential of the factors underlying PMT even more than could the risk genes for schizophrenia (whose essence is not disorder of mood but of attention, thought, and ego boundary).

From the observations of Benedek and Rubenstein (1939), Gottschalk (1961), and others, it would appear that periodic shifts in mood and thought content are part of being a female, during menstrual life and perhaps beyond and are more pronounced in neurotic women, less pronounced in normal women. If a woman is prone to preoccupation with themes of hostility, self-depreciation, disappointment, loss, etc., these will tend to surface in the premenstrual and menstrual phases. Benedek, as Frank had earlier, believed these changes could be ascribed to hormonal fluctuations, although both sets of rhythmically recurring phenomena could be epiphenomena of a circummensual (occurring at monthly intervals) biologic clock located in the central nervous system, whose effects are simply more discernible in (menstruating) women than in men (Stone, 1976).

The euphoria of the ovulative phase seldom reaches hypomanic proportions. But the dysphoria of the preovulative and especially of the paramenstrual phases often does reach such proportions as either to mimic a serious depressive disorder or aggravate a genuine, genetically predisposed depressive diathesis. That the depressive tendency should outweigh the euphoric is not surprising. Two factors may be of importance: one biologic, the other psychological. On the biologic side, bipolar conditions are rarer than (unipolar) depressive—and this may in part be a reflection of the higher degree of genetic liability some believe is necessary before the threshold is reached for a bipolar condition to manifest itself (Gershon et al., 1975). The more common occurrence of low to moderate liability for affective disorder apparently predisposes more to depression than to mania. On the psychological side, there is life in general, which usually is conducive more to depression than to elation. Lovers part; parents die; breadwinners lose jobs; children may disappoint. We often have more setbacks in our lives than triumphs. Genes, hormones, and life, may combine to render many women affectively ill, irritable, and depressed around the time of their period. Strong constitutional factors (for primary affective disorder or for the PMT syndrome itself) and preexisting neurotic (or worse) maladaptation may accentuate "premenstrual tension" to ominous proportions. Certain vulnerable women will become borderline, by one or more sets of criteria; others will appear borderline phasically, as the sensitive days of their cycle are approached and passed through.

The premenstrual and other factors discussed here may account, in large measure, for the disproportionately high percentage of women among borderline patients. No student of the borderline syndromes can ignore the "premenstrual" factor operating in many instances. Likewise no clinician specializing in menstrual disorder can afford to ignore the likelihood that many of his or her patients will be or appear borderline and will require psychological and psychopharmacologic interventions appropriate to these more serious psychiatric conditions.

References

Akiskal, H. S., A. H. Djenderedjian, R. H. Rosenthal, and M. K. Khani (1977). Cyclothymic disorder: Validating criteria for inclusion in the bipolar affective group. *Am. J. Psychiatry* 134:1227-1233.

Beaumont, P. J. V., D. H. Richards, and M. G. Gelder (1975). A study of minor psychiatric and physical symptoms during the menstrual cycle. *Br. J. Psychiatry* 126:431-434.

Benedek, T., and B. B. Rubenstein (1939). The correlations between ovarian activity and psychodynamic processes: I. The ovulative phase. *Psychosom. Med.* 1:245-270.

Brierre de Boisment, A. (1956). *Du Suicide et de la Folie Suicide.* Baillière, Paris, pp. 243-244.

Brooks, B. (1980). Familial influences in father-daughter incest. (Unpublished manuscript).

Brooks, B., and M. H. Stone (1980). Unpublished data.

Bychowski, G. (1953). The problem of latent psychosis. *J. Am. Psychoanal. Assoc.* 4:484-503.

Cancro, R. (1975). Genetics, dualism and schizophrenia. *J. Am. Acad. Psychoanal.* 3:353-360.

Carroll, B. J., J. F. Greden, M. Feinberg, N. Lohr, N. James, M. STeiner, R. F. Haskett, A. A. Albala, J. deVigne, and J. Tarika (1980). Evaluation of depression in borderline patients. (Unpublished manuscript).

Coppen, A. (1965). The prevalence of menstrual disorders in psychiatric patients. *Br. J. Psychiatry* 111:155-167.

Coppen, A., and N. Kessel (1963). Menstruation and personality. *Br. J. Psychiatry* 109:711-721.

Coppen, A., and D. M. Shaw (1963). Mineral metabolism in melancholia. *Br. Med. J.* 2:1439-1444.

Culberg, J. (1972). Mood changes and menstrual symptoms with different gestagen/estrogen combinations. *Acta Psychiatr. Scand. [Suppl.]* 236:9-86.

Dalton, K. (1959). Menstruation and acute psychiatric illnesses. *Br. Med. J.* 1:148-149.

Daly, C. D. (1935). The menstruation complex in literature. *Psychoanal. Q.* 4:307-340.

Deutsch, H. (1942). Some forms of emotional disturbance and their relationships to schizophrenia. *Psychoanal. Q.* 11:301-321.

Deutsch, H. (1965). *Neurosis and Character Types.* International Universities Press, New York.

American Psychiatric Association (1980). *Diagnostic and Statistical Manual of Mental Disorders* (Third Edition) (*DSM-III*). A.P.A., Washington, D.C.

Diamond, S. B., A. A. Rubinstein, D. L. Dunner, and R. R. Fieve (1976). Menstrual problems in women with primary affective illness. *Compr. Psychiatry* 17:541-548.

Dunner, D. L., J. L. Fleiss, and R. R. Fieve (1976). The course of development of mania in patients with recurrent depression. *Am. J. Psychiatry* 133:905-908.

Ekstein, R. (1955). Vicissitudes of the "internal image" in the recovery of a borderline schizophrenic adolescent. *Bull. Menninger Clin.* 19:86-92.

Esquirol, E. (1938). *Maladies Mentales.* Baillière, Paris, p. 585.

Feighner, J. P., E. Robins, S. B. Guze, R. A. Woodruff, G. Winokur, and R. Munoz (1972). Diagnostic criteria for use in psychiatric research. *Arch. Gen. Psychiatry* 26:57-63.

Frank, R. T. (1931). The hormonal causes of premenstrual tension. *Arch. Neurol. Psychol.* 26:1053-1057.

Friedman, R. C., S. W. Hurt, M. S. Aronoff, and J. Clarkin (1980). Behavior and the menstrual cycle. *Signs.*

Frosch, J. (1964). The psychotic character. *Psychiatr. Q.* 38:81-96.

Gershon, E. S., M. Baron, and F. Leckman (1975). Genetic models of the transmission of affective disorders. *J. Psychiatr. Res.* 12:301-317.

Glass, G. S., G. R. Heninger, M. Lansky, and K. Talan (1971). Psychiatric emergency related to the menstrual cycle. *Am. J. Psychiatry* 128:705-711.

Gordon, J. H., R. L. Borison, and B. I. Diamond (1980). Modulation of dopamine receptor sensitivity by estrogen. *Biol. Psychol.* 15:389-396.

Gottschalk, L. A., G. C. Gleser, E. B. Magliocco, and T. L. D'Zmura (1961). Further studies on the speech patterns of schizophrenic patients. *J. Nerv. Ment. Dis.* 132:101-113.

Graff, H., and R. Mallin (1967). The syndrome of the wrist cutter. *Am. J. Psychiatry* 124:74-80.

Grant, E. C. G., and J. Pryse-Davies (1968). Effect of oral contraceptives on depressive mood changes and on endometrial monoamine oxidase and phosphatases. *Br. Med. J.* 3:777-780.

Gray, L. A. (1941). The use of progesterone in nervous tension states. *South. Med. J.* 34:1004-1006.

Greene, R., and K. Dalton (1953). The premenstrual syndrome. *Br. Med. J.* 1:1007-1014.

Grinker, R. R., B. Werble, and R. C. Drye (1968). *The Borderline Syndrome.* Basic Books, New York.

Grunebaum, H. U., and G. L. Klerman (1967). Wrist slashing. *Am. J. Psychiatry* 4:113-120.

Gunderson, J. G., and J. E. Kolb (1978). Discriminating features of borderline patients. *Am. J. Psychiatry* 135:792-796.

Gunderson, J. G., and M. T. Singer (1975). Defining borderline patients: An overview. *Am. J. Psychiatry* 132:1-10.

Haskett, R. F., M. Steiner, J. N. Osmun, and B. J. Carrol (1980). Severe premenstrual tension: Delineation of the syndrome. *Biol. Psychol.* 15:121-139.

Hoch, P. H., and P. Polatin (1949). Pseudoneurotic forms of schizophrenia. *Psychiatr. Q.* 23:248-276.

Ivey, M. E., and J. M. Bardwick (1968). Patterns of affective fluctuation in the menstrual cycle. *Psychosom. Med.* 30:336-345.

Jacobson, E. (1953). Contribution to the metapsychology of cyclothymic depression. In *Affective Disorders* (P. Greenacre, ed.). International Universities Press, New York, pp. 49-83.

Kashiwagi, T., J. N. McClure, and R. D. Wetzel (1976). Premenstrual affective syndrome and psychiatric disorder. *Dis. Nerv. Syst.* 37:116-119.

Kernberg, O. F. (1967). Borderline personality organization. *J. Am. Psychoanal. Assoc.* 15:641-685.

Kernberg, O. F. (1977). The structural diagnosis of borderline personality organization. In *Borderline Personality Disorders* (P. Hartocollis, ed.). International Universities Press, New York, pp. 87-121.

Klein, D. F. (1977). Psychopharmacological treatment and delineation of borderline disorders. In *Borderline Personality Disorders: The Concept, the Syndrome, the Patient* (P. Hartocollis, ed.). International Universities Press, New York, pp. 365-383.

Klein, D. F., and R. I. Shader (1975). The borderline state. In *Manual of Psychiatric Therapeutics* (R. I. Shader, ed.). Little, Brown, Boston, pp. 281-293.

Knight, R. P. (1953). Borderline states. *Bull. Menninger Clin.* 17:1-12.

Kraepelin, E. (1921). *Manic-Depressive Insanity and Paranoia.* E. and S. Livingstone, Edinburgh.

Kramp, J. L. (1968). Studies on the premenstrual syndrome in relation to psychiatry. *Acta Psychiatr. Scand. [Suppl.]* 203:261-268.

May, R. R. (1976). Mood shifts and the menstrual cycle. *J. Psychosom. Res.* 20:125-130.

McClure, J. N., Jr., T. Reich, and R. Wetzel (1971). Premenstrual symptoms as an indicator of bipolar affective disorder. *Br. J. Psychiatr.* 119:527-528.

MacKinnon, P. C. B., and I. L. MacKinnon (1956). Hazards of the menstrual cycle. *Br. Med. J.* 1:555.

MacKinnon, I. L., P. C. B. MacKinnon, and A. D. Thomson (1959). Lethal hazards of the luteal phase of the menstrual cycle. *Br. Med. J.* 1:1015-1017.

Mead, R. (1748). *Opera Medica.* Antonio Bortoli, Venice, pp. 48-49.

Moos, R. H. (1968). The development of a menstrual distress questionnaire. *Psychosom. Med.* 30:853-867.

O'Connor, J. F., E. M. Shelley, and L. O. Stern (1973). Behavioral rhythms related to the menstrual cycle (Unpublished manuscript).

Paige, K. E. (1971). Effects of oral contraceptives on affective fluctuations associated with the menstrual cycle. *Psychosom. Med.* 33:515-537.

Parlee, M. B. (1973). The premenstrual syndrome. *Psychol. Bull.* 80:454-465.

Pattie, F. (1956). Mesmer's medical dissertation and its debt to Mead's *De Imperio Solis ac Lunae. J. Hist. Med.* 11:275-287.

Perr, I. N. (1958). Medical, psychiatric and legal aspects of premenstrual tension. *Am. J. Psychiatry* 115:211-219.

Perry, J. C., and G. L. Klerman (1978). The borderline patients. *Arch. Gen. Psychiatry* 35:141-150.

Pinel, P. (1799). *Nosographie Philosophique ou La Méthode de l'Analyse Appliqué a la Médecine.* Maradan, Paris.

Prichard, J. C. (1835). *A Treatise on Insanity.* Sherwood, Gilbert and Piper, London.

Rado, S. (1956). *Psychoanalysis of Behavior: Collected Papers.* Grune & Stratton, New York.

Rees, L. (1953). The premenstrual tension syndrome and its treatment. *Br. Med. J.* 1:1014-1016.

Rodrigue, E. M. (1955). Notes on menstruation. *Int. J. Psychoanal.* 36:328-334.

Rosenthal, R. J., C. Rinzler, R. Wallsh, and E. Dlausner (1972). Wrist-cutting syndrome: The meaning of a gesture. *Am. J. Psychiatry* 128:47-52.

Sampson, G. A. (1979). Premenstrual syndrome: A double-blind controlled trial of progesterone and placebo. *Br. J. Psychiatry* 135:209-215.

Schuckit, M. A., V. Daly, G. Herrman, and S. Hineman (1975). Premenstrual symptoms and depression in a university population. *Dis. Nerv. Syst.* 36:516-517.

Simon, B. (1978). *Mind and Madness in Ancient Greece.* Cornell University Press, Ithaca, New York.

Singer, K., R. Cheng, and M. Schou (1974). A controlled evaluation of lithium in the premenstrual tension syndrome. *Br. J. Psychiatry* 124:50-51.

Sletten, I. W., and S. Gershon (1966). The premenstrual syndrome: A discussion of its neurophysiology and treatment with lithium ion. *Compr. Psychiatry* 7:197-206.

Smith, S. L. (1975). Mood and the menstrual cycle. In *Topics in Psychoendocrinology* (E. J. Sachar, ed.). Grune & Stratton, New York, pp. 19-59.

Spitzer, R. L., J. Endicott, and M. Gibbon (1979). Crossing the border into borderline personality and borderline schizophrenia. The development of criteria. *Arch. Gen. Psychiatry* 36:17-24.

Spitzer, R. L., J. Endicott, and E. Robins (1975). Clinical criteria for psychiatric diagnosis and DSM-III. *Am. J. Psychiatry* 132:1187-1192.

Spurzheim, G. (1818). *Observations sur la Folie.* Treuttel & Würtz, Paris, pp. 190-191.

Steiner, M., R. F. Haskett, J. N. Osmun, and B. J. Carroll (1980). Treatment of premenstrual tension with lithium carbonate. *Acta Psychiatr. Scand.* 61:96-102.

Stern, A. (1938). Psychoanalytic investigation and therapy in the borderline group of neuroses. *Psychoanal. Q.* 7:467-489.

Stone, M. H. (1976). Madness and the moon revisited: Possible influence of the full-moon in a case of atypical mania. *Psychiatr. Ann.* 6:47-60.

Stone, M. H. (1977). The borderline syndrome: Evolution of the term, genetic aspects, and prognosis. Delivered at 17th Emil Gutheil Memorial Lecture, Association for the Advancement of Psychotherapy, New York City. *Am. J. Psychother.* 31:345-365.

Stone, M. H. (1979). Assessing vulnerability to schizophrenia or manic-depression in borderline states. (Discussion of Siever and Gunderson's article.) *Schizophr. Bull.* 5:105-110.

Stone, M. H. (1980). *The Borderline Syndromes: Constitution, Adaptation and Personality.* McGraw-Hill, New York.

Stone, M. H., B. Flye, and E. Kahn (1980). Unpublished manuscript.

Stone, M. H., and B. Oestberg (1979). Survey of borderline patients in Norway, using the Spitzer checklist. Dikemark Seminar. (Unpublished data).

Tonks, C. M. (1975). Premenstrual tension. *Br. J. Psychiatry* 9:399-408.

Torghele, J. R. (1957). Premenstrual tension in psychotic women. *Lancet* 77: 163-170.

Voisin, F. (1826). *Des Causes Morales and Physiques des Maladies Mentales.* Baillière, Paris.

Welner, A., J. L. Liss, and E. Robins (1973). Undiagnosed psychiatric patients: III. The undiagnosible patient. *Br. J. Psychiatry* 123:91-98.

Wetzel, R. D., and J. N. McClure (1972). Suicide and the menstrual cycle: A review. *Compr. Psychiatry* 13:369-374.

Wetzel, R. D., J. N. McClure, and T. Reich (1971a). Premenstrual symptoms in self-referrels to a suicide prevention service. *Br. J. Psychiatry* 119:525-526.

Wetzel, R. D., T. Reich, and J. N. McClure (1971b). Phase of the menstrual cycle and self-referrals to a suicide prevention service. *Br. J. Psychiatry* 119: 523-524.

Williams, E. Y., and L. R. Weekes (1952). Premenstrual tension associated with psychotic episodes. *J. Nerv. Ment. Dis.* 116:321-329.

Zilboorg, G. (1941). Ambulatory schizophrenia. *Psychiatry* 4:149-155.

17 Oral Contraceptives and the Menstrual Cycle

IRA D. GLICK   Cornell University Medical College, New York, New York, and The Payne Whitney Clinic, New York, New York

SUSAN E. BENNETT   Beth Israel Hospital, Boston, Massachusetts, and Harvard Medical School, Boston, Massachusetts

This chapter reviews the relationship of oral contraceptives (OCs) and mood/ behavior during the menstrual cycle. Available data are derived mainly from two sources: data collected when OCs are used for their contraceptive properties in patients without psychiatric illness and those collected when they are used as psychopharmacologic agents as in the treatment of depression. Our focus is on controlled studies; we have used uncontrolled data only if the ideas were novel.

I. Oral Contraceptives Used for Their Contraceptive Properties in Patients without Psychiatric Illness

A. Mood

What are the effects of oral contraceptives (OCs) on mood? Although early reports were largely anecdotal and were generally glowing in their descriptions of elevated mood (Table 1), more recent studies suggest that the situation is far more complex. What does seem clear is that *most* women using these drugs as OC agents experience *no* change in mood [1]. About one-sixth may note an elevation of mood and increased activity, manifested, for example, by doing

---

*Parts of this chapter are based on Glick, I. D., Psychotropic actions of oral contraceptives, in Itil, T. H. (ed.), *Psychotropic Action of Hormones,* Spectrum Publications, Inc., White Lake, New York, 1976.

Table 1 Summary of Studies of the Relationship Between Mood and Behavioral Change and Use of Oral Contraceptives (Reported by Gynecologists) [77]

Author	S_S	Drug	Clinical impression	Depression	Libido Inc. %	Dec. %	Unch. %	Coitus More satisfy. or incr. %	Less satisfy. or decr. %	Unch. %	Dysmenorrhea Imp. %	Wors. %	Unch. %	Premenstrual tension Imp. %	Wors. %	Unch. %
Lehberz and Fobes (1961)	112	Enovid or Norlutin	7 developed emotional distress	1 of 7 "severely depressed"												
Johnson (1962)	800	Enovid	"feel better and function better"											all		
Flowers (1964)	259	Enovid-E	"reduced discomfort of menstruation"											50		50
Guttmacher et al. (1965)	11,711	Enovid	Feel: Better 28%, Worse 6%, Unch. 66%	from 11% to 6% in "menstrually related depression"	32	8	60				75		25			
Zell and Crisp (1961)	250	Enovid	"No increase in emotional conflicts"					Impr.								
Sapir et al. (1965)	43	Enovid-E	Benefit psychologically	No increase noted after starting med.							"usually"					

Study	Preparation (No./Drug)	Notes										
Rice-Wray (1962)	364 Ortho-Novum					28	2	60 (10% unaccounted for)	60	27	13	
Tyler et al. (1961)	570 Ortho-Novum	1% nervous	18	3	79							
Hutcherson et al. (1963)	306 Ortho-Novum	"some"										"frequently"
Goldzieher et al. (1963)	211 Ortho-Novum		42	0	58				100			
Behrman (1964)	203 Ortho-Novum	5%	20	6	74				79	3	18	
Rovinsky (1964)	259 Ortho-Novum		43	0/5	50 (6% no report)							
Crocker et al.	185 Ortho-Novum								11 of 11			
Ringose (1965)	100 Ortho-Novum		22	13	55 (10% no report)	53	4 (8% uncertain)	35				
Provest Symposium – Provest (1963)		"better mood" and "sense of well being" / "no evidence"				75	17	8	"majority"			
Oracon Symposium – Oracon (1965)		"2 pts. of 95 became depressed"										
Goldzieher (1964)	C-Quens								80	10	10	"most"
Rice-Wray (1963)	2040 Several		54	5	41	54	3	43				
British Medical Society Symposium on Oral Contraceptives (1963)	Several	"Sense of well being"			"most"				"most"			"most" — 50 0 50 / 100 0 0

Source: Reprinted by permission from pages 156–164, Chapter 4 in *Psychotropic Action of Hormones* by Turan M. Itil, Gerhard Laudahn and Werner M. Herrmann (eds.) Copyright 1976, Spectrum Publications, Inc., New York.

more work than usual or initiating projects that have been chronically postponed.

This elevation has been attributed to a variety of causes. The first is estrogen, which has many properties in common with psychostimulants [2]; estrogen inhibits monoamine oxidase activity thereby increasing central nervous system catecholamine availability. A second possibility is that progestational agents may improve mood as a result of replacement in women with low blood levels [3] or of their sedative action in the presence of stress. In a controlled study with ovariectomized rats, Ladisich demonstrated that progesterone administered before stress resulted in higher cerebral concentrations of serotonin metabolites after stress [4]. Worsley studied 35 women on OCs with varying gestagen (synthetic progestational agent) content, and found that higher progesterone dosage correlated with improved automatization ability and mood scores. There was a significant increase in vigor and decrease in anger and fatigue symptoms in the OC group compared with controls [5]. Finally, improved mood has been attributed to a specific psychological factor associated with oral contraceptives: relief from the fear of pregnancy [6].

Data from two studies by Kutner [7,8] using a large population, and more recently by Fleming and Seager [9] have suggested that oral contraceptives do *not* produce depressive episodes or aggravate prepill depressive symptoms. Depressed mood has been reported in up to 50% of women taking oral contraceptives [10], but most studies report much lower figures. The depressant action of the OCs is thought to be due to a pharmacologic effect. By increasing hepatic tryptophan oxygenase activity, estrogen can enhance the metabolism of tryptophan to nicotinic acid in the liver, leaving less tryptophan available for conversion to serotonin and tryptamine in the brain [11,12]. Progesterone elevates monoamine oxidase at the synaptic junction, an effect that has been associated with depression [8]. Warnes and Fitzpatrick showed that changes in urinary serotonin and catecholamine metabolites associated with oral contraceptive use did not correlate with depressive symptoms [13]. This suggests that depressed mood may not be related to the pill at all or, alternatively, that a strong psychological effect may account for the lowered mood. Some women using OCs, although requesting them, may experience conflict about their role as mothers and become depressed when they cannot become pregnant [14]. A more likely explanation for conflicting reports is that study design affects the reporting of symptoms related to OC use [15].

Can changes in mood associated with various OC agents be predicted by a patient's previous history? In a prospective study, Cullberg [16] was able to demonstrate that patients with premenstrual irritability before starting OCs did significantly worse (became more depressed) when using more strongly estrogenic OCs. For them, the best OC was predominately progestational. Conversely, those patients without a history of premenstrual irritability became depressed with more gestogenic OCs, and noted fewer side effects when taking strongly estrogenic pills.

B. Sexuality

Do sexual drive, performance, and enjoyment change once a woman is using OCs? Earlier studies showed no change in long-standing patterns of sexual behavior for most women (see Table 1) with 10 to 20% of women reporting changes in sexual performance believed to reflect alterations in mood [11].

In a well-designed, prospective, controlled study, Adams et al. showed a significant increase in female-initiated sexual activity at the periovulatory time of the cycle. This change was not observed in women on OCs [17]; unfortunately there were no measurements of sex hormone levels [18]. The inference was that the OCs suppressed ovulatory increases in hormone secretion. Another study using a double-blind, crossover design, showed significantly decreased sexual responsivity without depressive symptoms in women on OCs [19]. In an equally well controlled study, however, Bancroft et al. demonstrated no significant difference in plasma levels of testosterone, androstenedione, and estradiol (measured longitudinally weekly over 4 weeks) between two groups of women with and without sexual problems (such as negative feelings during intercourse, lack of sexual arousal, orgasm, or sexual interest) on OCs [20]. Persky et al. found no relationship between plasma estradiol levels and sexual behavior [21].

Even more uncertainty exists regarding the role of hormones in regulating sexual behavior in the human being. The complex phenomena that are loosely termed gender identity and gender role are poorly understood and difficult to study, but it is believed by most students of the subject that cultural, social and psychiatric factors are primary determinants of sexual behavior and that hormonal factors, at best, act as secondary modifiers of the process. [22].

It is apparent that studies combining both behavioral and endocrinologic measures are needed to define the sexual changes occurring with OCs.

C. Amenorrhea

Could the amenorrhea that often follows discontinuation of the use of OCs result from psychological causes? Most investigators have presumed a physiological cause, i.e., failure of recovery from the inhibition of the cyclic release of gonadotropins caused by OCs. In two studies, Fries and Nillius [23,24] suggested a relationship between postpill amenorrhea and an emotionally stressful event leading to cessation of OC use. Although this association is correlative and not causal, the hypothesis that stressful events set off a chain of events in the hypothalamus that interact with biochemical factors resulting in amenorrhea is plausible. Further investigation seems warranted.

D. Postnatal Sexual Development in Males

Yalom et al. [25] have studied boys exposed prenatally to exogenous administration of estrogen and progesterone. They were studied on various parameters of psychosexual development and matched with controls for age and socioeconomic class. Results indicated that exposed 6-year-olds rated lower on several variables related to "general masculinity," assertiveness, and athletic ability. A more recent study defined significant personality differences between prenatal progesterone vs. estrogen exposure; those exposed to progesterone were more independent, sensitive, individualistic, self-assured, and self-sufficient than the estrogen or non-exposed control groups, whereas those exposed to estrogen were more group-oriented and group-dependent [26]. Another group of investigators has shown enhancement of female sexually dimorphic behavior in 8-year-old girls prenatally exposed to high dose medroxyprogesterone acetate; the boys similarly exposed have so far demonstrated no alteration in sexually dimorphic behavior [27,28].

E. Vitamin Levels and Depression

OCs have been shown to raise the mean serum vitamin A level and reduce the mean serum vitamin B_2 (riboflavin), vitamin B_6 (pyridoxine), vitamin C, folic acid, and vitamin B_{12} levels. Biochemical evidence of coenzyme deficiency has been reported for vitamin B_2, vitamin B_6, and folic acid. Depression has been reported as the end result of the biochemical changes secondary to the vitamin B_6 deficiency. Specifically, a defect in serotonin production resulting from competitive inhibition of pyridoxal phosphate by estrogen has been postulated [29]. It has been estimated that approximately 80% of women taking OCs are functionally vitamin B_6-deficient [12]. In a double-blind crossover study of 22 depressed women with an absolute vitamin B_6 deficiency, the administration of pyridoxine hydrochloride 40 mg daily produced a significant improvement [30].

II. Oral Contraceptives Used as Psychotropic Hormones

The data in the previous section suggest that OCs might be used for treatment of psychiatric disorders as discussed below (Table 2).

A. Depression

Women are twice as likely as men to experience a depressive illness, but the cause of this increased risk may be more socioeconomic than endocrinologic [31]. Over the past 20 years there has been a great upsurge of interest in treating recurrent affective disorder characterized by depressive episodes. Psychotherapy has been relatively ineffective in changing the long-term course of some of the affective disorders [32], and a variety of psychotropic agents has been used based in part on the rationale that some types of depression are caused by relative unavailability of monoamines at synaptic junctions. Uncontrolled pilot work with a small series of patients suggested to us that OCs might have a mood-stabilizing effect. For treatment of "depression," (1) estrogen has been used alone [33] and as an adjunct to tricyclic treatment [34], (2) progesterone seemed to have a "mood-stabilizing" effect [3,5], and (3) the risk of emotional illness decreases during pregnancy when estrogen and progesterone levels are high [35,36]. Enovid (norethylnodrel and mestranol) in doses up to 40 mg was administered to four women with periodic depressions who had at least two or more episodes of symptoms with an intervening period of at least 3 asymptomatic months. Although there was relatively little modification of affective state for two of the patients, the other two showed an elevation in mood. We believe that OCs deserve further controlled investigation [37].

Another study that bears on this issue is that of Paige [38]. In a study of changes in affect in a sample of 102 women, she found that women with natural menstrual cycles have a U-shaped pattern of negative affect. Affect was most negative at the beginning and end of the cycle. Women using combination OCs showed no cyclic affective changes, however. She ruled out a number of other variables that might account for these findings and suggested that the results might be due to the effects of the OCs on monoamine oxidase activity. Warren et al. recently developed a theoretical model correlating cyclic changes in mood and behavior with fluctuating serotonin levels in the brain [39]. These studies would certainly lend support to the mood stabilizing effects of OCs. Two recent uncontrolled studies, however, found only minimal cyclic changes in psychological state during the menstrual cycle of healthy women [40,41]. Further complicating the picture is the recent study of somatic symptoms recorded from the health diaries of 151 women; increased symptom-reporting occurred among women on OCs, with a higher symptom rate during the menstrual phase [41].

In a double-blind experiment, Klaiber et al. administered either placebo or high dose oral, conjugated estrogens (with medroxyprogesterone acetate 2.5 mg/day) to hospitalized premenopausal women with major depressive disorder who were resistant to treatment. A Hamilton Rating Scale was administered intermittently over a 3 month period, and blood samples were obtained to measure plasma monoamine oxidase activity. The estrogen-treated group had significantly lower ratings of depression compared with controls, but no relationship was found between improvement of depression and the diminished plasma monoamine oxidase activity in the estrogen group [43].

So far there have been no studies of OCs as psychotropic agents in males with depression. In one study [44], normal men were given 600 mg progesterone followed by 75 mg lysergic acid diethylamide (LSD). Progesterone had little ef-

Table 2 Psychotropic Actions of (Hormones) Oral Contraceptives

Year	Author	No. of Ss	Drug	Syndromes Studied	Results
1942	Blumberg & Billig [78]	1	Estradiol dipropianate 2 mg 1M, Insulin shock	Postpartum psychosis	Improved
1946	Billig & Bradley [79]	12	Progesterone 2 mg 1M, EST, Insulin shock	"Psychoses" (symptoms exacerbating premenstrually and postpartum)	"Alleviation of psychotic symptoms"
1956	Bower & Altschule [80]	39	Progesterone 100 mg 1 M, EST, Psychotherapy	Postpartum psychosis	100% remission
1962	Simpson et al. [61]	28	Enovid 10-30 mg O.D.	Symptoms exacerbating at time of menstruation	4 Ss temporarily improved with 3 of these relapsing
1964	Simpson et al. [62]	10	Enovid 30 mg for 30 days	Schizophrenia (regular menstruation)	4 Ss improved
		12	Enovid 30 mg for 30 days	Schizophrenia (irregular menstruation)	No change
1964	Swanson et al. [63]	21 4 1	Enovid 30 mg for 30 days for cycles, phenothiazine &/or psychotherapy	Misc. psychoses	Improved No change Worse
1965	Kane et al. [64]	1 6 2	Enovid or Orthonovum or Ovulen	Misc. psychoses Postpartum psychosis Involutional depression	Improved 5 Ss improved Improved
1969	Wieczarek et al. [56]	Unspecified	Chlormadinone and mestranol	Cyclic psychoses that were menstrual dependent	Some got complete relief, others got worse
1970	Herzberg & Coppen (study with 40 control Ss)	152	6 different OCs	Premenstrual tension	Significant decrease in depression and irritability, no change in headaches and swelling

Year	Author	N	Treatment	Condition	Results
1970	Baumblatt & Winston [81]	52	Pyridoxine	Unipolar depressive disorder associated with OC	"Complete resolution of sx in 18, considerable improvement in 26 and no change in 14
1970	Glick et al. [37]	3	Enovid, 40 mg	Unipolar depression	2 Ss improved
		1	Enovid, 40 mg	Involutional depression	Unimproved
1972	Prange et al. [33,34]	20	Imipramine and 25 µg Ethinyl Estradiol	Unipolar depression	Elevation in mood
1972	Cullberg [16]	20	50 µg Ethinyl Estradiol	Unipolar depression	Depression in mood
		322	0.05 mg Ethinyl Estradiol + gestagen in varying doses	Dysmenorrhea Premenstrual syndrome	Relieved by gestagen Trend to relief by gestagen
1973	Adams et al. [30]	22	Pyridoxine 40 mg/day	Unipolar depression associated with OC use—of whom, 11 of 22 had absolute B_6 deficiency	Significant improvement in 11 of 11 Ss with absolute deficiency of vitamin B_6
1975	Glick & Goldfein [49]	4	Medroxyprogesterone acetate 10-20 mg orally 10 days prior to period	Severe premenstrual syndrome	Improved in global outcome
1979	Klaiber et al. [43]	40	Oral, conjugated, estrogen, 5-25 mg/day (plus Provera 2.5 mg from 21-26th day in premenopausal women) compared with placebo group	Major depressive disorder	Significant decrease in depression compared to placebo treated group
1980	Felthous et al. [58]	1	Ortho-Novum 1/50-21	Recurrent menstrual psychosis	Complete cessation of symptoms
1980	Glick & Stewart [57]	3	Antipsychotics, lithium and OC	Recurrent menstrual psychosis	Marked decrease of symptoms

Source: Reprinted by permission from pages 156-164, Chapter 4 in *Psychotropic Action of Hormones* by Turan M. Itil, Gerhard Laudahn and Werner M. Herrmann (eds.). Copyright 1976, Spectrum Publications, Inc., New York.

fect on behavior, but did elicit irritability, slowness, and depression in certain subjects. The author noted that progesterone "seemed to inhibit the behavioral deterioration induced by LSD," suggesting an antipsychotic role (or more likely a sedative effect) of progesterone.

Another group tested the hypothesis that fluctuations of progesterone levels could account for the psychophysiological changes occurring during the luteal phase of the menstrual cycle. They administered 10 mg medroxyprogesterone acetate daily to six men on a double-blind basis. Results showed a significant rise in temperature and reaction time and increase in heart rate variability which returned to baseline soon after the drug was stopped. Interestingly, although there were no significant changes in the mood scales there was a trend ($P < 0.10$) toward better concentration ability [45].

B. Premenstrual Syndrome

Do women experiencing a premenstrual syndrome improve after being treated with OCs? The answer depends, in part, on whether there is concurrent psychiatric illness. Marinari et al. demonstrated that the increased adrenocortical reactivity to stress observed in the premenstruum (compared with midcycle) is blocked by OCs [46]. Controlled data using large samples in three studies suggest that patients with dysmenorrhea or the premenstrual syndrome without other significant psychiatric illness improve with gestagen-dominant pills [7,11, 47]. In such patients, estrogen-dominated OCs make the syndrome worse [11]. In that group of patients in whom the premenstrual syndrome is associated with other psychiatric illness, response to OCs as psychotropic agents (whether estrogen- or gestagen-dominated) has not been shown to result in improvement [11]. Studies using questionnaires may be biased in that labeling symptoms as "menstrual" has been shown to decrease the reporting of stress [48].

In 1970, we conducted a study [49] treating, over a period of 35 cycles, four subjects who had severe premenstrual syndromes (characterized by a broad range of psychologic and physiologic symptoms) without other psychiatric illness. We used Provera (medroxyprogesterone acetate) in oral doses of 10 to 20 mg, 10 days before the expected onset of menstruation. Our results indicated a mean improvement of 1.29 (on the three-point positive side of a seven-point global rating scale) above each individual's baseline levels (measured over two to four cycles. Dalton [50], based on her clinical experience, recommends progesterone therapy for severe premenstrual syndromes when symptoms are incapacitating, or social or vocational functioning is severely impaired. The suggestion that OCs improve global functioning and mood during the premenstrual syndrome is important in suggesting a role for OCs as psychotropic agents. Replication at different centers with larger numbers of subjects is desirable.

C. Postpartum Depression

Anecdotal reports [51] suggest that OCs may be useful in the treatment of postpartum psychiatric illness. The rationale is based on exogenous replacement of falling estrogen and progesterone levels during the postpartum period. However, no controlled studies test this idea. Steiner recently reviewed the literature on the psychobiology of postpartum psychiatric illness, and concluded that physiology of the puerperium is not a cause in itself of (postpartum psychosis) but a contributing or triggering factor acting upon an underlying predisposition" [52].

D. Involutional Psychiatric Illness

Various uncontrolled, anecdotal reports have also suggested that involutional psychiatric illness has been improved with estrogen and OCs [51,53]. Here, too, there are no controlled studies. Rationale is likewise based on exogenous replacement of endogenously decreased estrogen and progesterone levels in the involutional period. In a controlled study of 20 recently menopausal women, Ballinger et al. showed a significant relationship between stress secondary to depression and decreased urinary estrogen metabolite excretion. Estrogen levels increased over time as patients recovered from depression. The authors concluded that stress contributes to the estrogen deficiency of the menopause [54].

E. Recurrent Menstrual Psychosis

Recurrent menstrual psychosis is defined here as those episodes of psychosis (usually schizophrenia) that occur (or are intensified) in close association with the menstrual period. Endo et al. reported seven women with menstrual psychoses, two of whom showed signs of the premenstrual syndrome. These two women were also found to have unusually low plasma pregnanediol levels [55]. One group [56] has treated menstrual-dependent psychosis with OCs, in this case, Oviston (chlormadinone and mestranol), which produced in some women complete alleviation of the psychosis and in others increased the severity of the illness. This suggests that at least two separate etiologies may exist for cyclic psychosis.

Glick and Stewart have successfully treated three women suffering from treatment-resistant premenstrual exacerbation of their schizophrenic symptoms with a combination of lithium, antipsychotics, and OCs [57]. Felthous et al. successfully utilized a combination OC, Ortho-Novum 1/50-21, to control a patient with menstrually related psychosis who was refractory to high doses of antipsychotic medication and lithium [58].

III. Side Effects of Oral Contraceptives

We have chosen here to avoid a systematic review of the psychiatric side effects of OCs. These have been reviewed by Kane [59], Weissman and Slaby [60], and others. Kane suggested that, on the basis of a review of the literature, "a syndrome of mild to moderate depression, with tiredness, irritability, and some alteration in libido is the clinical picture most often found associated with the use of the combination" OCs [59]. He has also pointed out that there may be an increased risk of psychosis after discontinuation of OCs in those patients with preexisting psychiatric illness. Weissman and Slaby asserted that, "As yet there are few data to justify the belief that OCs cause psychiatric symptoms on a pharmacological basis" [60] and we agree.

The following case report in which depression is associated with the use of OCs illustrates how difficult it is to interpret the meaning of this association in the clinical situation.

A married 30-year-old woman who had two children experienced progressive symptoms of depression after her gynecologist switched her from Ovulen (0.1 mg mestranol and 1.0 mg ethynodial diacetate), which she had used for 6 years, to Ovral (0.05 mg ethinyl estradiol and 0.5 mg norgestrel). The change was made to lower the hormonal content of the pills. She told the senior author that she had begun to experience her symptoms about a week before her menses were to begin and for about 1 week thereafter. This pattern occurred over two cycles. Her depression was characterized by irritability (stimuli which would normally not make her upset now would), crying, and acute awareness of unhappy childhood memories. There were no recent changes in her life situation. Before using oral contraceptives, she had had what she described as "mild irritability" (compared with present symptoms) before the onset of her menses. The patient had been adopted at age 4 after the death of both her parents within a year of each other. Possibly because of this and because she had lost a limb in a childhood accident, she experienced some feelings of inadequacy as a wife and mother. The initial impression was that the symptoms were a result of a pharmacologic effect of oral contraceptives, but she was encouraged to continue another cycle since it has been noted that such symptoms have sometimes been known to spontaneously disappear within the first five cycles. The next month the patient reported she was much better, with symptoms markedly reduced in intensity. However, 3 months later she reported that she had had three cycles of symptoms of marked irritability and suspiciousness lasting 1 day on the day after stopping the medication. She had had no depressive symptoms. Stopping medication 1 day earlier on the next cycle did not reproduce the symptoms, but she developed irritability 3 days after cessation of medication, which lasted 5 days. At this time, oral contraceptive medication was discontinued and an intrauterine device was inserted.

She has had no recurrence of symptoms over an 8-month follow-up period, feeling "like my old self prior to starting oral contraceptives" [From Ref. 3] .

This case illustrates the difficulty the physician has in determining the etiology of the symptoms associated with oral contraceptive use. It is not clear whether there was a direct pharmacologic effect of the estrogen component or progesterone component (although the dosage of both was lowered when she switched medication), or a disturbance in endogenous production of estrogen or progesterone, or cumulative deficiency of the endogenous and exogenous hormones. In other cases, it is equally likely that the symptoms are related to psychological factors, e.g., the inability to conceive while on oral contraceptives reactivates conflicts about femininity. However, here the change to nonhormonal contraception resulted in a dramatic improvement in the patient's symptoms.

IV. Progesterone Used as a Psychopharmacologic Agent

To our knowledge, there have been no controlled studies of the use of progesterone to alter disturbed behavior over a prolonged period (5 or more months). Historically, studies of the behavioral effects of estrogenic and progestational compounds have gone through two phases. The early phase, from 1942 to 1964, comprised studies in which natural estrogens and progestins were used individually for possible adjunct psychopharmacologic effects in patients with neurotic, psychotic, and psychophysiologic reactions.

In this first phase, after discovery and isolation of the gonadal hormones, clinicians recommended their use for various psychiatric conditions based on an "endocrine deficiency or disturbed endocrine balance" theory of emotional illness. Doses used then were small compared with currently accepted dosages, and it is likely that spontaneous recovery rather than the drugs accounted for the observed changes.

Most of the studies in the second phase were uncontrolled. One such study [61] reported a series of 28 hospitalized psychiatric patients whose psychiatric symptoms were exacerbated at menstruation. Norethynodrel with mestranol was administered in doses of 10 to 30 mg/day for an unspecified length of time. Only four patients improved, and all but one patient failed to maintain the improvement. The same investigators reported further studies [62] on the use of norethynodrel with mestranol, again with chronic psychotic hospitalized patients. The patients included 22 schizophrenics, two psychotics with mental deficiency, and one neurotic. Of these patients, 12 menstruated irregularly. The dose regimen was 30 mg/day for 30 days. Four of the regularly menstruating patients showed improvement but relapsed within several months, and no improvement occurred among any of the patients in the irregularly menstruating group.

Twenty-one psychotic women whose symptoms exacerbated around the

time of menstruation were treated with norethynodrel with mestranol [62].
They were mostly schizophrenics, with a small number of "mental defectives
with psychosis," and involutional psychotics. The drug was given in 5 mg doses
twice a day for 20 days in two cycles. In addition, five psychotic patients whose
symptoms were unrelated to the menstrual cycle were included in the study. All
patients were concurrently receiving phenothiazines and/or psychotherapy. Results showed that 21 of the 26 improved, and 13 of these 21 left the hospital,
with the others being more easily managed in the hospital. Of the remaining
eight patients, three relapsed when the drug was discontinued, but all improved
when therapy was restarted. There was no change in four patients, and one became worse on the hormone therapy.

   Norethynodrel with mestranol was once again utilized as the experimental
drug in the treatment of nine patients with psychiatric illnesses possibly related
to "hormonal factors" [64]. One was a borderline patient with marked exacerbation of illness premenstrually; she improved with therapy. Five out of six patients with postpartum illness showed benefit. Finally, the two postmenopausal
depressed patients showed symptomatic improvement.

   Nine female psychiatric inpatients, ranging in age from 25 to 45, received
400 mg intramuscular progesterone over 48 h [65]. They were chronic patients,
who were prone to "anxiety and depression" (diagnosis not further defined) and
had been hospitalized for at least 1 year. Each patient served as her own control,
receiving saline and progesterone on alternate months in a double-blind fashion.
They were observed from 6 days before to 10 days after administration of progesterone or saline. Each filled out a Green-Nowlis checklist of mood, including
premenstrual symptoms, and each kept a diary of unusual events. Findings included drowsiness as a common side effect, beginning on the second or third day
after injections. A mild decrease in anxiety and depression and a modest decrease
in the responses to provocative stimuli also occurred. One patient went into a
depression similar to her premenstrual depression, but more severe.

   A study by Kyger and Webb [66] of psychological state in three groups of
10 women, each with progressively higher progesterone peaks (one at normal
cycle calculated progesterone peak, one during the height of Enovid therapy, and
one during the third trimester of pregnancy) failed to show worsening of cognitive or affective measures. A conservative conclusion was that "serious psychological disturbances are unlikely hazards with increased progesterone levels in
normal women."

V. Discussion

There are some major problems in interpreting the data now available.

A. Controlled vs. Uncontrolled Data

Most of the experiments reported have been uncontrolled. Although these experiments have been helpful in providing possible new clinical approaches and in providing leads for further research, their findings and postulates *have been generally misunderstood and taken as facts.*

B. Animal Studies

Most of the data collected in systematic, controlled fashion have been on animals. Extrapolating from animals to humans in the field of "mood and behavior" is hazardous, to say the least. As Richardson [67] has said in discussing ovarian physiology,

It is probably true that there are more species differences in the area of reproductive physiology than anywhere else, and it is impossible to know how much of the vast research effort that has been applied to rodents and to farm animals will prove applicable to humans . . . for the present purposes, it seems probable that interspecies variation is greatest at the level of the ovary itself.

In our opinion, interspecies behavioral differences are equally great or greater.

C. Measurement Techniques

Measurements of both cerebral physiology and mood and behavior are at present quite insensitive, and it is extremely difficult to measure drug-induced change directly. Therefore, most of the data are inferential. However, recent work has been more qualitative and replicable.

Dalton [68], Hamburg [69], and many others [37,65,70-74] have suggested a common etiologic thread in their studies (i.e., premenstrual tension, postpartum disorders, periodic depressions, and other affective disorders) and other disorders in this same group. The mechanism could be based on a genetic factor (e.g., disturbance in a particular metabolic pathway of progesterone), in part on an environmental factor (e.g., a disturbed feminine identity) [75], and in part on an immediate, precipitating stress (e.g., loss of spouse during pregnancy). Each may be a necessary, but not solely sufficient cause of the syndrome.

D. Psychological vs. Pharmacologic Effects

Because measurement techniques in psychiatry and endocrinology are still relatively crude, but becoming more precise, it has been difficult to distinguish the psychological effects of taking a "sex hormone" such as progesterone from the pharmacologic effects. For example, in descriptions of oral contraceptive effects, it is unclear whether depression is the result of a direct pharmacologic effect of progesterone or a specific psychodynamic effect (e.g., guilt about sexual relations), or a combination of other factors. Even more problematic is the fact that not only are there a variety of circulating, fluctuating hormones, but also marked individual differences in hormone secretion patterns [76].

E. Exogenous vs. Endogenous Effects

Both exogenous and endogenous hormones are metabolized and secreted in a similar way. This makes it extremely difficult to distinguish the effects induced by the exogenous drug vs. the endogenous hormone and complicates results of experiments in which OCs are administered.

VI. Summary

To sum up this mass of unwieldy, cross-disciplinary data in our present state of ignorance of the relative weights of physiological, pharmacological and psychological variables on mood and behavior is difficult indeed.

For now, our interpretation is that *most* women using OCs for their contraceptive properties can expect minimal change in mood and sexual behavior. Whether OCs cause depression is unknown at this time, but our interpretation does not support such an association. For women who have had *severe* premenstrual tension in the absence of other psychiatric illness, OCs may be useful [49]. The choice of OC would depend on the presence or absence of a history of premenstrual irritability [16]. OCs may be useful for a small subgroup of women with recurrent depressive disorder, but treatment should be considered experimental. For women with psychoses with premenstrual exacerbation, OCs may have a place as part of a regimen including lithium and/or antipsychotic medications.

Carefully controlled experiments with OCs in humans, on a prospective basis, over a long period of time (at least a year), and employing crossover and double-blind techniques are needed. Although difficult, and time-consuming, it is the only way to advance our knowledge in this field, which is currently inferential, speculative, and lacking enough controlled data to untangle the effects of physiological from psychological variables.

References

1. N. M. Morris and J. R. Udry, Contraceptive pills and day-by-day feelings of well-being. *Am. J. Obstet. Gynecol.* 113:763-765 (1972).

2. W. M. Herrmann and R. C. Beach, The psychotropic properties of estrogens. *Pharmakopsychiatr. Neuropsychopharmakol.* 11:164-176 (1978).

3. I. D. Glick and S. Bennett, Psychiatric effects of progesterone and oral contraceptives, in *Psychiatric Complications of Medical Drugs* (R. Shader, ed.). Raven Press, New York, 1972, pp. 295-332.

4. W. Ladisich, Influence of progesterone on serotonin metabolism: A possible causal factor for mood changes. *Psychoneuroendocrinology* 2:257-266 (1977).

5. A. Worsley, A prospective study of the effects of the progestagen content of oral contraceptives on measures of affect, automatization, and perceptual restructuring ability. *Psychopharmacology (Berlin)* 67:289-296 (1980).

6. J. Kutner and T. Duffy, A psychological analysis of oral contraceptives and the intrauterine device. *Contraception* 2:284-296 (1970).

7. S. J. Kutner and W. L. Brown, History of depression as a risk factor for depression with oral contraceptives and discontinuance. *J. Nerv. Ment. Dis.* 155:163-169 (1972).

8. S. J. Kutner and W. L. Brown, Types of oral contraceptives, depression and premenstrual symptoms. *J. Nerv. Ment. Dis.* 155:153-162 (1972).

9. O. Fleming and C. P. Seager, Incidence of depressive symptoms in users of the oral contraceptive. *Br. J. Psychiatry* 132:431-440 (1978).

10. F. J. Kane, Iatrogenic depression in women, in *Phenomenology and Treatment of Depression* (W. E. Fann, I. Karcan, and A. Polorny, eds.). Spectrum, Pub., New York, 1977, pp. 69-80.

11. F. Winston, Oral contraceptives, pyridoxine, and depression. *Am. J. Psychiatry* 130:1217-1221 (1973).

12. B. L. Parry and A. J. Rush, Oral contraceptives and depressive symptomatology: Biologic mechanisms. *Compr. Psychiatry* 20:347-358 (1979).

13. H. Warnes and C. Fitzpatrick, Oral contraceptives and depression. *Psychosomatics* 20:187-189 (1979).

14. R. W. Lidz, Emotional factors in the success of contraception. *Fertil. Steril.* 20:761-771 (1969).

15. P. P. Talwar and G. S. Berger, A prospective, randomized study of oral contraceptives: The effect of study design on reported rates of symptoms. *Contraception* 20:329-337.

16. J. Cullberg, Premenstrual symptom patterns and mental reactions to medication—a latent profile analysis. *Acta Psychiatr. Scand. [Suppl.]* 236, (1972).

17. D. B. Adams, A. R. Gold, and A. D. Burt, Rise in female-initiated sexual activity at ovulation and its suppression by oral contraceptives. *N. Engl. J. Med.* 21:1145-1150 (1978).

18. R. M. Tose, Psychoendocrinology of the menstrual cycle. Editorial. *N. Engl. J. Med.* 299:1186-1187.

19. J. Leeton, R. McMaster, and A. Worsely, The effects on sexual response and mood after sterilization of women taking long-term oral contraception: Results of a double-blind cross-over study. *Aust. NZ J. Obstet. Gynecol.* 18:194-197 (1978).

20. J. Bancroft, D. W. Davidson, P. Warner, and G. Tyrer, Androgens and sexual behaviour in women using oral contraceptives. *Clin. Endocrinol. (Oxf.)* 12:327-340 (1980).

21. H. Persky, N. Charney, H. I. Lief, C. P. O'Brien, W. R. Miller, and D. Strauss, The relationship of plasma estradiol level to sexual behavior in young women. *Psychosom. Med.* 40:523-535 (1978).

22. J. D. Wilson, Sex hormones and sexual behavior. *N. Engl. J. Med.* 300: 1269-1270 (1979).

23. H. Fries and S. J. Nillius, Psychological factors, psychiatric illness and amenorrhea after oral contraceptive treatment. *Acta Psychiatr. Scand.* 49:653-668 (1973).

24. S. Friedman and A. Goldfien, Amenorrhea and galactorrhea following O.C. therapy. *JAMA* 210:1883-1891 (1969).

25. I. D. Yalom, R. Gren, and N. Fisk, Prenatal exposure to female hormones. *Arch. Gen. Psychiatry* 28:554-561 (1973).

26. J. M. Reinisch, Prenatal exposure of human foetuses to synthetic progestin and oestrogen affects personality. *Nature* 266:(5602) 561-562 (1977).

27. A. A. Ehrhardt, G. C. Grisanti, and H. F. Meyer-Bahlburg, Prenatal exposure to medroxyprogesterone acetate (MPA) in girls. *Psychoneuroendocrinology* 2:391-398 (1977).

28. H. F. Meyer Bahlburg, G. C. Grisanti, and A. A. Ehrhardt, Prenatal effects of sex hormones on human male behavior: Medroxyprogesterone acetate (MPA). *Psychoneuroendocrinology* 2:383-390 (1977).

29. V. Wynn, Vitamins and oral contraceptive use. *Lancet* i:561-564 (1975).

30. P. W. Adams, V. Wynn, D. P. Rose, J. Folkard, M. Seed, and R. Strong, Effects of pyridoxine hydrochloride (vitamin B_6) upon depression associated with oral contraception. *Lancet* i:897-904 (1973).

31. M. M. Weissman and G. L. Klerman, Sex differences and the epidemiology of depression. *Arch. Gen. Psychiatry* 34:98-111 (1977).

32. G. Klerman, A. DiMascio, M. Weissman, B. Prusoff, and E. S. Paykel, Treatment of depression by drugs and psychotherapy. *Am. J. Psychiatry* 131: 186-191 (1974).

33. E. L. Klaiber, D. M. Broverman, W. Vogel, Y. Kobayashi, and D. Moriarty, Effects of estrogen therapy on plasma M.A.O. activity and E.E.G. driving responses of depressed women. *Am. J. Psychiatry* 128:1492-1498 (1972).

34. A. J. Prange, I. Wilson, A. Rabon, and M. A. Lipton, Enhancement of imipramine antidepressant activity by thyroid hormone. *Am. J. Psychiatry* 126:457-469 (1969).

35. T. Pugh, B. Jarath, W. Schmitt, and R. Reed, Rates of mental disease related to childbearing. *N. Engl. J. Med.* 268:1224-1228 (1963).

36. A. Rosenberg and E. Silver, Suicide, psychiatrists and therapeutic abortion. *Calif. Med.* 102:407-411 (1965).

37. I. D. Glick, B. Hauptman, and D. F. Klein, Pseudopregnancy treatment of periodic psychiatric illness: A pilot study. *Psychiatr. Q.* 44:403-407 (1970).

38. K. Paige, Effects of oral contraceptives on affective fluctuations associated with the menstrual cycle. *Psychosom. Med.* 33:515-537 (1971).

39. D. E. Warren, W. H. Tedford, Jr., and W. E. Flynn, Behavioral effects of cyclic changes in serotonin during the human menstrual cycle. *Med. Hypytheses* 3:359-364 (1979).

40. J. M. Abplanalp, R. M. Rose, A. F. Donnelly, and L. Livingston-Vaughan, Psychoendocrinology of the menstrual cycle: II. The relationship between enjoyment of activities, moods, and reproductive hormones. *Psychosom. Med.* 41:605-615 (1979).

41. J. M. Abplanalp, A. F. Donnelly, and R. M. Rose, Psychoendocrinology of the menstrual cycle: I. Enjoyment of daily activities and moods. *Psychosom. Med.* 41:587-604 (1979).

42. M. H. Banks and S. A. Beresford, The influence of menstrual cycle phase upon symptom recording using data from health diaries. *J. Psychosom. Res.* 23:307-313.

43. E. L. Klaiber, D. M. Broverman, W. Vogel, and Y. Kobayashi, Estrogen therapy for severe persistent depressions in women. *Arch. Gen. Psychiatry* 36:550-554 (1979).

44. D. N. Krus, S. Wapner, J. Bergen, and H. Freeman, The influence of progesterone on behavioral changes induced by lysergic acid diethylamide (LSD-25) in normal males. *Psychopharmacology* 2:177-184 (1961).

45. B. C. Little, R. J. Matta, and T. P. Zahn, Physiological and psychological effects of progesterone in man. *J. Nerv. Ment. Dis.* 159:256-262 (1974).

46. K. T. Marinari, A. I. Leshner, and M. P. Doyle, Menstrual cycle status and adrenocortical reactivity to psychological stress. *Psychoneuroendocrinology* 1:213-218 (1976).

47. B. Herzberg and A. Coppen, Changes in psychological symptoms in women taking oral contraceptives. *Br. J. Psychiatry* 116:161-164 (1970).

48. M. E. Chernovetz, W. H. Jones, and R. O. Hansson, Predictability attentional focus, sex role orientation, and menstrual-related stress. *Psychosom. Med.* 41:383-391 (1979).

49. I. D. Glick and A. Goldfein, Treatment of severe premenstrual syndromes with medroxyprogesterone acetate. Unpublished data (1978).

50. K. Dalton, *The Premenstrual Syndrome and Progesterone Therapy.* Yearbook Med. Pub., Inc., Chicago, 1977.

51. F. J. Kane and M. Keeler, The use of Enovid in postpartum mental disorders. *South. Med. J.* 58:1089-1092 (1965).

52. M. Steiner, Psychobiology of mental disorders associated with childbearing. An overview. *Acta Psychiatr. Scand.* 60:449-464 (1979).

53. H. J. Kantor, L. J. Milton, and M. L. Ernst, Comparative psychologic effects of estrogen administration on institutional and noninstitutional elderly women. *J. Am. Geriatr. Soc.* 26:9-16 (1978).

54. S. Ballinger, D. Cobbin, J. Krivanek, and D. Saunders, Life stresses and depression in the menopause. *Maturitas* 1:191-199 (1979).

55. M. Endo, M. Daiguji, Y. Asano, I. Yamashita, and S. Takahashi, Periodic psychosis recurring in association with menstrual cycle. *J. Clin. Psychiatry* 39:456-466 (1978).

56. V. Wieczarek, R. Bock, and H. Kluge, Use of ovulation inhibitors in female epileptics and psychiatric patients. *MMW* 111:254-259 (1969).

57. I. D. Glick and D. Stewart, A new drug treatment for premenstrual exacerbation of schizophrenia. *Compr. Psychiatry* 21:281-287 (1980).

58. A. R. Felthous, D. B. Robinson, and R. W. Conroy, Prevention of recurrent menstrual psychosis by an oral contraceptive. *Am. J. Psychiatry* 137:245-246 (1980).

59. F. Kane, Clinical psychiatric symptoms accompanying O.C. use. *Comments Contemp. Psychiatry* 1:7-16 (1971).

60. M. M. Weissman and A. E. Slaby, Oral contraceptives and psychiatric disturbance: Evidence from research. *Br. J. Psychiatry* 123:513-518 (1973).

61. G. Simpson, N. Radinger, D. Rochlin, and N. Kline, Enovid in the treatment of psychic disturbances associated wtih menstruation. *Dis. Nerv. Syst.* 23:589-590 (1962).

62. G. Simpson, D. Rochlin, and N. Kline, Further studies of enovid in the treatment of psychiatric patients. *Dis. Nerv. Syst.* 25:484-496 (1964).

63. D. Swanson, A. Barron, A. Floren, and J. Smith, The use of norethynodrel in psychotic females. *Am. J. Psychiatry* 120:1101-1103 (1964).

64. F. Kane, R. Daly, J. Ewing, and M. Keeler, Mood and behavioral changes with progestational agents. *Br. J. Psychiatry* 113:265-268 (1967).

65. B. S. Kopell, The role of progestins and progesterone in brain function and behavior, in *Metabolic Effects of Gonadal Hormones and Contraceptive Steroids* (H. A. Salhanick, D. M. Kipnis, and R. L. Vande Wells, eds.). Plenum, New York, 1969, pp. 649-667.

66. K. Kyger and W. W. Webb, Progesterone levels and psychological state in normal women. *Am. J. Obstet. Gynecol.* 113:759-762 (1972).

67. G. Richardson, Ovarian physiology. *N. Engl. J. Med.* 274:1008-1015 (1966).

68. K. Dalton, *The Premenstrual Syndrome.* Heineman, London, 1964.

69. D. A. Hamburg, Effects of progesterone on behavior. In *Endocrines and the Central Nervous System* (R. Levine, ed.). Williams & Wilkins, Baltimore, 1966, pp. 251-263.

70. D. Janowsky and J. Davis, Ovarian hormones, monoamines and mental illness. Presented at the Annual Meeting of the American Psychiatric Association, 1970.

71. F. Kane, Postpartum psychosis in identical twins. *Psychosomatics* 9:278-281 (1968).

72. R. Moos, Psychological aspects of oral contraceptives. *Arch. Gen. Psychiatry* 19:87-95 (1968).

73. J. R. Udry and N. M. Morris, Distribution of coitus in the menstrual cycle. *Nature* 220:593-596 (1968).

74. I. Yalom, D. Lunde, R. Moos, and D. Hamburg, "Postpartum blues" syndrome. *Arch. Gen. Psychiatry* 18:16-27 (1968).

75. N. Shainess, Psychiatric evaluation of premenstrual tension. *N.Y. State J. Med.* 62:3523-3579 (1962).

76. R. E. Whalen, Cyclic changes in hormones and behavior. *Arch. Sex. Behav.* 4:313-314 (1975).

77. I. D. Glick, Mood and behavioral changes associated with the use of the oral contraceptive agents. A review of the literature. *Psychopharmacology (Berlin)* 10:363-374 (1967).

78. A. Blumberg and O. Billig, Hormonal influence upon "puerperal psychosis" and neurotic conditions. *Psychiatr. Q.* 16:454 (1942).

79. O. Billig and J. Bradley, Combined shock and corpus luteum hormone therapy. *Am. J. Psychiatry* 102:783-787 (1946).

80. W. Bower and M. Altschule, Use of progesterone in the treatment of postpartum psychosis. *N. Engl. J. Med.* 254:157-160 (1956).

81. M. J. Baumblatt and F. Winston, Pyridoxine and the pill. *Lancet* i:832-833 (1970).

18 Recent Trends in the Treatment of Premenstrual Syndrome: A Critical Review

JUDITH GREEN   William Paterson College of New Jersey, Wayne, New Jersey

I. Overview

At least one-third of women are affected to some degree by unpleasant and at times disruptive symptoms in the days preceding the menses [1-6]. These somatic and psychological symptoms occur in clusters sufficiently well-defined to justify the term premenstrual syndrome (PMS). The physical symptoms typically include swollen, tender breasts; abdominal bloating and discomfort; and headaches; while the most common emotional symptoms are adverse mood changes consisting primarily of irritability, depression, and tension. Although the intensity of symptoms may fluctuate from month to month, a high degree of consistency has been found in the profile of symptoms reported by individual women over successive cycles [3]. Moreover, the cyclic nature of the subjective symptoms has been firmly established in several studies utilizing nonretrospective techniques [7-10], and numerous objectively measured cyclic physiological changes have been documented [11]. Thus, the reality of the premenstrual syndrome seems undeniable.

Although the symptoms of PMS are severe enough to impair normal functioning in a minority of women, the absolute numbers of individuals in this category, and the total amount of personal suffering involved, are large. The impact of these recurrent symptoms on the family, other social groups, and the economy cannot be dismissed [12,13]. In need of treatment also are women who suffer exacerbation of chronic illness during the premenstruum. Intensification of psychosis [14]; epilepsy [15,16]; suicidal tendencies [17]; and asthma and allergic manifestations [13] have all been observed.

II. Some Methodologic Considerations

The half-century of medical literature on premenstrual syndrome includes a vast array of treatments advocated on the basis of etiologic hypotheses. Although useful therapeutic approaches would enhance our understanding of the etiology of premenstrual symptoms, the results of clinical trials have on the whole been erratic, with causal factors of premenstrual symptoms not clearly indicated through treatment avenues. In view of the inconsistent clinical findings, the need for rigorously controlled double-blind treatment studies cannot be overemphasized. As Smith [18] noted, regardless of the therapeutic agent, improvement has been found in most uncontrolled studies, whereas therapeutic benefit has been far more difficult to demonstrate with any approach when conditions are adequately controlled. This discrepancy and the significant placebo effect observed in the majority of placebo-controlled investigations underscore the perplexing interaction between physiological and psychic factors in the experience of premenstrual symptoms.

Other issues which bear on the interpretation of clinical trials are the criteria used to define both the premenstrual symptoms and their improvement; and the methods for the assessment of symptoms. In particular, the validity of retrospective assessment as compared with daily monitoring of symptoms has been questioned on empiric grounds [19,20]. Measures sensitive not only to symptom kind and intensity, but also to timing during the menstrual cycle are critical in the resolution of etiologic and treatment issues.

Because older treatment studies have been the subject of several fine reviews [18,21], research findings during the last decade will constitute the major focus of this discussion. Particular emphasis will be given to findings emerging from controlled trials in an effort to interrelate etiologic hypotheses with reliable treatment outcomes.

III. Diuretic Therapy

A. Rationale

Since certain obvious somatic aspects of premenstrual syndrome, such as swollen breasts, abdominal distension, and weight gain, appear easily referable to alterations in fluid and electrolyte metabolism, it has seemed reasonable to surmise that other premenstrual symptoms could share this basis. However, somatic and emotional symptoms are not consistently correlated [3], and studies of fluid and electrolyte variables have provided weak theoretic justification for the use of diuretics in PMS. Moreover, studies have shown that only some affected women gain weight during the premenstruum [22,23] and in those who do, the increases have failed to correlate with premenstrual symptom severity [22,24]. O'Brien et al. [25] reported similar slight weight gains in patients with PMS and in symptom-free controls. Weight lability in the premenstruum in one study [24] was found related to the occurrence of symptoms, suggesting the contribution of fluid and electrolyte fluxes to symptom development. Conceivably, even slight shifts of fluid and electrolytes in the brain in association with alterations in the balance or distribution of these substances in the body [23,26] could explain the relatively nonspecific mood and behavioral changes typifying the premenstrual syndrome

B. Treatment Studies

The efficacies of several kinds of diuretics in the treatment of PMS have been investigated with the application of formal controls although, as discussed below, the usefulness of these methods in relation to diuretics is uncertain.

In a three-way double-blind comparison of placebo, norethisterone, and the diuretic combination, triamterene and benzthiazide, in 27 women with moderate to severe PM symptoms [27], the diuretic was associated with significantly greater relief of depression and irritability than placebo. Relief of pain, anxiety, nervousness, headache, and, interestingly, body swelling, was not superior to that obtained with placebo.

Conflicting outcomes resulted from two controlled studies of sulfonamide diuretics with thiazide-like actions. In one [28], chlorthalidone, lithium chloride, and placebo were compared using a three-way double-blind crossover design in 25 women experiencing mild to moderate PM symptoms. The treatments were administered in random order for 2 months each with symptoms rated during the anticipated late premenstrual phase of each cycle. All but two patients claimed to improve with placebo and it was the treatment preferred most often (10 of 25 women). Placebo provided the best relief of the symptom clusters anxiety-tension, depression-neurasthenia, and irritability-explosivity. Only four patients reported feeling better during the diuretic cycles, as compared with six during lithium treatment and 10 while taking placebo. Whether, as the authors suggested, differential responses to lithium, diuretic, and placebo reflected etiologically distinct subgroups of PMS or chance fluctuations in symptom intensity is not clear.

In contrast, Werch and Kane [29] reported a high degree of efficacy of the diuretic metolazone in the treatment of 33 women selected for PMS and substantial weight gain (3 pounds or more). Diuretic and placebo were each administered for two consecutive cycles, during the premenstrual week and the menses. Graded symptom scales completed on the estimated fourth day before menstrual onset showed significant decreases in irritability, depression, tension, nervousness, anxiety, edema and swelling of the breasts and abdomen during the diuretic as compared with baseline cycles. Placebo ratings for symptoms of negative affect and water retention were intermediate between those of pretreatment and metolazone cycles.

The conflicting findings of these diuretic trials are probably related to methodologies used, since age of subjects, symptom intensity, and manner of reporting symptoms differed greatly. In particular, low symptom intensity in the negative chlorthalidone study left little margin for improvement; and the unpleasant side effects of lithium, which initially induces diuresis, may have prejudiced some subjects. What becomes evident in analyzing these studies is the weakness of the double-blind design in a placebo-controlled diuretic trial. Increased frequency of urination provides a clear indicator of the independent variables under investigation.

Thus, while there was evidence that women with intense premenstrual symptoms have benefited from diuretics of the thiazide type [27,29,30], methodologic considerations prevent firm conclusions about the efficacy of these agents.

Spironolactone, an inhibitor of the sodium-retaining effects of aldosterone in the distal nephron, could act as a specific antidote to elevated luteal levels of this adrenocorticosteroid [31,32]. O'Brien et al. [33] reported that mean plasma aldosterone levels were higher in 28 women in the luteal than in the follicular phase, but failed to find significant differences in aldosterone levels between women with and without PMS. Despite the lack of empiric support for an aldosterone hypothesis of PMS, spironolactone as compared with placebo was associated with a significant decline in negative affect in women experiencing PMS in this double-blind crossover study. Mood variables were assessed daily for four cycles. It was concluded that although their mechanisms differ, spironolactone was as effective as metolazone in the treatment of PMS. Since women in both PMS and non-PMS groups lost similar and insignificant amounts of weight during spironolactone trials, neither specific aldosterone antagonism at the renal level (women in the PMS group might have been more sensitive to aldosterone effects) nor general diuretic action appear, in some easily measurable way, to underlie the clinical improvement. As in the case of other diuretics, the rigorous double-blind control may not have prevented women from correctly distinguishing active drug from placebo. On the other hand, some women may be more sensitive than others to slight changes in fluid and electrolyte balance or distribution, and even modest changes related to diuresis may exert a beneficial effect on symptoms. Where diuretics prove useful, spironolactone, because it does not provoke secondary aldosteronism, is preferable to agents of the thiazide type.

A subgroup of women experiencing "carefully documented" premenstrual depression appeared to obtain no relief when treated with spironolactone in a palcebo-controlled study [18]. Perhaps women who experience predominantly depressive symptoms in the premenstruum represent a subgroup etiologically distinct from those characterized by irritability or mixed irritable and depressive symptoms.

Taylor and James [16] claimed that spironolactone permitted a reduction of up to 50% in anticonvulsant medication when administered adjunctively in the premenstrual exacerbation of epilepsy. Similar claims have been made for progesterone [13], which promotes diuresis among its many actions. Although a reduction in central nervous system irritability is implied in the Taylor and James statement, no specific supporting data were provided.

Help in clarifying some of the inconsistencies in diuretic treatment outcomes may be provided by a recent study [25]. A definite trend toward earlier and more elevated postovulatory progesterone peaks was found in women with premenstrual symptoms compared with symptom-free controls. The changes in progesterone concentration correlated with a pattern of diuresis and natriuresis. This was followed by a premenstrual decrease in salt and water excretion to preovulatory levels, an effect ascribed to aldosterone. Symptoms followed the onset of the initial fluid and electrolyte changes. The authors concluded that "treatment should be aimed at preventing the natriuretic effect of progesterone in the postovulatory phase and the sodium-retaining effects of aldosterone in the premenstrual phase." Treatment timed specifically to ameliorate the opposing postovulatory and premenstrual electrolyte fluxes has not yet been carried out but might contribute to the refinement of etiologic concepts more productively than standard diuretic therapy has yet done. The result of this refinement might be a multiple stage treatment incorporating diuretics and other agents in a properly sequenced regimen that would be more effective than diuretic therapy alone.

IV. Progesterone

A. Rationale

A lack of progesterone alone or in relation to estrogen in the luteal phase of the menstrual cycle has been proposed as etiologic since the initial discussions of premenstrual tension [34,35]. Decreased sedative, diuretic, and glucocorticoid transport properties resulting from a lack of progesterone have been claimed as important in causing PMS [13]. In addition, a relative excess of estrogen has been described as pathogenetic [see 18], acting to promote renal salt and water retention, changes in capillary permeability, epithelial proliferation in breasts and pelvic organs [36], central nervous system irritability, and potentially relevant changes in biogenic amine metabolism [37,38].

Direct evidence related to differences in ovarian steroid levels in women with and without PMS has presented an unclear picture. For example, Taylor [39] found that mean progesterone levels did not differ significantly between 39 women classified into high and low premenstrual symptom groups. In women experiencing premenstrual anxiety and irritability, Backstrom and colleagues found elevated plasma estrogen to progesterone ratios in the late premenstruum [40,41]. These investigators attributed greater etiologic importance to increased plasma estrogen than decreased progesterone [42], although estrogen administration has often been associated with decreased negative affect and increased feelings of well-being [43]. Munday et al. [44] reported significantly lower plasma progesterone levels on the eighth to fifth days before the menses in a group of eight women with PMS. However, in six of the eight [45], the onset of the symptoms preceded the low progesterone levels, suggesting that other factors were operative. Also, since the PMS and control subjects in Munday's studies were not matched in age, the hormonal differences seen could represent normal age-related variations in secretory patterns. In a group of 58 women selected for severe premenstrual symptoms, luteal plasma progesterone deficiencies occurred in only 30% [45]. Although women selected for premenstrual depression showed a slight but significant reduction in progesterone levels, no correlation was found between blood levels of this hormone in any given cycle and the degree of premenstrual depression experienced [18].

Although some of these findings are provocative, it is important to note that if low progesterone levels or elevated estrogen to progesterone ratios were of primary etiologic importance, typical symptoms would occur in the preovulatory rather than the premenstrual phase of the menstrual cycle [46]. Recently, O'Brien and colleagues [33] reported that women with PMS had significantly higher, not lower, postovulatory plasma progesterone concentrations than control subjects, and that there was a weak but significant correlation between negative mood and progesterone level during this period. As discussed in the preceding section, O'Brien and co-workers [25] postulated that the diuresis produced by progesterone leads to a secondary aldosterone increase with consequent salt and water retention later in the luteal phase. "This flux in electrolyte state is coincident with the onset of psychological symptoms, and [is] probably causative" [45]. Thus, subtle progesterone-aldosterone interactions may occur during the luteal phase; depending on the precision of compensatory mechanisms, small but physiologically significant electrolyte fluxes may occur. Because of the variability of individual physiological mechanisms, the timing of related therapies would be of the utmost importance.

B. Treatment Studies

Despite the absence of controlled studies, Dalton [13,47,48] has been an enthusiastic advocate of the use of progesterone to correct the deficiencies which, in her view, underlie premenstrual symptom formation. Because a variety of causal factors may lead to functionally inadequate progesterone levels, therapeutic agents which address these factors would benefit only some women, whereas the efficacy of progesterone in PMS should be universal [13].

The widely held belief that, for reliable attainment of effective blood levels, progesterone must be administered parenterally or in pessary form has recently been challenged [49], but studies of PMS have not yet employed the more attractive oral route of administration. Dalton [13] recommended 25 to 100 mg progesterone intramuscularly daily or every second day; up to four 200 to 400 mg suppositories or pessaries per day from day 14 of the cycle; or the subcutaneous implantation of five to 12 pellets of 25 or 100 mg progesterone each. Most of these dosages have been shown to produce significant and prolonged elevations of plasma progesterone in normal women [50]. Using these regimens, Dalton [13] reported that 40 women experiencing premenstrual symptoms had been successfully treated with progesterone for more than 10 years without adverse effects. Thus progesterone treatment, regardless of its efficacy, is apparently safe.

Although the need for controlled studies of the usefulness of progesterone in PMS was made abundantly clear by the reported improvement of women receiving insignificant doses [51], only two placebo-controlled double-blind investigations are documented in the literature [9,52]. In both these studies, progesterone failed to prove superior to placebo in the reduction of premenstrual symptoms. In a regimen similar to Dalton's [13], Sampson's [9] subjects used 200 mg progesterone suppositories or pessaries twice daily during the 12 days preceding menstrual onset. Both daily symptom (menstrual distress questionnaire) and retrospective ratings failed to demonstrate a significant difference between progesterone and placebo in the relief of symptoms documented during a pretreatment cycle. While on global ratings 31% of subjects found progesterone more helpful than placebo, 43% found placebo more helpful than progesterone. Whether the 31% of subjects who preferred progesterone to placebo represented a particular subgroup of women with PMS, perhaps corresponding to the 30% of 58 women reported to have low luteal progesterone levels [44], is not clear because of the absence of actual measurements. Again, chance fluctuations in symptoms could account for an apparently therapeutic effect. Smith's [52] subjects were selected for premenstrual depression and received progesterone intramuscularly with a similar lack of overall therapeutic response.

In an uncontrolled trial, Dalton [48] claimed good or moderate relief of menstrual migraine in 83% of 65 women receiving progesterone pessaries or suppositories. In contrast, Somerville [53] reported that of six women with pretreatment documentation of premenstrual migraine headaches, four developed characteristic migraines and one a shortened headache at the usual time in the cycle despite progesterone administration. Progesterone was injected intramuscularly in doses producing typical midluteal plasma levels. None of the six women experienced migraines when progesterone was withdrawn to permit bleeding, even though progesterone concentrations fell rapidly. Thus, hypotheses of menstrual migraine based on low or falling levels of progesterone were not supported; estrogen withdrawal was implicated as a more probable etiologic factor.

Due to the recency of the findings, reports on dydrogesterone, an oral progestin which differs only slightly from the natural ovarian steroid, will be included here, although adequately controlled trials have not as yet been carried out. Taylor [54] claimed that more than 70% of 50 women with premenstrual symptoms and lower than normal progesterone levels in the luteal phase believed themselves cured or greatly improved by dydrogesterone. The drug was administered in an open protocol in 10 mg doses twice daily from the 12th to the 26th day of the cycle. Regardless of the progesterone level, however, the overall improvement rate remained at about 70% in more than 200 women with premenstrual symptoms [16]. Symptoms related to fluid retention were ameliorated most frequently (90%); and mental symptoms by about 80%; while breast symptoms were apparently not relieved by dydrogesterone [16,55]. Using dydrogesterone in a single-blind placebo-controlled study, Day [55] also found an improvement rate of about 70%. In more than 40% of patients, similar improvement occurred with placebo. Since women with low and normal progesterone levels responded similarly, these findings suggest that any therapeutic benefit attributable to dydrogesterone was due to pharmacologic effects rather than to a correction of deficient progesterone levels [56]. Accurate knowledge of the usefulness of dydrogesterone in the treatment of PMS, however, awaits well-controlled investigations.

V. Bromocriptine

A. Rationale

The semisynthetic ergot, bromocriptine, is a dopamine agonist which, among other actions, suppresses the secretion of prolactin (PRL) from the pituitary gland. Interest in the use of bromocriptine was stimulated by a dramatic case report [57]. A woman with severe PMS and large premenstrual weight gains (5 to 8 kg) due to fluid and electrolyte retention was found to have mean luteal prolactin levels twice those of the follicular phase. Bromocriptine appeared effective in the long-term reduction of both the PRL levels and the premenstrual symptoms. The authors believed this woman to be the first example of "a prolactin-induced fluid and electrolyte disorder."

Although major mood or behavioral effects have not been identified with prolactin, some evidence favors the role of PRL in premenstrual syndrome [58]. The plasma level of this pituitary hormone, which has been shown to promote the retention of water, sodium and potassium in human beings [59], was elevated throughout the menstrual cycle in women with PMS and was further elevated parallel with PM symptoms in the late luteal phase of the cycle [60]. Kullander and Svanberg [61] reported that 10 women with PMS had midluteal serum prolactin levels in the upper range of normal and that there appeared to be a correlation in these women between symptom severity and PRL level. Andersch et al. [30] found no difference between luteal PRL levels in women with and without PMS, although follicular phase PRL levels were significantly lower in the symptomatic group. In all these studies, compared with controls, women with PMS underwent a greater increase in prolactin level from follicular to luteal phase. On the other hand, Andersen et al. [62] found no follicular-luteal change in serum PRL levels in 21 women with PMS; and these investigators [63] concluded that women experiencing PMS "seem to have normal prolactin levels as well as normal thyrotrophin releasing hormone induced increments." Munday [44] reported that of 58 women with severe premenstrual symptoms, only two showed plasma prolactin concentrations beyond the normal range. Recently, O'Brien et al. [33] reported no differences in plasma PRL levels measured throughout the menstrual cycle in women with and without PMS. It was noted [63] that bromocriptine may be an effective therapeutic agent but for reasons other than its effects on prolactin.

B. Treatment Studies

Similarly to studies of other drugs used in the treatment of PMS, investigations into the usefulness of bromocriptine have yielded inconsistent results. In reviewing controlled trials of bromcriptine in a total of 119 women, Andersen and Larsen [63] pointed out that a major source of discrepancies in outcome was variation in dosages used. Total dosage of less than 5 mg per day was associated with short-lived reduction in plasma prolactin [64] and with lack of efficacy. Although the high incidence of side effects occurring with bromocriptine led to the use of low doses in some studies, in others a phase-in period at half dosage (e.g., 1.25 mg twice daily on days 14 to 16 of the cycle) permitted the administration of the full amount without notable side-effects during the remainder of each cycle [63,65].

A total of four controlled studies using adequate dosages of bromocriptine have led to reports of clinical improvement in somatic and psychological symptoms in women with PMS whereas two similarly designed studies have not.

1. Positive Studies

The much cited study of Benedek-Jaszmann and Hearn-Sturtevant [66] involved 10 women who completed two cycles in a double-blind crossover comparison of bromocriptine and placebo. This study is not without methodologic problems, however. For example, pretreatment symptom data were not obtained; instead each woman was asked during the treatment trial to score herself retrospectively "in relation to the cycle preceding the trial." Mood changes assessed were lability of mood, depression, and tiredness, with the cardinal symptom of irritability omitted. In addition, the subjects all were experiencing functional infertility. Since there is no general agreement as to the correspondence of premenstrual symptoms in anovulatory and normal menstrual cycles, the applicability of these findings is uncertain.

Andersch and colleagues [30] compared bromocriptine with bumetanid in a double-blind crossover study in 19 women with premenstrual symptoms. When compared with these patients' scores on a psychiatric inventory during two pretreatment months, bromocriptine administration was associated with a significant decline in "total rated score." Diuretic (bumetanid) treatment was associated with modest but significantly less improvement, particularly of psychological symptoms. Of the 19 subjects, 11 (58%) experienced "good" relief of irritability with bromocriptine whereas the corresponding number for the diuretic was only five (26%). Breast symptoms responded particularly well to the ergot. For reasons already discussed, choice of a diuretic rather than a placebo as a comparison agent may have negated the double-blind control in this study.

Somatic symptoms and irritability were reported to have improved significantly in 20 women with PMS compared with a randomly assigned parallel group receiving placebo under double-blind conditions [67]. Other psychological symptoms such as nervousness and depression did not improve significantly over subjects' remembered prestudy intensity levels. Accurate assessment of the treatment effects was somewhat compromised in this investigation by the choice of a retrospective symptom standard.

In an unusually well thought out study of eight affected women [65], bromocriptine administered during the luteal phases of two cycles compared with placebo was associated with significant improvement in feelings of bloatedness, depression, anxiety, and irritability. Symptoms were recorded daily during the last week of each cycle. Significant decreases in objectively measured breast swelling and weight gain were also reported.

2. Negative Studies

A similarly designed study of bromocriptine in 10 women resulted in a negative therapeutic outcome [61]. Although retrospectively obtained symptom scores tended to correlate positively with serum prolactin levels, and the higher prolactin levels were significantly lowered by bromocriptine, statistically significant improvement in symptoms was not achieved. The greatest improvement observed was a strong trend toward reduction in mastodynia. Similarly negative results were reported by Andersen et al. [62] except that with bromocriptine treatment the relief of mastodynia achieved significance. It bears noting that the patients in this study reported only slight premenstrual symptoms during the baseline month, except for a moderate degree of mastodynia, which was the only symptom relieved. Clearly the subjects did not constitute a well-defined PMS sample and, therefore, the outcome of this trial cannot be construed as evidence against the effectiveness of bromocriptine.

In sum, although the evidence marshalled to provide a rationale for the use of bromocriptine in the treatment of PMS is not definitive, the results of treatment studies are relatively positive. Of the six controlled trials employing adequate doses of bromocriptine, four had positive and two had negative outcomes. Only a single study [65] had no discernible design factors which created difficulties in accepting the authors' conclusions. The greater number of positive outcome studies and subjects, the possible non-PMS population investigated in one of the negative studies [62], and the positive outcome of the best designed trial

[65] together suggest that bromocriptine is effective in the reduction or premenstrual symptoms, and particularly mastodynia [68]. However, because of the high incidence of side effects associated with bromocriptine administration in doses likely to be helpful, its use must be justified by symptom intensity and failure to respond to alternative, less toxic medications. Even where bromocriptine administration appears justified, clinicians have been advised to avoid potential risks associated with its long-term use [68].

Whatever the degree of efficacy of bromocriptine, most investigators concur that the mechanism by which it may alleviate dysphoria is not the suppression of prolactin secretion. Even if plasma PRL levels were definitely elevated in women with premenstrual symptoms, the significance of this condition would be unclear. Elevated circulating PRL levels occur in a variety of pathologic states not associated with the mood and behavioral changes typical of PMS. Perhaps the same neurophysiological conditions which suppress prolactin-inhibiting factor (PIF; dopamine), and thereby permit enhanced prolactin secretion, independently alter metabolic, mood, or behavioral variables. Accordingly, direct dopaminergic action at central nervous and peripheral (e.g., renal) sites has most often been suggested as bromocriptine's alternative mode of action.

VI. Lithium Salts

A. Rationale

Two lines of reasoning led to testing of lithium salts as possible agents in the treatment of PMS. First, lithium was noted to cause a diuresis which "promotes sodium, potassium and water excretion and is thus directly opposite to prolactin in effect" [59]. However, the sodium-potassium diuresis is transient, generally lasting no more than 24 h, and is followed during the next 4 to 5 days of lithium treatment by normal potassium excretion and sodium retention [69]. Consequently, any beneficial effects lithium may have on premenstrual symptoms cannot be due to antagonizing the renal effects of prolactin. Second, because PMS is a cyclic condition involving affective symptoms, it seemed reasonable that it might share an etiologic basis with the cyclic affective disorders for which lithium is a treatment. When research diagnostic criteria were applied, however, premenstrual depression, when it occurred, was found to be not of the endogenous type [70]. In addition, premenstrual "state anxiety and depression mean scores were . . . much lower than those of patients with psychiatric disorders" [71]. Thus, it is difficult to find rational grounds in affective symptoms for the use of lithium in PMS.

B. Treatment Studies

Two double-blind crossover studies of lithium are documented in the literature. Mattsson and von Schoultz [28] found lithium inferior to placebo in a study which also included a diuretic. Of the three treatments, the highest incidence of symptom worsening and side effects occurred with lithium. The six patients who felt better with lithium treatment (10 felt better with placebo) were not previously more depressed than the other women. In the other study [72], a psychiatrically heterogeneous group of 19 Chinese outpatients with moderate to severe symptoms were found to improve considerably with both lithium and placebo. Four patients dropped out of the study due to the side effects of lithium.

Of four open studies, only one claimed treatment success with lithium. Sletten and Gershon [73] reported that eight women with bizarre premenstrual symptoms, resembling psychotic excitement states, improved during 12 to 18 months of lithium treatment. Fries [74] reported a "good effect" of lithium in only two of five patients with severe PMS. Both women who appeared to improve were considered to have affective personality disturbances. In the most recent study, Steiner and colleagues [75] treated 15 women with severe PMS with 600 to 900 mg per day lithium carbonate continuously throughout three cycles. As in other studies, side effects were marked: three women dropped out and six women who remained in the study experienced significant adverse effects. Of the nine patients who continued in the study, five "seemed to benefit from lithium therapy" but only three (with probable 'subsyndromic' affective disorders) were willing to continue on lithium beyond the formal study period. The authors concluded that lithium "was ineffective in most women, and caused side effects even in low dose (reminiscent of observations in normal volunteers)."

Thus it seems clear that with the possible exception of some women whose underlying affective symptoms are exacerbated during the premenstruum, lithium has no place in the treatment of premenstrual syndrome. The use of these salts for ordinary premenstrual tension not only lacks a rational basis but would also expose women to unjustifiable risks with no greater promise of benefit than has been obtained with placebo or minor tranquilizers.

VII. Progestins and Oral Contraceptive Combinations

A. Rationale

Some clinicians view hormonal changes rather than absolute hormone levels during the luteal phase as causal factors in PMS [76]. By suppressing gonadotrophin secretion and ovulation, oral contraceptives (OCs) induce a relatively constant hormonal environment throughout the menstrual cycle. Presumably, therefore, the cyclic physiologic changes which occur in response to endogenous hormonal oscillations are minimized. Based on the findings of Johansson [77], Dalton [13] has contended, however, that progestins, a component of oral contraceptives, cause a decrease in already low progesterone levels in women with PM symptoms while failing to provide the protective physiologic actions (natriuresis,* glucocorticoid transport) of the natural hormone. Thus, in her view, synthetic progestins have no place in the treatment of premenstrual syndrome.

B. Treatment Studies

A variety of pharmacologically diverse oral contraceptives in different doses, combinations, and schedules have been used in clinical trials. Few controlled studies have been carried out, perhaps in part because, as in the case of diuretics, the validity of the placebo control in studies of steroidal agents with overt physiological effects is questionable [78]. Adequate controls may not be available. Moreover, Cullberg [78] has noted that the use of progestins as contraceptive agents introduces confounding variables in clinical investigations of mood effects. Because of these and other factors discussed below, definite conclusions cannot be drawn as to the efficacy of oral contraceptives in the treatment of premenstrual symptoms, although large survey studies have strongly suggested a positive role.

1. Oral Contraceptive Users and Nonusers Compared

Several studies compared the symptoms of women who were taking steroidal oral contraceptives with those of women who were not. Since pretreatment symptom baselines and drop-out rates were lacking in most of these studies, the comparability of the groups and the degree of drug effect were not discernible. Nevertheless, the data from comparison studies involving large numbers of women suggest a beneficial effect of oral contraceptives for premenstrual difficulties.

Moos [79] reported that 420 women using OCs scored lower than 298 controls on menstrual distress questionnaire (MDQ) scales measuring pain, concentration, behavioral change, water retention, and negative affect variables related to the premenstruum. Negative affect included irritability, mood swings, depression, and tension. Since the two groups had equivalent intermenstrual symptom scores, the results could not be explained by a nonuser group with a generally high tendency to complain. Findings support the changing physiology hypothesis of PMS: women taking sequential OC preparations reported greater premenstrual symptoms than women taking combinations preparations. Moos concluded that "there seems to be little doubt that progestin-estrogen combinations relieve a number of symptoms associated with premenstrual tension" [79]. Several subsequent studies supported this conclusion [80-83]. The results of a survey of more than 5,100 women enrolled in the Kaiser Foundation Health Plan [81] suggested that OCs protected against moodiness and irritability in the women

---

*The natriuretic effect of progesterone has been implicated in the genesis of PMS [25].

who were then using them (one-third of survey). Importantly, the current users, past users, and women who had never used oral contraceptives were found to have equivalent mean scores on the MMPI depression scale, indicating that the reduced prevalence of premenstrual depression among the OC users was independent of the general level of this trait. In one study, when depressive symptoms did occur during OC use, they were associated with the monthly withdrawal period (a period of physiological change) rather than with the agents themselves [84].

2. Double-Blind Studies

Several double-blind studies of oral contraceptives and placebo have led to inconsistent findings. Silbergeld et al. [7] compared Enovid and placebo in eight young women in a crossover manner. While patients were taking the contraceptive, premenstrual somatic symptoms (water retention, breast tenderness, nausea) were worse and extended throughout much of the cycle whereas, on the whole, mood symptoms improved or were not affected. Self-rated irritability and aggression, in particular, were reduced and the cyclic variation in Free Association Test (FAT) anxiety was abolished. The subjects in this study were not selected for premenstrual symptoms, however. In 27 patients with moderate to severe symptoms [27], irritability was reportedly improved with norethisterone and with a diuretic compared with placebo. Somatic and other mood variables were not relieved. Cullberg [78] compared placebo with combinations of steroids in separate groups of women in a double-blind fashion. In the three active drug groups, the dose of synthetic estrogen (etinyl estradiol) was constant (0.05 mg per day) while the progestin dose varied (norgestral, 1.0, 0.5, and 0.06 mg per day). Compared with the placebo group, the hormone-treated groups showed significantly more adverse mental changes throughout the cycle. The premenstrual symptoms of irritability and depression were not significantly relieved by any of the hormone combinations utilized, "though there was a trend toward relief with gestagen, and an increase of symptoms with estrogen dominated treatment."

Some criticisms of the Cullberg study should be considered. These include the lack of a crossover design, the subjects' acknowledged awareness of the drugs being used, and the use of retrospective symptom assessment. Adverse effects appeared to occur throughout the cycle, but without daily appraisal of symptoms, their fluctuations could not be accurately determined nor related to premenstrual events. In sum, the crucial nature of the relationships of the steroidal combinations to premenstrual phenomena remained unclarified.

In another controlled study, the progestin medroxyprogesterone in combination with a diuretic was found to be no different from placebo in relieving premenstrual symptoms [85]. Although frequently cited in this context, the study of Morris and Udry [86] did not specifically address the issue of effects of oral contraceptives on premenstrual symptoms.

An important distinction between the survey comparisons of oral contraceptive users and nonusers and the double-blind OC studies was in the duration of use of the steroidal preparations. Not only do women with adverse reactions tend to discontinue the use of these agents [87], but also in the majority of cases in which unpleasant side effects occur, they subside within a few months [88]. Thus, the controlled studies, which represented only initial months of use, reflected the highest incidences of adverse change. The relationships to normal hormonal physiology and premenstrual symptoms of the adverse changes and the typical adaptational changes that follow warrant further investigation.

In conclusion, despite initial side effects of a predominantly somatic nature, chronically administered oral contraceptives tend to alleviate the somatic and emotional symptoms characteristic of the premenstruum. It would be useful to determine whether women who discontinue OCs because of adverse side effects comprise a subpopulation with a higher baseline prevalence or unique pattern of premenstrual symptoms.

VIII. Pryidoxine

A. Rationale

The rationale for using pyridoxine in the treatment of PMS is based on two interrelated lines of reasoning. Pyridoxine is a cofactor in the synthesis of the monoamine (MA) neurotransmitters serotonin and dopamine and it was found to have a dopaminergic effect on the hypothalamus [89]. Mood and behavioral variables could be affected by pyridoxine deficiency through reduced central nervous system (CNS) levels of these MAs while enhanced prolactin levels due to decreased neuronal dopamine (prolactin inhibiting factor) could be associated with some premenstrual somatic symptoms. Unfortunately, no evidence indicates differences in pyridoxine absorption or metabolism in women with and without PMS [56] and studies of monoamine levels in women have been largely indirect, and have focused with scant reward on possible cyclic changes of MAs in women not selected for PMS [38,90-94].

The second line of reasoning is based on the empiric finding of a functional pyridoxine deficiency in women taking combination oral contraceptives [95] which was manifest in the shunting of the serotonin precursor, tryptophan, into non-serotonin-producing pathways. Some evidence suggests that large doses of pyridoxine correct not only the abnormality in tryptophan metabolism but also the depression that develops in a small subgroup of women who take oral contraceptives [96], thus indirectly supporting the low serotonin hypothesis of depression [97]. Since the functional pyridoxine deficiency was subsequently found to be related to high estrogen levels (reviewed by Winston [98]), elevated luteal levels of this hormone may occur in a subgroup of women, resulting in functional pyridoxine deficiency, decreased serotonin synthesis, and premenstrual depression. There is, however, no direct support for these relationships.

B. Treatment Studies

Although pyridoxine has low toxicity, causes no overt physiological changes, and is thus well-suited to study in a placebo-controlled double-blind protocol, few investigations using this approach are documented. In studies lacking adequate controls, pyridoxine has reportedly produced high rates of improvement of PM symptoms but, as we have seen, this is not an uncommon feature of such investigations. Preliminary results of an open study [99] suggested that 40 to 100 mg pyridoxine administered daily during the luteal phase was an "effective and well-tolerated form of treatment" in 70 women with premenstrual tension. Improvement rates of 50 to 60% were reported for depression, irritability, breast tenderness, and bloatedness, while headaches appeared to sustain an 80% improvement rate. In another recent open study [16], the pyridoxine-related improvement rate (40 mg twice daily) was similar. Breast tenderness was reported to be particularly responsive to the B vitamin.

Day [55] studied pyridoxine in a single-blind placebo-controlled manner and reported that 63% of women experiencing PMS claimed improvement in their symptoms when taking the vitamin (100 mg per day) from days 10 through 3 preceding menstruation. The corresponding placebo response rate was 43%.

In the one recent double-blind placebo-controlled study [100], pyridoxine was not found to be superior to placebo in relieving premenstrual symptoms throughout 8 months of randomized treatments.

Thus despite a promising rationale for the use of pyroxidine, its low toxicity, and its amenability to double-blind placebo controls, adequate investigation of its potential efficacy in the treatment of PMS is still lacking.

IX. Other Treatments

The dearth of recent studies using androgens, hormonal sensitization, high carbohydrate diets, and vitamin A may be due to the failure of prior reports to provide encouraging conclusions as to the efficacy, safety, or acceptability of these methods in the treatment of PMS. For a review of these approaches, see Tonks [21].

A. Physical Activity

Although physical activity was claimed to be therapeutic for or preventive of premenstrual syndrome, convincing documentation was not provided [101,102]. Even if women engaged in manual jobs or athletic lifestyles were found to have an indisputably low prevalence of PMS, these women could be self-selected for the absence of interfering menstrual difficulties. In a recent large survey, however,

Wood et al. [83] reported no relationship between premenstrual symptoms and physical activity levels at work.

B. Neuroleptics and Psychotherapy

There is no acceptable rationale for the use of neuroleptic agents in the treatment of premenstrual tension that is uncomplicated by the concurrence of a major psychiatric disorder. Even in severe form, the symptoms of this condition may occur in women in the absence of chronic psychopathology [70]. The two reports encountered in the literature [103,104] in which neuroleptics were used contributed neither to the understanding nor to the useful pharmacotherapy of premenstrual symptoms.

It is widely acknowledged that the high placebo response rates among women with PMS reflect the important role of psychological factors in the experience and reporting of premenstrual symptoms. Since the personal interpretation of the symptoms can be influenced by external factors, education and reassurance concerning PMS is apparently of therapeutic value [13,52,105,106]. Stress can intensify premenstrual symptoms through physiological means and may alter the individual's ability to accommodate the symptoms, which are themselves a form of stress. Thus minor tranquilizers, short-term counseling, and relaxation techniques may have a place in the treatment of PMS, although adequately controlled trials have not as yet been carried out in these areas. In one study, systematic desensitization was found not to be useful in diminishing premenstrual symptoms [107].

C. Bellergal

A placebo-controlled double-blind trial of ergotamine, belladonna alkaloids, and phenobarbital in combination (Bellergal) was carried out in 32 hospitalized and general practice patients [108]. When Bellergal was administered for the last 10 days of the cycle, a significant decrease in "fatigue, tender breasts, nervousness, irritability, lethargy and listlessness" was reported. It is impossible to discern which of the many pharmacologic actions was responsible for the salient effects on premenstrual symptoms. These actions might include interactions with central and peripheral monoamines, including decreased prolactin secretion; other peripheral autonomic effects; and central sedation. It remains to be shown that this combination of drugs has greater efficacy than any one used alone.

X. Discussion

There is a great need to clarify etiologic issues in premenstrual syndrome and to generate clinically reliable data which can provide indicators for appropriate treatment and for discrimination among etiologic concepts. Despite the many rational treatment approaches pursued in recent years, definitive studies have

failed to emerge in any of the areas investigated. Uncontrolled trials have generally led to positive therapeutic outcomes regardless of the agent, the strength of
the rationale, or the population sample involved. Of clinical importance is the
marked interplay between psychological and physiological factors in premenstrual
experiences underscored by this phenomenon. In contrast, placebo-controlled
double-blind methods have yielded inconsistent results across studies and no single
therapeutic agent has shown unique efficacy.

Despite the planned controls, the primary causes for the outcome inconsistencies in double-blind studies have been methodologic.

Symptom assessment techniques have varied greatly, differing with respect to
the specific symptoms evaluated, the symptom intensity gradations sought, and
especially important, the timing of the symptom reports. The continuing (nonretrospective) assessment of symptoms is crucial in minimizing memory distortions. Moreover, because the psychological symptoms of the premenstruum are
to a large extent not continuously manifest but occur as a heightened tendency
to react with negative emotional responses to life events [20], only frequent reporting can sensitively reflect the degree and precise timing of many of the symptoms in any given cycle.

In only some studies were drug free baseline data obtained from women prior
to treatment, although such information, gathered nonretrospectively, is important (1) as a screening device to provide documentation of premenstrual symptoms and their intensity; and (2) in providing a standard of comparison for the
effects of active treatment and placebo.

Failure of the double-blind control contributed greatly to outcome inconsistencies when drugs producing noticeable physiological effects were used. The
diuretic and steroid studies suffered particularly from this problem. Adequate
controls which meet both experimental and ethical standards may not be available for pursuing the effects of these agents. With oral contraceptives, comparisons of symptoms gathered nonretrospectively from large numbers of women
involved in the long term use of steroidal and other means of contraception would
provide a reasonable alternative. A possibility for further study of diuretics could
utilize this approach, comparing premenstrual symptoms of normally menstruating
women who take these drugs for reasons other than premenstrual tension with
those of an appropriately matched control group.

Timing of treatments had differed among studies. Schedules have included primarily treatment throughout the luteal phase or during various portions of it, although administration throughout the cycle has occasionally been used. In some
cases basal body temperature has been recorded to document phase for treatment
and symptom evaluation purposes while in others less acceptable data have been
based on crude estimations of phase. When administering drugs such as progesterone and diuretics [25], timing of pharmacotherapy may be particularly important.

Population samples have not been consistent. Considerable variation across studies both in etiologic findings and in response to therapeutic agents can probably be ascribed to the pronounced differences in degree and predominant manifestations of baseline symptomatology. Other variables such as age, marital status, and parity may also affect treatment responses.

References to possible subtypes of PMS [58,78,99,109] without the delineation of clinically useful profiles suggests that clinical and etiologic investigation would benefit from two strategies. The first focuses on treatment responses in a cross-section of women, with the goal of distinguishing placebo effects, chance fluctuations in symptoms, and consistent responses to therapies amenable to well-controlled protocols. In contrast with the 1 and 2 months of active drug and placebo administration typical of studies to date, controlled trials extended sufficiently to permit chance fluctuations to cancel out and placebo responses to "wear off" could help to discriminate potential subtypes of women who consistently benefit from particular therapeutic approaches. The symptom and hormonal profiles throughout the cycle of responders to a particular drug could be compared with those of nonresponders and thus an understanding of the relationship between etiologic factors and therapeutic responses could be developed in an integrated manner.

The second strategy is based on investigations of known subtypes of premenstrual syndrome and would entail thorough examination of the therapeutic responses of women presenting differing symptom and hormonal patterns. For example, although women with PMS usually gain little weight in the premenstruum, some regularly gain large amounts [29]. In these individuals, exactly when does the increase begin, reach a plateau, and reverse? What are the hormonal concomitants of these changes and how are the physiological and symptom variables affected by therapeutic agents? In women who experience primarily premenstrual depression, is pyridoxine more effective than in other subgroups of women; and if so, are differences in pyridoxine metabolism discernible? Is the constant internal milieu induced by oral contraceptives of greater benefit to women whose symptoms are largely psychological rather than either predominantly somatic or mixed? These and a great many more questions require answers through detailed studies which correlate hormonal, metabolic, and symptom changes throughout the cycle and which examine the manner in which various therapies alter these events.

One recently emerging area in the study of menstrual disorders which has been little investigated in relation to PMS concerns the role of endometrial prostaglandins. Prostaglandin $F_{2\alpha}$ ($PGF_{2\alpha}$), produced in high concentration by the endometrium, induces the smooth muscle activity which initiates menstruation and is used clinically to induce therapeutic abortions. In women with dysmenorrhea as compared with those without, significantly greater intrauterine pressures [110] and levels of $PGF_{2\alpha}$ in menstrual fluid [111,112] have been found. Inhibitors of PG synthesis, such as ibuprofen [112,113] and naproxen-sodium [114]

have been shown highly effective compared with placebo in reducing both endometrial PGF concentrations and menstrual cramps.

The production of endometrial prostaglandins corresponds to the timing of
premenstrual symptoms. Endometrial prostaglandin levels increase markedly during the luteal phase of the menstrual cycle, peaking at the onset of menstruation
[115]. The exceedingly short half-life of prostaglandins (PGs) and their spontaneous formation during sampling and storage, make plasma levels difficult to
measure. Recently, however, plasma levels of the more stable PGF_{2a} metabolite
PGFM (13,14-dihydro-15-oxoprostaglandin F_{2a}) was studied daily throughout
the menstrual cycle in five healthy women [116]. Two PGFM peaks were found
in all cycles. One short-lived peak of about 24 h preceded ovulation by 2 to 4
days and was thought to be of nonendometrial origin. The second peak, occurring
in the premenstruum, probably reflected increased endometrial PGF_{2a} production,
was more protracted (about 72 h), and coincided with the falling levels of estrogen and progesterone. Chan and Hill [111] noted that PGs produced in the endometrium are apparently absorbed not only into the myometrium where smooth
muscle activity is stimulated and excessive activity produces cramping, but also
into the systemic circulation where they account for the additional somatic and
psychological symptoms of dysmenorrhea. "When injected intravenously, prostaglandin F_{2a} can reproduce virtually all the symptoms of dysmenorrhea, including
headache, irritability, difficulty with concentration, uterine cramping, nausea,
vomiting, diarrhea, and dizziness" [117]. Obviously, many of these symptoms
are also associated with the premenstruum.

Other work has shown that the prostaglandins act as mediators at pre- and
postsynaptic sites in the central nervous system [see 118], exerting a variety of
stimulant and depressant effects on neurons [see 119]. Convulsions are an adverse effect of pharmacologic doses of PGF_{2a}, suggesting that premenstrual
events such as irritability and the exacerbation of seizure disorders could be related to circulating PGF_{2a} of endometrial origin. Increased capillary permeability
and vasodilatory effects have been attributed to PGF_{2a} [see 119] and could account for edema during the premenstruum. In addition, premenstrual exacerbation of asthma [13] may be linked to PGF_{2a}, as its bronchoconstrictor effects
have been implicated in asthmatic attacks [120].

Thus, a role for prostaglandins in premenstrual syndrome is suggested by
the coincidence in the late premenstrual-early menstrual phases of peaks in
endometrial PG levels, plasma PGF metabolites, and premenstrual symptoms
(assessed nonretrospectively; [7,9,19]). The increase in PGs probably contributes
through vascular effects to the symptoms of fluid imbalance and the increase
coupled with the withdrawal of ovarian steroids, particularly the decline of the
sedative actions of progesterone, contributes through CNS effects to the mood
and behavioral changes of PMS. Although studies of plasma PGF metabolites in
women with premenstrual syndrome have not been carried out, such women, as
compared with controls, may have elevated premenstrual levels or extended peaks

of the prostaglandin. This would be compatible with a number of previous concepts and hypotheses concerning PMS: (1) the low progesterone hypothesis of PMS, since progesterone inhibits the release of PGs from the secretory endometrium; (2) the low incidence of PMS among women using oral contraceptives, since these agents seem to reduce endometrial PG synthesis [112]; and (3) the prolactin hypothesis, since $PGF_{2\alpha}$ increases the secretion of that pituitary hormone [see 119]. An efficient way of investigating whether PGs contribute importantly to premenstrual symptoms would entail administration during the premenstruum of an inhibitor of prostaglandin synthesis, such as ibuprofen, to women with PMS. Ibuprofen is ideally suited to a rigorously controlled clinical trial because in therapeutic doses it has no overt physiological effects. To date, side effects have been virtually absent when ibuprofen has been used to treat dysmenorrhea [116]. The results of the one study carried out in this area are encouraging [121].

XI. Summary

Over the years a variety of hypotheses concerning the causes of premenstrual tension have been proposed and have found some empiric support. Concurrently, treatment approaches have proliferated, but no single treatment has achieved unique standing. Although hormonal hypotheses of PMS have been the most prevalent, the roles of estrogen, progesterone, aldosterone, and prolactin individually and interactively remain to be clarified. Moreover, little is known about gonadotropin effects early in the cycle which might bear on subsequent endocrine events and symptom formation. To date, treatments directed to raising progesterone concentrations, antagonizing aldosterone, and suppressing prolactin secretion have yielded inconsistent outcomes. Bromocriptine appears effective in relieving PRL-related breast discomfort, as well as other symptoms, but marked side effects diminish the acceptability of this agent. By suppressing gonadotropin secretion and inducing a relatively constant hormonal environment, combination oral contraceptives seem to reduce the prevalence and intensity of premenstrual symptoms in a large subgroup of women. However, that these agents are not specific for premenstrual symptoms mitigates against their long-term use in this capacity outside of a contraceptive regimen.

Diuretic therapy has tried to correct presumed premenstrual fluid and electrolyte imbalances. Although diuretics are sometimes effective, much greater knowledge is needed of hormonally related fluid and electrolyte changes throughout the cycle and of the effects of properly timed and possibly multistaged therapy involving diuretics on these aspects of physiological functioning. On the basis of indirect evidence concerning serotonin and dopamine synthesis, pyridoxine deficiency has been implicated in PMS, but little is known of the metabolism or physiological effectiveness of the B vitamin in women with and without PMS [56]. Adequate justification is lacking for the use of lithium, neuroleptics, or antidepressants in the treatment of premenstrual symptoms per se. Unfortunately, the minor tranquilizers and relaxation techniques have not been studied sufficiently in controlled trials to determine their efficacies, although ample evidence exists for the role of psychological factors in the experience of premenstrual symptoms. A possible role for inhibitors of prostaglandin synthesis in the treatment of PMS is discussed. At present, positive attitude appears to be the most potent item in the premenstrual treatment armamentarium.

References

1. A. W. Clare, Psychological profiles of women complaining of premenstrual symptoms. *Curr. Med. Res. Opin.* 4(Suppl. 4):23-28 (1977).
2. N. Kessel and A. Coppen, The prevalence of common menstrual symptoms. *Lancet* 2:61-64 (1963).
3. R. H. Moos, Menstrual Distress Questionnaire Manual, Department of Psychiatry, Stanford University and Veterans Administration Hospital, Palo Alto, California, 1977.
4. H. Sutherland and I. Stewart, A critical analysis of the premenstrual syndrome. *Lancet* 1:1180-1183 (1965).
5. O. Widholm, Dysmenorrhea during adolescence. *Acta Obstet. Gynecol. Scand.* 87(Suppl.):61-66 (1979).
6. C. Wood, L. Larsen, and R. Williams, Menstrual characteristics of 2,343 women attending the Shepherd Foundation. *Aust. NZ J. Obstet. Gynecol.* 19:107-110 (1979).
7. S. Silbergeld, N. Brast, and E. P. Noble, The menstrual cycle: A double-blind study of symptoms, mood and behavior, and biochemical variables using Enovid and placebo. *Psychosom. Med.* 33:411-428 (1971).
8. M. E. Ivey and J. M. Bardwick, Patterns of affective fluctuations in the menstrual cycle. *Psychosom. Med.* 30:336-345 (1968).
9. G. A. Sampson, Premenstrual syndrome: A double-blind controlled trial of progesterone and placebo. *Br. J. Psychiatry* 135:209-215 (1979).
10. J. W. Taylor, The timing of menstruation-related symptoms assessed by a daily symptom rating scale. *Acta Psychiatr. Scand.* 60:87-105 (1979).
11. A. L. Southam and F. P. Gonzaga, Systemic changes during the menstrual cycle. *Am. J. Obstet. Gynecol.* 91:142-165 (1965).
12. J. N. Fortin, E. D. Wittkower, and F. Kalz, A psychosomatic approach to the menstrual syndrome: A preliminary report. *Canad. Med. Assoc. J.* 79:978-998 (1958).
13. K. Dalton, *The Premenstrual Syndrome and Progesterone Therapy.* Heinemann, London, 1977.
14. J. L. Kramp, Studies on the premenstrual syndrome in relation to psychiatry. *Acta Psychiatr. Scand.* 203(Suppl.):261-267 (1968).

15. R. Greene, Discussion on the premenstrual syndrome. *Proc. R. Soc. Med.* 48:337-338 (1954).

16. R. W. Taylor and C. E. James, The clinician's view of patients with premenstrual syndrome. *Curr. Med. Res. Opin.* 6(Suppl. 5):46-51 (1979).

17. P. C. B. MacKinnon and I. L. MacKinnon, Hazards of the menstrual cycle. *Br. Med. J.* 1:555 (1956).

18. S. L. Smith, Mood and the menstrual cycle. In *Topics in Psychoendocrinology* (E. J. Sachar, ed.). Grune & Stratton, New York, 1975, pp. 19-58.

19. M. B. Parlee, The premenstrual syndrome. *Psychol. Bull.* 80:454-465 (1973).

20. B. Sommer, Stress and menstrual distress. *J. Hum. Stress* 5-10 (1978).

21. C. M. Tonks, Premenstrual tension. *Br. J. Psychiatry Spec. No.* 9:399-408 (1975).

22. J. Bruce and G. F. M. Russell, Premenstrual tension—a study of weight changes and balances of water, sodium and potassium. *Lancet* 2:267-271 (1962).

23. B. Andersch, L. Hahn, M. Andersson, and B. Isaksson, Body water and weight in patients with premenstrual tension. *Br. J. Obstet. Gynaecol.* 85:546-550 (1978).

24. B. D. Reeves, J. E. Garvin, and T. W. McElin, Premenstrual tension: Symptoms and weight changes related to potassium therapy. *Am. J. Obstet. Gynecol.* 109:1036-1041 (1971).

25. P. M. S. O'Brien, C. Selby, and E. M. Symonds, Progesterone, fluid, and electrolytes in premenstrual syndrome. *Br. Med. J.* 1161-1163 (1980).

26. W. H. Wong, R. I. Freedman, N. E. Levan, C. Hyman, and E. J. Quilligan, Changes in the capillary filtration coefficient of cutaneous vessels in women with premenstrual tension. *Am. J. Obstet. Gynecol.* 114:950-953 (1972).

27. A. J. Coppen, H. B. Milne, D. H. Outram, and J. C. P. Weber, Dytide, norethisterone and a placebo in the premenstrual syndrome—a double-blind comparison. *Clin. Trials J.* 6:33-36 (1972).

28. B. Mattson and B. von Schoultz, A comparison between lithium, placebo and a diuretic in premenstrual tension. *Acta Psychiatr. Scand. [Suppl.]* 255:75-83 (1974).

29. A. Werch and R. E. Kane, Treatment of premenstrual tension with metolazone: A double-blind evaluation of a new diuretic. *Curr. Ther. Res.* 19:565-572 (1976).

30. B. Andersch, L. Hahn, C. Wendestam, R. Ohman, and L. Abrahamsson, Treatment of premenstrual tension syndrome with bromocriptine. *Acta Endocrinol.* 88(Suppl. 216):165-174 (1978).

31. W. D. Schwartz and G. E. Abraham, Corticosterone and aldosterone levels during the menstrual cycle. *Obstet. Gynecol.* 45:339-342 (1975).

32. D. S. Janowsky, S. C. Berens, and J. M. Davis, Correlations between mood,

weight and electrolytes during the menstrual cycle: A renin-angiotensin-aldosterone hypothesis of premenstrual tension. *Psychosom. Med.* 35:143-154 (1973).

33. P. M. S. O'Brien, D. Craven, D. Selby, and E. M. Symonds, Treatment of premenstrual syndrome by spironolactone. *Br. J. Obstet. Gynaecol.* 86:142-147 (1979).

34. R. T. Frank, Hormonal causes of premenstrual tension. *Arch. Neurol. Psychiatry* 26:1053-1057 (1931).

35. S. L. Israel, Premenstrual tension. *JAMA* 110:1721-1723 (1938).

36. J. H. Morton, Premenstrual tension. *Am. J. Obstet. Gynecol.* 60:343-352 (1950).

37. E. L. Klaiber, Y. Kobayashi, D. M. Broverman, and F. Hall, Plasma monoamine oxidase activity in regularly menstruating women and in amenorrheic women receiving cyclic treatment with estrogens and a progestin. *J. Clin. Endocrinol.* 33:630-637 (1971).

38. E. L. Klaiber, D. M. Broverman, W. Vogel, Y. Kobayashi, and D. Moriarty, Effects of estrogen therapy on plasma MAO activity and EEG driving responses of depressed women. *Am. J. Psychiatry* 128:1492-1498 (1972).

39. J. W. Taylor, Plasma progesterone, oestradiol 17 B and premenstrual symptoms. *Acta Psychiatr. Scand.* 60:76-86 (1979).

40. T. Backstrom and H. Carstensen, Estrogen and progesterone in plasma in relation to premenstrual tension. *J. Steroid Biochem.* 5:257-260 (1974).

41. T. Backstrom, L. Wide, R. Sodergard, and H. Carstensen, FSH, LH, TeBG-capacity, estrogen and progesterone in women with premenstrual tension during the luteal phase. *J. Steroid Biochem.* 7:473-476 (1976).

42. T. Backstrom and B. Mattsson, Correlation of symptoms in premenstrual tension to oestrogen and progesterone concentrations in blood plasma. A preliminary study. *Neuropsychobiology* 1:80-86 (1975).

43. I. Schiff and K. J. Ryan, Benefits of estrogen replacement. *Obstet. Gynecol. Surv.* 35:400-411 (1980).

44. M. Munday, M. G. Brush, and R. W. Taylor, Progesterone and aldosterone levels in the premenstrual tension syndrome. *J. Endocrinol.* 73:21P (1977).

45. M. Munday, Hormone levels in severe premenstrual tension. *Curr. Med. Res. Opin.* 4(Suppl. 4):16-22 (1977).

46. S. O'Brien, Premenstrual tension. *Br. Med. J.* 1:754 (1979).

47. K. Dalton, *The Premenstrual Syndrome.* Chas. C Thomas, Springfield, 1964.

48. K. Dalton, Progesterone suppositories and pessaries in the treatment of menstrual migraine. *Headache* 12:151-159 (1973).

49. M. I. Whitehead, P. T. Townsend, D. K. Gill, W. P. Collins, and S. Campbell, Absorption and metabolism of oral progesterone. *Br. Med. J.* 825-827 (1980).

50. S. J. Nillius and E. D. B. Johansson, Plasma levels of progesterone after

vaginal, rectal, or intramuscular administration of progesterone. *Am. J. Obstet. Gynecol.* 110:470-477 (1971).

51. L. A. Gray, The use of progesterone in nervous tension states. *South. Med. J.* 34:1004-1006 (1941).

52. S. L. Smith, The menstrual cycle and mood disturbances. *Clin. Obstet. Gynecol.* 19:391-397 (1976).

53. B. W. Somerville, The role of progesterone in menstrual migraine. *Neurology* 21:853-859 (1971).

54. R. W. Taylor, The treatment of premenstrual tension with dydrogesterone ("Duphaston"). *Curr. Med. Res. Opin.* 4(Suppl. 4):35-40 (1977).

55. J. B. Day, Clinical trials in the premenstrual syndrome. *Curr. Med. Res. Opin.* 6(Suppl. 5):40-45 (1979).

56. M. G. Brush, Endocrine and other biochemical factors in the aetiology of the premenstrual syndrome. *Curr. Med. Res. Opin.* 6(Suppl. 5):19-27 (1979).

57. E. N. Cole, D. Evered, D. F. Horrobin, M. S. Manku, J. B. Mtabji, and B. A. Nassar, Is prolactin a fluid and electrolyte regulating hormone in man? *J. Physiol.* 252:54-55 (1975).

58. B. J. Carroll and M. Steiner, The psychobiology of premenstrual dysphoria: The role of prolactin. *Psychoneuroendocrinology* 3:171-180 (1978).

59. D. F. Horrobin, M. S. Manku, B. Nassar, and D. Evered, Prolactin and fluid and electrolyte balance. In *Human Prolactin* (J. L. Pasteels and C. Robyn, eds.). Excerpta Medica, Amsterdam, 1973, pp. 152-155.

60. U. Halbreich, M. Ben-David, M. Assael, and R. Bornstein, Serum prolactin in women with premenstrual syndrome. *Lancet* 2:654-656 (1976).

61. S. Kullander and L. Svanberg, Bromocriptine treatment of the premenstrual syndrome. *Acta Obstet. Gynecol. Scand.* 58:375-378 (1979).

62. A. N. Andersen, J. F. Larsen, O. R. Steenstrup, B. Svendstrup, and J. Nielsen, Effect of bromocriptine on the premenstrual syndrome. *Br. J. Obstet. Gynecol.* 84:370-374 (1977).

63. A. N. Andersen and J. F. Larsen, Bromocriptine in the treatment of the premenstrual syndrome. *Drugs* 17:383-388 (1979).

64. K. Ghose and A. Coppen, Bromocriptine and premenstrual syndrome: Controlled study. *Br. Med. J.* 1:148-149 (1977).

65. J. J. Graham, P. E. Harding, P. H. Wise, and H. Berriman, Prolactin suppression in the treatment of premenstrual syndrome. *Med. J. Aust.* 2(Suppl. 3):18-20 (1978).

66. L. J. Benedek-Jaszmann and M. D. Hearn-Sturtevant, Premenstrual tension and functional infertility. Aetiology and treatment. *Lancet* 1:1095-1098 (1976).

67. E. Philipp, Zur behandlung des praemenstruellen syndroms. Klinische erfahrungen mit dem prolaktinhemmer bromokriptin zur behandlung des praemenstruellen syndroms. *Therapie Woche* 27:7296-7301 (1977).

68. A. N. Andersen, J. F. Larsen, P. C. Eskildsen, M. Knoth, S. Micic, B. Svend-
     strup, and J. Nielsen, Treatment of hyperprolactinaemic insufficiency with
     bromocriptine. *Acta Obstet. Gynecol. Scand.* 58:379-383 (1979).
69. M. J. Peach, Cations: Calcium, magnesium, barium, lithium, and ammo-
     nium. In *The Pharmacological Basis of Therapeutics,* (L. S. Goodman and
     A. Gilman, eds.). Macmillan, New York, 1975, pp. 782-797.
70. R. F. Haskett, M. Steiner, J. D. Osmun, and B. J. Carroll, Severe premen-
     strual tension: Delineation of the syndrome. Presented at 34th Annual
     Meeting, Society of Biological Psychiatry, Chicago, Illinois, May 10-13,
     1979.
71. S. Golub, The magnitude of premenstrual anxiety and depression. *Psycho-
     som. Med.* 38:4-12 (1976).
72. K. Singer, R. Cheng, and M. Schou, A controlled evaluation of lithium in
     the premenstrual tension syndrome. *Br. J. Psychiatry* 124:50-51 (1974).
73. J. W. Sletten and S. Gershon, The premenstrual syndrome: A discussion
     of its pathophysiology and treatment with lithium ion. *Compr. Psychiatry*
     7:197-206 (1966).
74. H. Fries, Experience with lithium carbonate treatment at a psychiatric de-
     partment in the period 1964-1967. *Acta Psychiatr. Scand. [Suppl.]* 207:
     41-43 (1969).
75. M. Steiner, R. F. Haskett, J. D. Osmun, and B. J. Carroll, Treatment of pre-
     menstrual tension with lithium carbonate: A pilot study. Presented at the
     34th Annual Meeting, Society for Biological Psychiatry, Chicago, Illinois,
     May 10-13, 1979.
76. J. Studd, Premenstrual tension syndrome. *Br. Med. J.* 1:410 (1979).
77. E. D. B. Johansson, Depression of the progesterone levels in plasma in wo-
     men treated with synthetic gestagens after ovulation. *Acta Endocrinol.*
     68:779-792 (1971).
78. J. Cullberg, Mood changes and menstrual symptoms with different gestagen/
     estrogen combinations. *Acta Psychiatr. Scand. [Suppl.]* 236:1-84 (1972).
79. R. H. Moos, Assessment of psychological concomitants of oral contracep-
     tives. In *Metabolic Effects of Gonadal Hormones and Contraceptive Ster-
     oids* (H. A. Salhanick, D. M. Kipnis, and R. L. Vande Wiele, eds.). Plenum,
     New York, 1969, pp. 676-705.
80. B. Herzberg and A. Coppen, Changes in psychological symptoms in women
     taking oral contraceptives. *Br. J. Psychiatry* 116:161-164 (1970).
81. S. J. Kutner and W. L. Brown, History of depression as a risk factor for
     depression with oral contraceptives and discontinuance. *J. Nerv. Ment. Dis.*
     155:163-169 (1972).
82. P. Rouse, Premenstrual tension: A study using the Moos Menstrual Distress
     Questionnaire. *J. Psychosom. Res.* 22:215-222 (1978).
83. C. Wood, L. Larsen, and R. Williams, Social and psychological factors in

relation to premenstrual tension and menstrual pain. *Aust. NZ J. Obstet. Gynecol.* 19:111-115 (1979).

84. B. N. Herzberg, A. L. Johnson, and S. Brown, Depressive symptoms and oral contraceptives. *Br. Med. J.* 4:142-145 (1970).

85. O. Jordheim, The premenstrual syndrome—clinical trials of treatment with a progestogen combined with a diuretic compared with both a progestogen alone and with a plaecbo. *Acta Obstet. Gynecol. Scand.* 51:77-80 (1972).

86. N. M. Morris and J. R. Udry, Contraceptive pills and day-by-day feelings of well-being. *Am. J. Obstet. Gynecol.* 113:763-765 (1972).

87. B. N. Herzberg, K. C. Draper, A. L. Johnson, and G. C. Nicol, Oral contraceptives, depression, and libido. *Br. Med. J.* 3:495-500 (1971).

88. F. Murad and R. C. Haynes Jr., Estrogens and progestins. In *The Pharmacological Basis of Therapeutics,* (A. G. Gilman, L. S. Goodman, and A. Gilman, eds.). Macmillan, New York, 1980, p. 1443.

89. G. Delitala, A. Masala, S. Alagna, and L. De Villa, Effect of pyridoxine on human hypophyseal trophic hormone release: A possible stimulation of hypothalamic dopaminergic pathway. *J. Clin. Endocrinol. Metab.* 42:603-606 (1976).

90. R. H. Belmaker, D. L. Murphy, R. J. Wyatt, and D. L. Loriaux, Human platelet monoamine oxidase changes during the menstrual cycle. *Arch. Gen. Psychiatry* 31:553-556 (1974).

91. F. Lamprecht, R. J. Matta, B. Little, and T. P. Zahn, Plasma dopamine-beta-hydroxylase (DBH) activity during the menstrual cycle. *Psychosom. Med.* 36:304-310 (1974).

92. P. Patkai, G. Johansson, and B. Post, Mood, alertness and sympathetic-adrenal medullary activity during the menstrual cycle. *Psychosom. Med.* 36:503-512 (1974).

93. H. A. Zacur, J. E. Tyson, M. G. Ziegler, and C. R. Lake, Plasma dopamine-B-hydroxylase activity and norepinephrine levels during the human menstrual cycle. *Am. J. Obstet. Gynecol.* 130:148-151 (1978).

94. W. Feichtinger, P. Kemeter, H. Salzer, E. Euller, A. Korn, R. Fulmek and F. Friedrich, Daily epinephrine and norepinephrine excretion in urine of normal cyclic women compared with prolactin, LH, FSH, estradiol, progesterone, testosterone and cortisol. In *Psychoneuroendocrinology in Reproduction* (L. Zichella and P. Pancheri, eds.). Elsevier/North Holland Biomedical Press, Amsterdam, 1979.

95. J. M. Price, M. J. Thornton, and L. M. Mueller, Tryptophan metabolism in women using steroid hormones for ovulation control. *Am. J. Clin. Nutrition* 20:452-456 (1967).

96. P. W. Adams, V. Wynn, D. P. Rose, M. Seed, J. Folkard, and R. Strong, Effect of pyridoxine hydrochloride (Vitamin B_6) upon depression associated with oral contraception. *Lancet* 1:897 (1973).

97.   A. Coppen, The biochemistry of affective disorders. *Br. J. Psychiatry*
      113:1237-1264 (1967).
98.   F. Winston, Oral contraceptives, pyridoxine, and depression. *Am. J. Psychiatry* 130:1217-1221 (1973).
99.   G. D. Kerr, The management of the premenstrual syndrome. *Curr. Med. Res. Opin.* 4(Suppl. 4):29-34 (1977).
100. J. Stokes and J. Mendels, Pyridoxine and premenstrual tension. *Lancet* 1:1177-1178 (1972).
101. J. Navratil, The pathogenesis of the premenstrual tension. *Act. Nerv. Super. (Praha)* 17:304-305 (1975).
102. S. Timonen and B.-J. Procope, The premenstrual syndrome and physical exercise. *Acta Obstet. Gynecol. Scand.* 50:331-334 (1971).
103. J. Hrbek and J. Navratil, Pharmacotherapy in the premenstrual tension. *Act. Nerv. Super. (Praha)* 13:189-190 (1971).
104. R. I. Schader and J. S. Harmatz, Molindone: A pilot evaluation during the premenstruum. *Curr. Ther. Res.* 17:403-406 (1975).
105. R. A. Kinch, Premenstrual tension: Etiology and treatment. *Clin. Invest. Med.* 1:7-8 (1978).
106. P. F. H. Giles, Recent research on the treatment of premenstrual syndrome. *Curr. Med. Res. Opin.* 6(Suppl. 5):28-34 (1979).
107. M. A. Chesney and D. L. Tasto, The effectiveness of behavior modification with spasmodic and congestive dysmenorrhea. *Behav. Res. Ther.* 13:245-253 (1975).
108. K. Robinson, K. Huntington, and M. G. Wallace, Treatment of the premenstrual syndrome. *Br. J. Gynaecol.* 84:784-788 (1977).
109. M. Steiner and B. J. Carroll, The psychobiology of premenstrual dysphoria: Review of theories and treatments. *Psychoneuroendocrinology* 2:321-335 (1977).
110. M. O. Pulkkinen and A. I. Csapo, The effect of ibuprofen on the intrauterine pressure and menstrual pain of dysmenorrheic patients. *Prostaglandins* 15:1055-1062 (1978).
111. Y. W. Chan and J. C. Hill, Determination of menstrual prostaglandin levels in non-dysmenorrheic and dysmenorrheic subjects. *Prostaglandins* 15:365-375 (1978).
112. Y. W. Chan and M. Y. Dawood, Prostaglandin levels in menstrual fluid of nondysmenorrheic and of dysmenorrheic subjects with and without oral contraceptive or ibuprofen therapy. In *Advances in Prostaglandin and Thromboxane Research* (B. Samuelsson, P. W. Ramwell, and R. Paoletti, eds.). Raven Press, New York, 1980, pp. 1443-1447.
113. Y. W. Chan, M. Y. Dawood, and F. Fuchs, Relief of dysmenorrhea with the prostaglandin synthetase inhibitor ibuprofen; effect on prostaglandin levels in menstrual fluid. *Am. J. Obstet. Gynecol.* 135:102-108 (1979).

114. M. O. Pulkkinen, M. R. Henzl, and A. I. Csapo, The effect of naproxen-
      sodium on the prostaglandin concentrations of the menstrual blood and
      uterine "jet washings" in dysmenorrheic women. *Prostaglandins* 15:543-
      550 (1978).
115. M. O. Pulkkinen and A. I. Csapo, Effect of ibuprofen on menstrual blood
      prostaglandin levels in dysmenorrheic women. *Prostaglandins* 18:137-142
      (1979).
116. E. N. Koullapis and W. P. Collins, The concentration of 13,14-dihydro-
      15-oxo-prostaglandin $F_{2\alpha}$ in peripheral venous plasma throughout the
      normal ovarian and menstrual cycle. *Acta Endocrinol.* 93:123-128 (1980).
117. Editorial, The menstrual cycle and its disorders. *Obstet. Gynecol. Surv.*
      172 (1980).
118. H. A. Gross, D. L. Dunner, D. Lafleur, H. L. Meltzer, H. L. Muhlbauer,
      and R. R. Fieve, Prostaglandins. A review of neurophysiology and psy-
      chiatric implications. *Arch. Gen. Psychiatry* 34:1189-1196 (1977).
119. S. Moncada, R. J. Flower, and J. R. Vane, Prostaglandins, prostacyclin,
      and thromboxane A_2. In *The Pharmacological Basis of Therapeutics* (A.
      G. Gilman, L. S. Goodman, and A. Gilman, eds.). Macmillan, New York,
      1980, pp. 668-681.
120. C. W. Parker and D. E. Snider, Prostaglandins and asthma. *Ann. Intern.
      Med.* 78:963-965 (1973).
121. C. Wood and D. Jacubowicz, The treatment of premenstrual symptoms
      with mefenamic acid. *Br. J. Obstet. Gynecol.* 87:627-630 (1980).

19 Premenstrual Tension: Etiology

JEFFREY L. RAUSCH AND DAVID S. JANOWSKY   University of California,
San Diego, La Jolla, California

The regular occurrence of symptoms related to the premenstrual-menstrual phases of the menstrual cycle is well-documented. In a review of the literature, Moos [1] reported more than 150 different symptoms which fluctuate with the menstrual cycle, the most common of which include anxiety, irritability, depressed affect, altered sexual drive, aches and pains, and fluid retention.

The incidence of premenstrual-menstrual psychologic symptoms (premenstrual tension) has been estimated as between 25 and 100% of all women [2], with severity ranging from mild irritability to frank psychotic episodes [3,4]. Symptoms are usually confined to the 5 days before menstruation, and abate with the onset of menses or shortly thereafter [3]. However, increases in negative affect have been found to occur as early as 11 days before menstruation, and to continue well into the menstrual phase [5], although these symptoms are to be distinguished from dysmenorrhea, a syndrome of menstrual pain etiologically associated with prostaglandin levels [6,7].

In addition to these affective and behavioral phenomena, several sensory, autonomic, and cognitive parameters have been found to vary with the menstrual cycle. Premenstrual impairments in auditory discrimination [8] and visual detection [9] have been reported. Olfactory sensitivity has been found to decrease between ovulation and menses [10], and sensitivity to taste perception has been found to vary with the menstrual cycle [11]. Greater reactivity to stress and higher levels of arousal in the premenstruum have been widely reported, as reviewed elsewhere [12].

Cognitive changes on standardized testing have been noted in comparisons of the pre- and postovulatory periods, with a trend noted in one report toward working faster and less accurately before ovulation, and slower with greater accuracy during the postovulatory period [13]. Conversely, other authors maintain that few, if any, decreases in cognitive or performance ability are related to the menstrual cycle [14]. Electroencephalographic (EEG) studies suggest premenstrual changes in a majority of women, with increases in alpha [15,16] and theta frequencies, paraoxysmal activity EEG driving [16], and abnormal responses to hyperventilation [16]. However, one earlier study did not find increases in alpha frequency or EEG driving in the premenstrual period [17]. Findings of premenstrual EEG changes are interesting in view of reports of female epileptics having increases cortical firing and number of seizures during the premenstrual period [18-20].

A variety of hypotheses have been employed to explain the etiology of premenstrual tension. Speculations have ranged from the psychosocial to the biochemical. To date, no single hypothesis is altogether satisfactory. The reason for such a variety of explanations can be understood, in part, by an examination of the phenomenology of the syndrome, whose existence has been criticized for being too broadly and inconsistently defined [21]. Although there is general agreement on the existence of premenstrual symptoms, there is less agreement as to the nature of the syndrome. Its definition blurs interdisciplinary boundaries when psychological, cultural, and biologic factors are taken into account.

Also, the nature of available research strategies used in the study of premenstrual tension may foster a tendency to multiple hypotheses. With many research techniques available to measure endocrine or other variables during the menstrual cycle, separate hypotheses tend to be constructed around individual variables, each of which may represent only a part of an entire psychophysiologic profile.

Each research strategy also has its own problems, and a brief discussion of these may be helpful before considering different hypotheses for the etiology of premenstrual tension.

A major research strategy used to study premenstrual tension is temporal correlations: measuring one or more endocrine or physiologic variables over time and correlating these temporally with the onset of emotional symptoms. Positive correlations are often used to imply etiology. However, since many psychobiologic, neuroendocrine, and psychophysiologic variables fluctuate during the menstrual cycle, temporal correlates of any one may be inadequate to suggest strongly any evidence of etiology, and may merely be epiphenomena.

Furthermore, failure to specify the dependent and independent variables before the experiment has been a problem with much previous research in the area of premenstrual tension. Through biased selection, occurring after the fact, when a number of measures have been included, one can take advantage of chance occurrences to support a favored hypothesis [22].

Much premenstrual tension research has also utilized retrospective reports. Whereas retrospective studies have demonstrated a very high incidence of increased emotional symptoms during the premenstrual and menstrual phases of the cycle, prospective studies have revealed less dramatic findings. Indeed, in several prospective studies normal women were asked to report their moods on a daily to weekly basis and no significant fluctuations in mood were shown across the menstrual cycle [21]. However, other prospective studies have reported cyclic fluctuation of mood in normal women, as measured by a variety of means [23].

From the perspective of understanding some of the problems inherent in premenstrual tension research, we will examine the various hypotheses formulated to explain premenstrual tension.

I. Psychological Hypotheses

As proposed by Benedek [24], the clinical, behavioral, and psychological findings characteristic of severe premenstrual tension may be considered to reflect intense conflicts concerning the female role. Helene Deutsch [25] and other psychoanalysts suggest that the perception of menstrual flow may intensify a woman's preexisting conscious and unconscious conflicts about pregnancy, childbearing, castration, feelings of uncleanliness, lack of control of bodily functions, aggression, penis envy, or masturbation. These investigators feel that, in the presence of a vulnerable ego structure, neurotic, psychotic, or characterologic reactions may occur. In many women it is postulated that the compensation for the hypothesized deprivations of being female is the process of pregnancy and bearing of a child [26], hence the common clinical, psychoanalytic observation that a menstrual period is experienced as a "lost child."

However, theories proposing that premenstrual symptoms occur as a response to the perception of menstrual flow do not account for the observation that psychological symptoms occur before the menstrual flow, and most commonly abate at or around the onset of menses. However, the arousal of intrapsychic conflict may not depend on the menses itself as a stimulus, but instead may involve anxiety associated with the somatic perception of impending menstruation. In one study [27], however, it was demonstrated that when women were tricked into thinking that their menstrual period was not about to occur, even though it was, they reported fewer premenstrual physical symptoms, although negative affect was still equal to that reported in women who thought and were about to have menstrual periods.

In a more general sense, Dalton [20] has pointed out that external stress in a patient's life at a given time is linked to the increase of premenstrual tension then. Coppen [28] and Rees [29] have correlated premenstrual tension with neuroticism scores, although Rees found that some very neurotic women had no premenstrual symptoms, and Coppen's study has been criticized for its methodology [30,31].

More recently, several studies have suggested that premenstrual affective changes may predict or be associated with episodes of psychiatric illness, especially affective disorders [31-33]. Some studies [31,32] have found premenstrual mood elevations in women with positive family histories of manic depressive illness. These reports are supported by the observations of Verghese [34], Ota [35], and others [36,37]. Thus, at least the more severe manifestations of premenstrual tension may be hypothesized to occur on the basis of vulnerability to premenstrual increases in reaction to stress [11,38], allowing for exacerbation of an underlying predisposition to psychiatric disorder.

II. Sociobiologic Hypothesis

Several authors have hypothesized that premenstrual tension may have survival value. Thus, we may consider premenstrual tension from the point of view of its survival value to the species, rather than limiting etiologic considerations to the individual organism. Wilson [39] states that the emotional centers of the brain may have evolved by natural selection, a process governed by methods which not only prolong individual survival, but also promote superior mating performance. Thus, the hypothalamic-limbic complex proliferates maximally only if it efficiently orchestrates behavioral responses between individuals.

Rosseinsky and Hall [40] contend that in primate colonies the thwarting of male sexual advances during the infertile period after ovulation may serve to increase male ardor during the next onset of fertility, thus increasing the chances of conception. He meets the anticipated objection that a male would only need turn to another female with the observation that colonies of cohabiting females tend toward menstrual cycle synchronicity, an assertion supported by some but not all studies.

A similar hypothesis may be derived from Gorney et al.'s suggestion [41] that menstrual avoidances may have served to protect vulnerable early communities from wasting a possible pregnancy due to a male mating with a temporarily infertile female. Morris and Keverne [42] have likewise postulated that premenstrual hostility toward the male may serve a survival function. They believe such rejections could become cumulative in the infertile pair, promoting dissolution of the relationship, and allowing for a new, fertile pair-bond to be formed with subsequent offspring, and thus greater survival value for the population. Indeed, Morris and Keverne point toward premenstrual tension as a possible factor in the increased rate of marital breakdown. This assertion may have profound implications for our present society where less frequent pregnancy because of contraception has resulted in women spending a greater proportion of time menstruating than did their ancestors [42].

III. Biologic Hypotheses

A. Ovarian Hormone Hypothesis

In 1931, Frank [43] first described the premenstrual tension syndrome and postulated its hormonal pathogenesis. This hypothesis is now widely accepted, and derives considerable support from animal as well as human studies. The ovarian hormones, progesterone and estrogen, have been most widely studied for their relation to premenstrual tension. Various theories have been proposed as to how alterations in these hormones may be etiologic.

Progesterone has behavioral effects which may parallel or be related to menstrual cycle emotional changes. Michael [44] has shown that some rhesus monkey pairs show significantly diminished sexual behavior during the luteal phase, when progesterone levels are highest. Likewise, diminished sexual activity in humans occurs during the luteal phase of the cycle [45], correlating with peak blood and urine progesterone levels [46]. A reduction in sexual activity is also seen when progesterone is administered to estrogen-pretreated, ovarectomized rhesus monkeys [47]. There is evidence that the degree of libido loss and depression occurring when oral contraceptives are administered in humans is directly related to the progestin content and inversely related to the estrogen content of the preparation used [48].

Other more direct evidence, however, implicates low or falling progesterone levels in the etiology of premenstrual tension, at least in the premenstrual phase of the cycle.

Low progesterone levels have been reported in women with premenstrual tension. Mundy et al. [49] have studied 16 women, eight of whom experienced premenstrual tension. At 5 to 8 days before menstruation, the mean plasma progesterone for the premenstrual tension group was 31 ± 10 (SEM) nmol/liter, compared with 45 ± 14 nmol/liter for controls. These findings are comparable with those of Bäckström and Carstensen [50], who found that in women with predominantly psychological symptoms, progesterone levels were reduced and estrogen levels increased compared with normal women during the week before menstruation. Smith [3] reported small but significant differences in progesterone levels in patients with menstrual depression. The symptomatic group showed slightly lower progesterone levels than those of normal women during the week preceding menstruation. O'Brien [51], however, reported significantly higher levels of progesterone 10 days before menstruation in symptomatic women, as compared with controls. However, 4 days before menstruation, the symptomatic group's mean progesterone level was lower than the mean for the control group, although the difference did not reach statistical significance.

Emitional symptoms may be related to decreasing levels of progesterone. Dysphoric emotional symptoms often begin in the luteal phase, intensifying as progesterone drops from its highest level (the luteal peak) during the menstrual cycle to its low premenstrual level. Also, dysphoria occurs in the third trimester of pregnancy, when progesterone is elevated, and increases postpartum as progesterone levels fall [52,53]. Also, induction of depressive symptoms has been reported after withdrawal of exogenous progesterone treatment [54]. These findings support the possibility that psychic symptoms may be secondary to the withdrawal of progesterone. Thus, premenstrual symptoms, as they relate to an ovarian hormone hypothesis, might be understood not in terms of absolute hormone levels but of hormone withdrawal.

As with progesterone, it has been suggested that premenstrual symptoms may be related to high estrogen levels. Occurrence of symptoms increases during the luteal phase when estrogen levels are high, intensifying as these levels fall. However, these symptoms do not consistently increase at midcycle when estrogen is most elevated, nor is there evidence of increased premenstrual symptoms in women with endogenously prolonged or increased estrogen levels such as in metropathia hemorrhagia [55]. However, Morton [56] reported production of a premenstrual tensionlike syndrome after intramuscular injection of estrogen.

As with progesterone, estrogen withdrawal has been postulated for the behavioral changes of premenstrual tension [23]. Increases in emotionality in the premenstrual phase correlate with falling estrogen levels [57]. However, the premenstrual fall in serum estrogen levels may not reflect central nervous system estrogen activity, since estrogen is selectively bound and concentrated in the limbic system and hypothalamus [50,58]. Absolute levels of estrogen may be less meaningful than the ratio of estrogen to progesterone.

The estrogen-progesterone ratio has been etiologically implicated as a cause of premenstrual tension since 1938, when Israel [59] suggested that premenstrual tension was caused by the presence of estrogen, unantagonized by progesterone, possibly secondary to deficient ovarian luteinization. This hypothesis was supported by evidence from vaginal smears. Greene and Dalton [60], more recently, have specifically hypothesized a high estrogen-progesterone ratio as etiologic of premenstrual tension. They substantiated this by noting that intramuscular progesterone alleviates the premenstrual syndrome [20,61], (a finding recently challenged in a well-controlled study [3]), and by citing evidence that the premenstrual tension syndrome was produced in castrated subjects after administration of large doses of estrogen.

In a study of mood changes and menstrual symptoms associated with oral contraceptives with varying estrogen-progesterone ratios, Cullberg [62] found that women with a history of premenstrual irritability who took progesterone-dominant contraceptive pills had significantly lower incidences of adverse mental changes, compared with those who took estrogen-dominant pills. Conversely, in women who did not report premenstrual irritability before treatment, Cullberg noted a tendency to higher incidences of adverse mental reactions with the progesterone-dominant pills, suggesting that these women may have been hormonally balanced before treatment, or possibly hiding an endogenous progesterone dominance. He suggested that premenstrual irritability is at least partly due to an endogenous estrogen dominance, or susceptibility to endogenous estrogen around the premenstrual phase. In a review of the literature, Cullberg noted three previous studies citing increased depressive symptoms after treatment with contraceptives with high progestational content. One study reported negative affect associated with estrogen dominance, and in two other studies different preparations did not show different mental effects.

Conflicting results in studies of the incidence of psychic symptoms after treatment with various oral contraceptives with different estrogen-progesterone ratios might be understood by considering the possibility that heterogeneous groups of women are being treated.

Similarly, Steiner and Carroll [23] have suggested that premenstrual irritability-anxiety-hostility may be a separate condition from premenstrual depression. The above studies of oral contraceptives seem to associate irritability-anxiety symptoms with a high estrogen-progesterone ratio, and depressive symptoms to a low estrogen-progesterone ratio.

As further support for an estrogen-progesterone ratio hypothesis, Bäckström and Carstensen [50] noted that women with anxiety as the main premenstrual symptom had significantly higher estrogen levels premenstrually than a group of healthy women. More specifically, estrogen-progesterone ratios in this study were significantly higher in the symptomatic group before menstruation. In a later publication by Bäckström and Mattsson [63], a positive correlation was found between the estrogen-progesterone ratio and anxiety in 15 women with premenstrual tension. Estrogen levels alone, however, correlated positively with irritability and anxiety, but progesterone levels did not.

Animal studies suggest that estrogen has behavioral effects which may be counteracted by progesterone. Estradiol implants in the anterior hypothalamus of female rats and cats have been shown to cause increased running and mating behaviors [64]. By contrast, exogenous progesterone decreases mating activity in estrogen-primed rabbits [65] and monkeys [43], and leads to sedative effects in many mammals [66]. Exogenous estrogen, administered to castrated female rhesus monkeys, restores attempts to initiate sexual encounters and increases male mounting and ejaculatory potential [67]. Although this implies a direct effect of these hormones on the female central nervous system, these hormones may also alter female "attractiveness." Local applications of estrogen to the vaginal wall of rhesus monkeys induces sexual excitation in the male partner without increasing the female's sexual interest. This effect may occur through the induction of vaginally emitted olfactory cues. Furthermore, progesterone given to a female rhesus monkey appears to decrease male sexual interest while increasing female sexual refusals [2].

In the same manner that estrogen and progesterone are seen to exhibit antagonistic actions in the behavioral and emotional spheres, there is evidence of apparent electrophysiological antagonism. Woolley and Timiras [68] found estrogen to decrease electroshock seizure thresholds in rats in a dose-dependent manner. With progesterone these investigators could, at least partially, counteract this estrogen effect. Timiras [69] has also shown that the excitability of the dorsal hippocampus is increased by estradiol. Logthetis et al. [18] found increased cortical firing and number of seizures in epileptic females in the premenstrual period, correlating with increased estrogen secretion which lowered seizure threshold. Selye [70] reported progesterone to have the opposite effect, being the most effective among the sedative steroid hormones, consistent with the observations of EEG slowing during the luteal phase in humans [71].

This evidence supports the psychoanalytic hypothesis employed by Benedek and Rubenstein [24] in 1951. They proposed that estrogen stimulates active heterosexual fantasies with progesterone producing passive, narcissistic thought content. Using this as a basis for prediction, they attempted to correlate the thematic content from psychoanalytically derived observations of women's speech with the actual estrogen-progesterone balance as measured by daily vaginal smears and basal body temperatures. Studying nine patients over the period of 75 cycles, Benedek was able to correlate her predictions of the day of ovulation with Rubenstein's analysis of vaginal smears with unusual accuracy. In several series the correlations approached 1.0. Serious criticism has been directed toward this study [72], however, with Benedek herself noting problems in defining precisely what in the records allowed her to make such precise predictions.

In summary, the ovarian hormone hypothesis holds that premenstrual symptoms are etiologically related to the ratios of progesterone and estrogen in the late luteal phase, or directly related to absolute or falling levels of progesterone or estrogen. A considerable amount of evidence supports this view. Several other considerations, however, make it difficult to implicate estrogen and progesterone completely in the ovarian-linked emotional disorders.

First and most importantly, Greene and Dalton [60] found 17% of their 84 premenstrual tension patients attributed the onset of cyclic menstrual symptoms to the menopause, when estrogen and progesterone are relatively low. Also, studies of endogenous variations often must rely on behavioral-temporal correlations which do not establish causality definitively. Conclusions from administration of synthetic hormones rest on the assumption that pharmacologic doses of these hormones have similar psychological effects to physiologic levels. Any estrogen-progesterone ratio hypothesis must account for the relative absence of symptoms during the preovulatory period, when serum estrogen levels are markedly higher than progesterone. Finally, no specific neurophysiologic mechanism for these hormones to effect mood changes has been definitively demonstrated, although several lines of evidence are discussed below. Thus, the premenstrual emotional disorders may not result directly from changes in estrogen or progesterone.

B. Mineralocorticoid Hypothesis

A major and enduring endocrine hypothesis suggests that mineralocorticoids may be etiologic. As mentioned above, premenstrual symptoms of an emotional and physical nature often begin or intensify after menopause or ovariectomy, suggesting an extraovarian etiologic focus [20].

Dalton [20] refers to Pellandra's hypothesis that symptoms of premenstrual emotional upsets may occur when there is an increase in mineralocorticoids and glucocorticoids in relation to ovarian steroids. Dalton postulated that aldosterone may be the hormonal cause, since it is a mineralocorticoid whose sodium-retaining properties are antagonized by the sodium wasting [73] effects of progesterone.

Studies of normal women indicate that fluctuations of aldosterone may parallel the emotional fluctuations of the menstrual cycle. Reich [74] reported a slight midcycle elevation of urinary aldosterone excretion, followed by a luteal rise which peaked during the premenstrual phase of the cycle, falling just before or soon after the onset of menses. Aldosterone elevations during the luteal phase, furthermore, were noted to be about twice that of the follicular phase. Gray [75] noted increased aldosterone secretory rates in the luteal phases of the cycle, and Katz and Romfh [76] found plasma aldosterone levels to be highest in normally menstruating women 9 to 10 days before menstruation. Sundsfjord and Aakvaag [73] reported a small preovulatory peak in plasma aldosterone. More importantly, they noted a much larger luteal peak of aldosterone which paralleled the plasma fluctuations of progesterone, both levels beginning to fall approximately 6 days before the onset of menstruation. Schwartz and Abraham [77] found serum aldosterone and corticosterone to be significantly higher in the luteal phase in four out of five normal subjects.

The stimulus for increased aldosterone in the late luteal phase is not completely understood, but progesterone and estrogen have been implicated. Progesterone has been found to antagonize aldosterone, and to cause a sodium diuresis with a secondary increase in plasma renin activity and aldosterone secretion rate [78]. Thus, the natriuretic effect of progesterone may be the stimulus for compensatory luteal increases in aldosterone. The findings of Sundsfjord and Aakvaag [73] support this idea. They found the pattern of increase and decrease in the plasma levels of aldosterone and plasma renin activity to be similar to those of plasma progesterone, suggesting that these fluctuations are causally related. It is notable, however, that the smaller preovulatory peak of aldosterone is not accompanied by an increase in plasma progesterone, although Sundsfjord and Aakvaag refer to the findings of Shott et al. who report a preovulatory peak of 17α-hydroxyprogesterone.

In 1937, Thorn and Harrop [79] reported that estrogen caused sodium retention, and several reports have since indicated that certain women are subject to hypertension in response to oral estrogen [78]. These effects may be partially due to a direct salt-retaining effect of the estrogen steroid, but there is evidence [80,81] that estrogen may stimulate the renin-angiotensin-aldosterone system. Estrogens have been reported to increase plasma aldosterone levels in one study [82], but this finding was unreplicated in two later studies [78,83].

Aldosterone secretion may be altered in women with premenstrual tension. Two early studies reported markedly increased premenstrual aldosterone excretion in symptomatic women [84,85]. However, more recent studies have failed to support these findings. Munday and Brush [48] found that the levels of plasma aldosterone in eight patients with premenstrual tension were not consistently different from those of eight controls. There was, however, a small surge of aldosterone in the late luteal phase of the premenstrual tension group which did not reach statistical significance. O'Brien [51], in a series of 28 women, found that the aldosterone level of symptomatic women on day 24 was nonsignificantly lower than the control group's.

Supportive evidence for a role for mineralocorticoids in the etiology of the cyclic emotional upsets comes from a series of reports which have noted a relationship between the phases of the menstrual cycle and expected changes in weight and/or sodium retention [86-91]. Generally, these studies have demonstrated midcycle and premenstrual-menstrual weight gains associated with sodium retention. Usually, these studies did not evaluate mood systematically.

A few studies of cyclic weight and sodium changes have utilized metabolic balance techniques and have been well-controlled. Bruce and Russell [89] studied 10 women with a history of premenstrual tension, keeping their hospitalized subjects on a fixed caloric, water, sodium, and potassium intake. They demonstrated small ovulatory and premenstrual increases in weight, associated with water and sodium retention. Thorn et al. [90] reported that of two obese and four normal subjects on a fixed intake of sodium, food, and water, one obese and two normal women gained weight and retained sodium in the premenstrum and during ovulation, and Landau and Lugibihl [91] noted premenstrual sodium retention in four women studied in the metabolic unit of a hospital.

By contrast, Andersch et al. [92], in a study of 20 pateints with premenstrual symptoms and 20 normal controls, found no significant changes in water or body weight in either group during the premenstrual period. Wong [93] has suggested that premenstrual symptoms may be due not to an absolute change in water balance but to a redistribution of fluid: a shift from the intravascular to the extravascular compartment.

Early hypotheses of the etiology of premenstrual tension postualted that increased sodium and water retention may lead to cerebral edema, with secondary neurologic findings including emotional instability. Investigators have therefore studied the efficacy of diuretics for treatment of premenstrual tension symptoms. Generally, controlled studies have found them ineffective in relieving the emotional upsets of premenstrual tension syndrome, slthough they do relieve the physical effects such as bloating and weight gain [3].

Janowsky et al. [5] evaluated changes in mood, weight, and urinary potassium-sodium (K^+-Na^+) ratio over a total of fifteen menstrual cycles in eleven women in order to investigate whether these changes correlated in the same patients. The urinary K^+-Na^+ ratio was measured, since there is evidence that, when dietary factors are controlled, this variable may in part reflect aldosterone and other mineralocorticoid effects. The data indicated that increases in negative affect, weight, and K^+-Na^+ ratio follow similar patterns in normal women when studied longitudinally. The changes in negative affect were consistent with the findings of others, who have evaluated cyclic emotional fluctuations, and reported luteal, premenstrual, and early menstrual increases in negative affect, such as depressed mood and increased anxiety, hostility, and aggressiveness. Similarly, the data were consistent with those of others in defining a small but definite progressive increase in weight during the luteal and premenstrual phases. It differed from some reports showing a large ovulatory weight increase; a relatively small mid-cycle weight gain was noted.

The data indicated that a statistically significant increase in urinary K^+-Na^+ ratio occurred in the premenstrual phase of the cycle. The curve of the K^+-Na^+ ratio noted in this study strikingly paralleled the aldosterone excretion curve noted by Reich [74]. The shift in the K^+-Na^+ ratio, with its implied increase in sodium retention, may in part underlie the weight changes described in other studies.

Netter [94] pointed out that aldosterone influences salivary electrolyte excretion similarly to renal excretion: decreasing the sodium concentration and increasing the potassium concentration and K^+-Na^+ ratio. In a study of saliva samples from 30 menstruating women, DeMarchi [95] found ovulatory and premenstrual increases in the K^+-Na^+ ratio. He noted that changes in salivary sodium and potassium composition have been observed in patients with depressive illness, and that increased intraocular pressure has been found in women with marked premenstrual tension.

The diuretic aldosterone antagonist, spironolactone, has been reported to be more effective than placebo in decreasing physical and psychological symptoms of premenstrual tension [51]. However, this study contains a standard regression artifact inherent in the method used to discriminate the symptomatic women from controls. Further studies will determine whether this single observation is valid and can thus be used to support a renin-angiotensin-aldosterone hypothesis for premenstrual tension.

Some data do not, however, support an aldosterone hypothesis of premsnstrual tension. As noted, evidence from some studies shows that aldosterone is not particularly elevated in patients with premenstrual tension compared with normals, although other studies do show such an increase. Steiner and Carroll [23] have noted that the renin-angiotensin-aldosterone system is not elevated during the luteal phase of anovulatory women. They refer to Adamopulous et al.'s observations that premenstrual emotional symptoms can occur in anovulatory cycles. Furthermore, the late luteal increase in serum aldosterone is not absolutely consistent, although it has been noted in a number of cases. Lastly, there is little evidence that the aldosterone changes noted during the menstrual cycle are directly causative of the cyclic emotional upsets, since other diseases with increased aldosterone levels are not necessarily associated with mental upsets. Specifically, in Conn's syndrome, where aldosterone is elevated, we find no reports of psychopathology.

Thus, it may be reasonable to hypothesize that a substance fluctuating in parallel with aldosterone may cause the cyclic behavioral changes. Angiotensin may be a reasonable candidate, since it is probably an endogenous compound which may stimulate aldosterone secretion, being activated itself by renin. Angiotensin is elevated during the luteal phase of the menstrual cycle, after progesterone administration, and during pregnancy, at all of which times the psychic upsets may be increased [2]. As for plasma renin activity, increases are found a few days before the increase in basal body temperature [90] and again during the second half of the luteal phase [96,97].

Angiotensin affects animal behavior, central neuroteansmitters, and autonomic functioning [2]. It causes increased drinking behavior when given by vertebral artery infusion or intraventricularly [98], a probable cholinergic effect antagonized by atropine [84]. It counteracts the anesthetic effects of amobarbital [99] and decreases exploratory activity in mice when given intraventricularly [100]. It disrupts learned passive avoidance responses in rats, possibly due to an effect on memory [101]. A central hypertensive effect has also been reported [102] which appears to have cholinergic and adrenergic components [103]. Immunohistochemical studies have revealed nerve fibers containing angiotensin in several different parts of the brain [104,105]. A brain enzyme with a reninlike activity has been demonstrated [106], and may be brain renin.

Other considerations, however, make less certain the notion of an angiotensin role in the etiology of premenstrual tension. The suggestion of a brain renin-angiotensin system has been criticized. Immunohistochemical localization of angiotensin in brain has been criticized on the basis of possible cross-immunoreactivity with other peptides [107]. Evidence of brain renin activity has been faulted as being nonspecific [107], and renin has not been obtained from brain in pure form [107]. Steiner and Carroll [23] note that the luteal peak of plasma renin activity is followed by a sharp drop occurring about 6 days before menstruation, although a minority of women in these studies [76,77] showed highest plasma renin activity around day 28 of the cycle.

C. Androgen Hypothesis

Steiner and Carroll [23] noted that plasma androgens have not been studied in the premenstrual tension syndrome. They find this surprising in view of the association between testosterone and both sexual drive and aggression, and the common observation of premenstrual exacerbations of acne.

In general, androgens tend to exhibit a midcycle peak and subsequent premenstrual trough [108-110]. This is most clearly seen with androstenedione, which is lowest during the premenstrual period. Thus the behavioral and psychological manifestations of premenstrual tension syndrome may be related to the fluctuations of androgens at the premenstrual phase of the cycle. However, available evidence is inadequate to implicate androgens strongly in the etiology of premenstrual tension.

D. Glucocorticoid Hypothesis

Some evidence supports the hypothesis that cyclic emotional upsets associated with the premenstruum are related to the secretion of serum cortisol. A recent study by Walker and McGilp [111] of the excretion of urinary free 11-hydroxy-corticosteroids and total estrogens in normal women indicated a peak in the corticosteroid excretion at 8 to 10 days after ovulation, synchronous with the second estrogen peak during the luteal phase. Similarly, Genazzani et al. [112] observed increased plasma concentrations of both cortisol and adrenocorticotropic hormone (ACTH) 10 days after ovulation. Previous studies, however, indicated cortisol secretion rates to be relatively stable over the course of the menstrual cycle [113,114].

Many patients with depressive illness exhibit increased levels of corticosteroid production and excretion [115], and depression has been described in many patients with Cushing's syndrome [116]. The neuropeptide stimulator for cortisol secretion, ACTH, has been implicated as having an anxiogenic effect in animals [117]. Adrenocorticol reactivity to psychological stress, as measured by serum cortisol levels, has been found to vary across the menstrual period in one study [38], with significantly greater cortisol secretion in response to stress being found in the premenstrual period than at midcycle. A similar study [118], however, found that cortisol responses to psychological stress were not related to the menstrual cycle. As mentioned above, several psychophysiologic measures of reactivity to stress are increased during the premenstrual period. Thus, increased stress reactivity with concomitant cortisol increases may be implicated in the causes of premenstrual tension. However, these increases may be secondary to some more primary etiologic focus, since there is no direct evidence that high cortisol produces premenstrual syndrome.

E. Insulin Hypothesis

Morton [61], in a study of premenstrual tension, found that a diagnosis of at least subclinical premenstrual hypoglycemia could be established in a majority of symptomatic patients. Recently, the specific binding of insulin to circulating monocytes and erythrocytes has been studied across the menstrual cycle [118]. An inverse relationship was found between the insulin binding to monocytes and levels of 17-β-estradiol, progesterone, and 17-α-hydroxyprogesterone, suggesting that sex steroids may play a role in the control of insulin receptors. This data may, in part, explain the reduction of glucose tolerance in the second half of the menstrual cycle reported by various authors. Positive relationships between insulin binding and glucose tolerance have been reported, and decreases in insulin receptor concentrations have been found after the administration of corticoid-steroids, gestagens, and in the third trimester of pregnancy, as well as when estrogen and progesterone levels are increased [119]. A common clinical observation associated with hypoglycemia is anxiety and irritability associated with the transient fall in serum glucose. Thus, symptoms in the premenstrual phase may be explainable, at least in part, by the changes in insulin receptor binding and glucose tolerance at that time.

F. Prolactin Hypothesis

Like estrogen and progesterone, the pituitary hormone prolactin has been proposed as a cause of the premenstrual tension syndrome [120-122]. Prolactin may cause sodium and water retention by potentiating the renal action of aldosterone and antidiuretic hormone [123]. Prolactin levels probably fluctuate throughout the menstrual cycle, with peaks occurring at ovulation and later in the mid- and late luteal phases [124,125]. However, some women show little change throughout the cycle [126]. Increases in prolactin have been reported in premenstrual tension patients compared with normal controls [120].

Bromocriptine, a dopamine agonist which decreases prolactin, may ameliorate premenstrual tension syndrome as well as premenstrual weight gain and breast enlargement [122]. This implicates prolactin in the etiology of premenstrual tension. However, at least one well-controlled study has shown beomocriptine only equal to placebo in its efficacy in treating premenstrual tension, and others have shown no efficacy [121,122]. Furthermore, the primary effects of bromocriptine, if it is effective, may rest in its dopaminergic rather than antiprolactin effects [127]. Lastly, at least one study [124] suggests that prolactin does not increase in the luteal phases in anovulatory women, and Adamopoulos et al. [128] have noted that premenstrual tension continues during anovulatory cycles, although their observations are limited to a very small number of subjects.

Conflicting with a prolactin hypothesis is the fact that elevations of prolactin from other causes, such as dopamine-blocking agents and pituitary tumors, do not seem to lead to psychological upset.

G. Melatonin

Fluctuations in the pineal hormone melatonin have been correlated with gonadal function [129,130], sleep changes [131], and limbic system electrophysiology [132]. Melatonin has been shown to inhibit pituitary gonadotropin secretion in animals, as well as increase synthesis of progesterone in the human corpus luteum [129].

One study [129] has measured human serum melatonin during the menstrual cycle, reporting highest melatonin values during the premenstrual and menstrual phases. In view of reports of increased sleep duration in women during the premenstrual phase [133], it is interesting to note that melatonin has been found to prolong sleep in humans when given exogenously [134].

Melatonin can improve mood in normal subjects, but has been reported to exacerbate dysphoira when given to depressed patients [135]. It is not known how premenstrual-menstrual elevations of melatonin may relate to premenstrual dysphoria. To date, melatonin has not been measured in women with premenstrual tension, although this is obviously desirable.

H. Monoamine Neurotransmitters

The monoamine neurotransmitters serotonin, norepinephrine, and dopamine have been widely implicated in psychiatric disorders [136]. Evidence also implicates them in the pathophysiology of premenstrual tension.

Animal studies indicate that ovarian hormones and monoamines show overlapping behavioral effects. Similarly to certain antidepressants, estrogen induces running behavior in rats [137] and, like reserpine, progesterone induces sedation in rats and other mammals [66].

Brain monoamines and sex steroids show overlapping effects in the regulation of sexual behavior in rats. Reserpine and tetrabenazine, both monoamine depletors, may be substituted for progesterone in activating sexual behavior in estrogen-primed castrated female rats. In contrast, tricyclic antidepressant drugs and monoamine oxidase (MAO) inhibitors decrease sexual activation in estrogen-progesterone primed castrated female rats, especially when brain serotonin is selectively increased [138]. Furthermore, selective depletion of rat brain serotonin induces sexual excitation, especially when brain catecholamines such as dopamine and norepinephrine are simultaneously elevated [139].

Ovarian hormones and monoamines also exhibit overlapping functions in regulating ovulation. Elevation of brain serotonin blocks superovulation in immature rats [140], and decreased norepinephrine levels inhibit physiological estrus as determined by vaginal smears [141]. Large doses of norepinephrine administered into the third ventricle induce ovulation. Reserpine administration inhibits ovulation in the rat, which is antagonized by the administration of MAO inhibitors or dopamine [142]. Reserpine induces pseudopregnancy in rats when given systematically and following local hypothalamic administration; this effect is also prevented by treatment with monoamine oxidase inhibitors (MAOI) [138, 142]. Dopamine appears to exhibit an important role in the regulation of gonado-tropin secretion. Small doses of dopamine, incubated in vitro in the presence of pituitary and hypothalamic tissue, induce the release of luteinizing hormone (LH) and follicle stimulating hormone (FSH) [138,143]. Kamberi and others [143, 144] have recently found that administration of small doses of dopamine or relatively high doses of norepinephrine or epinephrine significantly increases blood LH levels, while serotonin causes an opposite effect [139].

Evidence indicates that ovarian hormones exert an influence on MAO activity. Pharmacologic doses of estradiol are associated with decreased tissue MAO activity in rats [145,146]. Progesterone appears to increase tissue MAO activity in rats [146], and increase plasma MAO activity in amenorrheic females [147]. Increased endometrial monoamine oxidase occurs in the late luteal phase of the menstrual cycle and in direct proportion to the progestin content of oral contra-ceptives [148]. Conversely, Belmaker et al. [149] have noted a decrease in paltelet monoamine oxidase premenstrually and these findings have been repli-cated by Wirz-Justice [150].

Changes in brain monoamine levels have been found to occur cyclically throughout the estrous cycle of the rat. Greengrass and Toungue [151] reported that the concentration of all three monoamines decreased in the rat during estrus, when ovulation is being stimulated by luteinizing hormone. During metaestrus, under the influence of luteal progesterone, the monoamine neurotransmitters began to rise toward their maximum, achieved at dioestrus when estrogen and progesterone are low.

Thus, there is evidence that alterations in monoamines may be linked to ovarian and adrenal hormone fluctuations, as well as to behavioral changes. On this basis, a catecholamine (norepinephrine/dopamine) hypothesis, and a sero-tonin hypothesis of premenstrual tension have evolved.

1. Catecholamine Hypothesis

Various studies have found norepinephrine and dopamine to be influenced by exogenous ovarian and other steroid hormones. The effects of estrogen, proges-terone, and angiotensin on catecholamine activity have been demonstrated in a number of in vitro studies using neurophysiological preparations. Angiotensin has been found to accelerate the biosynthesis of norepinephrine by rat heart atrium [152] and to inhibit the uptake and reuptake of tritiated norepinephrine by brain stem slices and perfused rat brain ventricles [99]. Also, endogenous rat brain norepinephrine is lowered by intraventricular angiotensin administration [100]. Estrogen, progesterone, and deoxycorticosterone enhance the contractile effect of norepinephrine and epinephrine on aortic strips [150]. Estrogen decreases by more than 25% the amount of labeled preequilibrated tritiated norepinephrine released by electrically stimulated rat brain slices [153].

The uptake and passive release of various monoamines from nerve endings can be studied in vitro using isolated nerve endings (synaptosomes). Janowsky et al. [154] reported that progesterone and estradiol block the uptake of labeled norepinephrine by synaptosomes, and that the passive effux of preequilibrated norepinephrine from synaptosomes is slightly slowed by estradiol and increased by progesterone. Estradiol and progesterone inhibited the uptake of tritiated dopamine and norepinephrine by synaptosomes. Hydrocortisone caused minimal inhibition of norepinephrine uptake and no significant effects on dopamine uptake. Progesterone (1×10^{-4} M) increased the rate of passive effux of labeled dopamine and norepinephrine from synaptosomes, whereas estradiol (1×10^{-5} M) did not affect dopamine effux. Angiotensin amide (1×10^{-4} to 1×10^{-5} M) also blocked the uptake of tritiated norepinephrine, but did not affect the passive effux of preequilibrated tritiated norepinephrine [2].

In the intact female rat, exogenous estrogen ahs been shown to decrease hypothalamic norepinephrine. Increased norepinephrine and decreased dopamine turnover rates have been shown in the rat after castration, these effects being reversible with large doses of estradiol and progesterone [5]. Increased dopamine turnover has been shown in the tuberoinfundibular region after estradiol, progesterone have no effect [155].

Norepinephrine and dopamine are metabolized enzymatically, in part, by catechol-O-methyltransferase (COMT), and this enzyme's activity has been inhibited in vitro by estrogen, progesterone, and deoxycorticosterone [156]. In the rat midbrain, COMT has been found to decrease during estrus [157]. Dopamine-β-hydroxylase, which converts dopamine to norepinephrine, has shown decreases in the premenstrual-menstrual phases of the cycle [158].

Several studies in humans have investigated measures of catecholamine metabolism from peripheral sources during the menstrual cycle. Wiener [159] in 1962, and Patkai [133] in 1974, reported increases in urinary norepinephrine excretion during the premenstruum. The later study also measured urinary epinephrine excretion and found small nonsignificant decreases during the 5 days before menstruation. However, these measures do not differentiate central norepinephrine metabolism from peripheral norepinephrine. A more recent study [160] measured the urinary metabolite of central norepinephrine, MHPG, daily in four healthy women. A statistically significant increase in MHPG was found during the late luteal phase, followed by a rapid decline 2 days before menstruation, and a subsequent elevation during the menses. This premenstrual drop is interesting in view of previous findings of decreased MHPG in some individuals with depressive illness [161].

During the premenstrual-menstrual phase of the cycle, sensitivity increases to tyramine, a measure of noradrenergic receptor sensitivity or increased presynaptic neuronal norepinephrine activity [162]. In view of the premenstrual decreases in urinary MHPG, tyramine sensitivity may be more a reflection of increased receptor sensitivity complimenting decreased norepinephrine activity.

Cyclic fluctuations in catecholamine and/or sodium balance may be linked to early observations of the possible usefulness of lithium carbonate as a treatment for premenstrual tension, since lithium affects both of these systems and is efficacious in the treatment of affective disorders. However, subsequent well-controlled trials of lithium in the treatment of premenstrual tension show it to be no better than placebo and possibly worse, at least in most cases [23].

2. Serotonin Hypothesis

Several lines of evidence, in addition to that described above, would support a role for indoleamine in premenstrual tension. Rats treated with a series of injections of progesterone showed increased serotonin uptake [163] and turnover [164] in several areas of brain. Brain serotonin uptake decreased 24 h after withdrawal of the last progesterone injection [163].

Ladisich [164] reported increased brain serotonin concentrations in the rat after stress. In a clinical component of the same report, he found that reactivity to stress in women was greater 1 day before menstruation than at 8 days before when progesterone is at its peak. Thus, we may hypothesize that a decrease in brain serotonin may occur secondary to progesterone withdrawal, with subsequent increased reactivity to stress. Sicuteri [165] has related the decreased pain threshold associated with administration of serotonin-depleting drugs (e.g., PCPA) to the idea that fluctuations in monoamine turnover during the menstrual cycle may provoke lowering of the pain threshold. An induction of depressive symptoms has been reported following withdrawal of exogenous progesterone [54], and depression is common during the postpartum period, when progesterone is falling [52,53]. Greengrass and Toungue [166] reported lower serotonin concentrations in mouse brain during the postpartum period.

The uptake of serotonin into platelets has been found in several studies [167, 168] to be decreased in patients with depressive illness. Variations in platelet serotonin uptake, after chlorimipramine treatment, have been found to occur across the menstrual cycle, with premenstrual decreases [169]. The amino acid precursor of serotonin, tryptophan, has shown menstrual variations in the plasma, with premenstrual increases [150]. Most other amino acids have demonstrated premenstrual decreases, according to one study of two menstruating women [170], although tryptophan was not measured.

The urinary metabolite of serotonin, 5-hydroxyindole acetic acid (5-HIAA) has been measured across the menstrual period in normal women. The 5-HIAA excretion has been found to be higher during the secretory phase than the proliferative phase, with the final descent occurring during the premenstrual phase [171]. This would be consistent with the notion that luteal progesterone secretion increases serotonin turnover, with subsequent premenstrual progesterone withdrawal resulting in lowered serotonin turnover.

The serotonin hypothesis may bear some relevance to the mineralocorticoid hypothesis discussed above, since administration of the serotonin precursors tryptophan and 5-hydrosytryptophan have been found to stimulate renin in dogs. Stress can lead to increases in both plasma renin and brain serotonin [172]. Deoxycorticosterone, the sodium-retaining precursor of aldosterone, shares sedative properties with progesterone [20,66] and corticosterone itself can increase or decrease serotonergic function depending on the dosage [113].

Oral contraceptives cause a functional decrease in pyridoxine, a coenzyme essential in the regulation of serotonin and nicotinic acid formation. Shunting of the serotonin precursor tryptophan toward the formation of nicotinic acid and possibly away from the formation of serotonin may occur in the presence of oral contraceptives. Pyridoxine deficiency has been documented in a subgroup of women taking oral contraceptives and oral pyridoxine has relieved symptoms of depression in these women. Pyridoxine has been shown to improve the impaired glucose tolerance curve observed in women taking oral contraceptives. Pyridoxine has therefore been explored as a treatment for premenstrual tension, and found to be effective in early studies. However, a later, more well-controlled study could not demonstrate its therapeutic efficacy [173].

I. Acetylcholine Hypothesis

Cholinergic mechanisms may be etiologic in premenstrual-menstrual emotional upsets. As reviewed elsewhere [5], angiotensin increases brain acetylcholine content in rat and mouse and causes an increase in the output of acetylcholine from the parietal cortex of cats. It causes an increase in the secretion of antidiuretic hormone, which appears to be cholinergically mediated and itself is water-retaining. Consistent with these observations, the uterine hyperemia which precedes menstruation is due to increased acetylcholine activity, and neostigmine, a cholinesterase inhibitor, can induce menstruation in nonpregnant women who have delayed menstruation, presumably by increasing uterine acetylcholine activity. Furthermore, a variety of ovarian hormones and other steroids can increase acetylcholine activity in physiologic preparations and can increase sensitivity to acetylcholine in muscle preparations.

Menstrually related remission of symptoms has been demonstrated in patients with myasthenia gravis, and is associated with cyclic variations of red cell acetylcholinesterase activity, suggesting a hormonal influence on acetylcholinesterase activity [174]. Physostigmine, a centrally acting cholinominetic drug, alleviates manic symptoms and causes withdrawal, lethargy, dysphoria, psychomotor retardation, and, in some cases, depression in normal, remitted, schizophrenic, and manic patients [175]. The premenstrual-menstrual emotional upset may represent in part a relative predominance of central cholinergic activity caused by angiotensin or a variety of endogenous steroid compounds. Finally, a proprietary combination drug containing an ergot, a barbiturate, and an anticholinergic agent can alleviate premenstrual tension more effectively than placebo [176]. If this finding is valid, and if the effects are due to the anticholinergic agent, a role for acetylcholine in the ovarian-linked emotional disorders would be supported.

IV. Discussion

Changes in human and primate emotional behavior are in part correlated with, and possibly regulated by, fluctuations in the menstrual cycle. Not enough information exists to define precisely a neurohormone, hormone, or combination of hormones actually causative of menstrual cycle-linked behavioral changes. Elevated or rapidly falling levels of estrogen, progesterone, aldosterone, and angiotensin, or a potential myriad of undiscovered or unstudied compounds, seem to be associated with emotional instability. These would include compounds that fluctuate during the third trimester and postpartum phases of pregnancy, during or after progestin ingestion, and in the late luteal and premenstrual-menstrual phase of the cycle.

Hormones which fluctuate in the menstrual cycle-linked emotional disorders, and in the regulation of female sexual behavior, alter neurotransmitters in the brain. Cyclic emotional, and possibly sexual, changes occur through this mechanism. It is important to note that the serotonin, catecholamine, and acetylcholine hypotheses of mental illness in general remain unproven and await further direct studies. However, even if the neurotransmitter hypotheses are valid, it is still uncertain how specific neurotransmitters or combinations of neurotransmitters actually affect emotions. Similarly, although much evidence indicates that neurotransmitters are affected by the hormones previously considered, the actual occurrence of these changes in women under physiological conditions is uncertain.

Lastly, although it has been implied that circulating hormones or neurohormones alter neurotransmitters, thus leading to cyclic emotional changes, it is at least as possible that cyclic fluctuations in neurotransmitters cause ovarian and adrenal changes. These could lead to temporal correlates of disturbed behavioral changes, but may be in no way etiologic of these changes. Conversely, the neurotransmitter changes themselves may be primary in regulating mood and hormonal fluctuations. However, it is more likely that the cyclic hormonal, neurotransmitter, and behavioral changes are mutually interactive, regulating each other in a variety of ways.

Despite a number of unanswered questions, alternate possibilities, and conflicting facts and paradoxes, the proposed etiologic relationship of endocrine-related neurotransmitter alterations to menstrual-cycle-linked emotional and sexual behavioral changes remains a possibility worthy of continued investigation. Furthermore, since the cyclic emotional upsets are of ubiquitous and serious psychiatric significance, their continued study represents a very important direction for psychiatric research.

References

1. R. H. Moos, Typology of menstrual cycle symptoms. *Am. J. Obstet. Gynecol.* 103:390-402 (1969).
2. D. S. Janowsky, W. E. Fann, and J. M. Davis, Monoamines and ovarian hormone-linked sexual and emotional changes. *Arch. Sex. Behav.* 1:205-218 (1971).
3. S. L. Smith, The menstrual cycle and mood disturbances. *Clin. Obstet Gynecol.* 19:391-397 (1976).
4. M. Endo, M. Daiguji, Y. Asano, I. Yamashita, and S. Takahasi, Periodic psychosis recurring in association with menstrual cycle. *J. Clin. Psychiatry* 39:456-466 (1978).
5. D. S. Janowsky, S. C. Berens, and J. M. Davis, Correlations between mood, weight, and electrolytes during the menstrual cycle: A renin-angiotensin-aldosterone hypothesis of premenstrual tension. *Psychosom. Med.* 35:143-152 (1973).
6. W. Y. Chan and M. Yusoff Dawood, Prostaglandin levels in menstrual fluid of nondysmenorrheic and of dysmenorrheic subjects with and without oral contraceptive or ibuprofen therapy. *Adv. Prostaglandin Thromboxane Res.* 8:1443-1447 (1980).
7. V. R. Pickles, Prostaglandins and dysmenorrhea. *Acta Obstet Gynecol. Scand. [Suppl.]* 87:7-12 (1979).
8. M. Haggard and J. B. Gaston, Changes in auditory perception in the menstrual cycle. *Br. J. Audiol.* 12:105-118 (1978).
9. M. M. Ward, S. C. Stone, and C. A. Sandman, Visual perception in women during the menstrual cycle. *Physiol. Behav.* 20:239-243 (1978).
10. R. G. Mair, J. A. Bouffard, T. Engen, and T. Morton, Olfactory sensitivity during the menstrual cycle. *Sens. Processes* 2:90-98 (1978).
11. E. V. Glanville and A. P. Kaplan, Task perception and the menstrual cycle. *Nature* 205:930-931 (1965).
12. D. Asso, Levels of arousal in the premenstrual phase. *Br. J. Soc. Clin. Psychol.* 17:47-55 (1978).
13. M. Cormack and P. Sheldrake, Menstrual cycle variations in cognitive ability: A preliminary report. *Int. J. Chronobiol.* 2:53-55 (1974).
14. B. Sommer, The effect of menstruation on cognitive and perceptual-motor behavior: A review. *Psychosom. Med.* 35:515-534 (1973).

15. O. D. Creutzfelt, P. M. Arnold, D. Becker, S. Langenstein, W. Tirsch, H. Wilhelm, and W. Wuttke, EEG changes during spontaneous and controlled menstrual cycles and their correlations with psychological performance. *Electroencephalogr. Clin. Neurophysiol.* 40:113-131 (1976).

16. P. M. Leary and K. Batho, Changes in the electroencephalogram related to the menstrual cycle. *S. Afr. Med. J.* 55:666-668 (1979).

17. W. Vogel, D. M. Broverman, and E. L. Klaiber, EEG responses in regularly menstruating women and in amenorrheic women treated with ovarian hormones. *Science* 172:338-391 (1971).

18. J. Logothetis, R. Harner, F. Morrell, and F. Torres, The role of oestrogen and catamenial exacerbations of epilepsy. *Neurology* 9:352-360 (1959).

19. J. Laidlaw, Catamenial epilepsy. *Lancet* 2:1235-1237 (1956).

20. K. Dalton, *The Premenstrual Syndrome.* Heineman, London, 1964.

21. M. B. Pardee, The premenstrual syndrome. *Psychol. Bull.* 80:454-465 (1973).

22. B. Sommer, Stress and menstrual distress. *J. Hum. Stress* 4:5-47 (1978).

23. M. Steiner and B. J. Carroll, The psychobiology of premenstrual dysphoria; a review of theories and treatment. *Psychoneuroendocrinology* 2:321-335 (1977).

24. T. Benedek, *Studies in Psychosomatic Medicine: Psychosexual Functions in Women.* Roland Press, New York, 1952.

25. H. Deutsch, *The Psychology of Women.* Grune & Stratton, New York, 1944.

26. S. Freud, *Some Psychical Consequences of the Anatomical Distinction Between the Sexes.* Standard Edition XIX. Hogarth Press, London, 1961.

27. D. N. Ruble, Premenstrual symptoms: A reinterpretation. *Science* 197: 291-292 (1977).

28. A. Coppen and N. Kessel, Menstrual disorders and personality. *Acta Psychother. (Basel)* 11:174-180 (1963).

29. L. Rees, Psychosomatic aspects of the premenstrual tension syndrome. *Br. J. Psychiatry* 99:62-73 (1953).

30. S. L. Smith, Mood and the menstrual cycle, in *Topics in Psychoendocrinology* (E. J. Sachar, ed.). Raven Press, New York, 1975.

31. R. D. Wetzel, T. Reich, J. N. McClure Jr., and J. Wald, Premenstrual affective syndrome and affective disorder. *Br. J. Psychiatry* 127:219-221 (1975).

32. J. N. McClure Jr., T. Reich, and R. D. Wetzel, Premenstrual symptoms as an indication of bipolar affective disorder. *Br. J. Psychiatry* 119:527-528 (1971).

33. M. A. Schuckit, V. Daly, G. Herrman, and S. Hineman, Premenstrual symptoms and depression in a university population. *Dis. Nerv. Syst.* 36:516-518 (1975).

34. A. Verghese, The syndrome of premenstrual psychosis. *Indian J. Psychiatry* 5:160-163 (1963).
35. J. Ota and T. Mukai, Studies on the relationship between psychotic symptoms and sexual cycle. *Folia Psychiatr. Neurol. Jpn.* 8:207-217 (1954).
36. J. L. Kramp, Studies on the premenstrual syndrome in relation to psychiatry. *Acta Psychiatr. Scand. [Suppl.]* 203:261-267 (1968).
37. E. Y. Williams and L. R. Weekes, Premenstrual tension associated with psychotic episodes. *J. Nerv. Ment. Dis.* 116:321-329 (1952).
38. K. T. Marinari, A. I. Leshner, and M. P. Doyle, Menstrual cycle status and adrenocortical reactivity to stress. *Psychoneuroendocrinology* 1:213-218 (1976).
39. E. O. Wilson, *Sociobiology: The New Synthesis.* Belknap Press (Harvard University Press), Cambridge, 1975.
40. D. R. Rosseinsky and P. G. Hall, An evolutionary theory of premenstrual tension. *Lancet* 2:1024 (1974).
41. R. Gorney, D. S. Janowsky, and B. Kelley, The curse—vicissitudes and variations of the female fertility cycle: Part II. Evolutionary aspects. *Psychosomatics* 7:283-287 (1966).
42. G. M. Morriss and E. B. Keverne, Premenstrual tension. *Lancet* 2:1317-1318 (1974).
43. R. T. Frank, The hormonal causes of premenstrual tension. *Arch. Neurol. Psychiatry* 26:1053 (1931).
44. R. P. Michael, Gonadal hormones and the control of primate behavior, in *Endocrinology and Human Behavior.* Oxford University Press, London, 1968.
45. J. R. Udry and N. M. Morris, Distribution of coitus in the menstrual cycle. *Nature* 220:593-596 (1968).
46. J. A. Loraine and E. T. Bell, Hormone excretion during the normal menstrual cycle. *Lancet* 1:1340-1342 (1963).
47. R. P. Michael, G. Saayman, and D. Zumpe, Inhibition of sexual receptivity in rhesus monkeys. *J. Endocrinol.* 39:309-310 (1967).
48. E. C. G. Grant and J. Pryse Davies, Effect of oral contraceptives on depressive mood changes and on endometrial monoamine oxidase and phosphates. *Br. Med. J.* 3:777-780 (1968).
49. M. Munday, M. G. Brush, and R. W. Taylor, Progesterone and aldosterone levels in the premenstrual tension syndrome. *J. Endocrinol.* 73:21P (1977).
50. T. Bäckström and H. Corstensen, Estrogen and progesterone in plasma in relation to premenstrual tension. *J. Steroid Biochem.* 5:257-260 (1974).
51. P. M. S. O'Brien, D. Craven, C. Selby, and E. M. Symonds, Treatment of premenstrual syndrome by spironolactone. *Br. J. Obstet. Gynaecol.* 86:142-147 (1979).
52. R. C. Treadway, F. J. Kane, A. Jarreh-Zadeh, and M. A. Lipton, A psycho-

endocrine study of pregnancy and puerperium. *Am. J. Psychiatry* 125: 1380-1386 (1969).

53.   O. M. Helmer and W. E. Judson, Influence of high renin substrate levels on the renin-angiotensin system in pregnancy. *Am. J. Obstet. Bynecol.* 99:9-17 (1967).

54.   D. Hamburg, Effects of progesterone on behavior. *Res. Publ. Assoc. Res. Nerv. Ment. Dis.* 43:251-265 (1966).

55.   R. W. Taylor, The treatment of premenstrual tension with dydrogesterone. *Curr. Med. Res. Opin.* 4(Suppl. 4):35-40 (1977).

56.   J. H. Morton, Premenstrual tension. *Am. J. Obstet. Gynecol.* 60:343-352 (1950).

57.   D. T. Baird and A. Guevara, Concentration of unconjugated estione and estradiol in peripheral plasma in nonpregnant women throughout menstrual cycle, castrate, and post-menopausal women and men. *J. Clin. Endocrinol.* 29:149-156 (1969).

58.   C. H. Anderson and G. S. Greenward, Autoradiographic analysis of estradiol uptake in the brain and pituitary of the female rat. *Endocrinology* 85: 1160-1165 (1969).

59.   S. L. Israel, Premenstrual tension. *JAMA* 110:1721-1723 (1938).

60.   R. Greene and K. Dalton, The premenstrual syndrome. *Br. Med. J.* 1:1007-1013 (1953).

61.   L. Rees, The premenstrual tension syndrome and its treatment. *Br. Med. J.* 1:1014-1016 (1953).

62.   J. Cullberg, Mood changes and menstrual symptoms with difficult gestagen/estrogen combination. *Acta Psychiatr. Scand. [Suppl.]* 236:1-86 (1972).

63.   T. Bäckström and B. Mattsson, Correlation of symptoms in premenstrual tension to oestrogen and progesterone concentrations in blood plasma. *Neuropsychogiology* 1:80-86 (1975).

64.   G. B. Colvin and C. H. Sawyer, Induction of running activity by intracerebral injections of estrogen in ovarectomized rats. *Neuroendocrinology* 4: 309-320 (1969).

65.   C. Beyer, N. Vidal, and P. G. McDonald, Interaction of gonadal steroids and their effect on sexual behavior in the rabbit. *J. Endocrinol.* 45:407-413 (1969).

66.   H. Selye, Spironolactone actions independent of mineralocorticoid blockade. *Steroids* 13:803-808 (1969).

67.   R. P. Michael, G. S. Saayman, and D. Zumpe, The suppression of mounting behavior and ejaculation in male rhesus monkeys by administration of progesterone to their female partners. *J. Endocrinol.* 41:421-431 (1968).

68.   D. E. Woolley and P. S. Timeras, The gonad-brain relationship. Effects of female sex hormones on electroshock convulsions in the rat. *Endocrinology* 70:196-209 (1962).

69. P. S. Timeras, Estrogen as 'organizers' of CNS function. Influences of hormones on the nervous system. Kargel, Basel, 1971, pp. 242-245.

70. H. Selye, Correlations between the chemical structure and pharmacological actions of the steroids. *Endocrinology* 30:437-453 (1942).

71. F. Gibbs and D. Reich, The electroencephalogram in pregnancy. *Am. J. Obstet. Gynecol.* 44:672-675 (1952).

72. M. Bleuler, *Endokrinologische Psychiatrie.* Georg Thieme Verlag, Stuttgart, 1954.

73. J. A. Sundsfjord and A. Aakvaag, Plasma renin activity, plasma renin substrate and urinary aldosterone excretion in the menstrual cycle in relation to the concentration of progesterone and oestrogens in the plasma. *Acta Endocrinologica* 71:519-529 (1972).

74. M. Reich, The variations in urinary aldosterone levels of normal females during the menstrual cycle. *Aust. Ann. Med.* 11:41-49 (1962).

75. M. J. Gray, K. S. Strausfeld, M. Wantanabe, E. A. H. Sims, and S. Solomon, Aldosterone secretory rates in the normal menstrual cycle. *J. Clin. Endocrinol. Metab.* 28:1269-1275 (1968).

76. F. H. Katz and P. Romfh, Plasma aldosterone and renin activity during the menstrual cycle. *J. Clin. Endocrinol. and Metab.* 34:819-821 (1972).

77. U. D. Schwarz and G. E. Abraham, Corticosterone and aldosterone levels during the menstrual cycle. *Obstet. Gynecol.* 45:339-342 (1975).

78. M. G. Crane and J. J. Harris, Estrogens and hypertension. *Am. J. Med. Sci.* 276:33-54 (1978).

79. G. W. Thorn and G. A. Harrop, The sodium-retaining effect of the sex hormones. *Science* 86:40-41 (1937).

80. O. M. Helmer and W. E. Judson, Influence of high renin substrate on the renin-angiotensin system in pregnancy. *Am. J. Obstet. Gynecol.* 99:9-17 (1967).

81. S. L. Skinner, E. R. Lumbers, and E. M. Symonds, Alterations by oral contraceptives on normal menstrual changes in plasma renin activity concentration and substrate. *Clin. Sci.* 36:67-76 (1969).

82. R. Beckerhoff, H. Armbruster, W. Vetter, J. Luetscher, and W. Siegenthaler, Plasma aldosterone during oral contraceptive therapy. *Lancet* 1: 1218-1220 (1973).

83. F. H. Katz and P. Beck, Plasma renin activity, renin substrate and aldosterone during treatment with various oral contraceptives. *J. Clin. Endocrinol.* 39:1001-1004 (1974).

84. D. S. Janowsky, R. Gorney, and A. J. Mandell, The menstrual cycle. *Arch. Gen. Psychiatry* 17:459-469 (1977).

85. N. Perrini and N. Piliego, The increase of aldosterone in the premenstrual syndrome. *Minerva Med.* 50:2897-2899 (1959).

86. L. I. Golub, H. Menduke, and S. S. Conley, Weight changes in college

women during the menstrual cycle. *Am. J. Obstet. Gynaecol.* 91:89-94
(1965).

87. P. E. Watson and M. Robinson, Variations in body weight of young women
during the menstrual cycle. *Br. J. Nutr.* 19:237-238 (1965).

88. M. Abramson and J. R. Torghele, Weight, temperature changes and psychosomatic symptomatology in relation to the menstrual cycle. *Am. J.
Obstet. Gynecol.* 81:223-232 (1961).

89. J. Bruce and G. F. M. Russel, A study of weight changes and balances of
water, sodium and potassium. *Lancet* 2:267-271 (1962).

90. G. W. Thorn, K. R. Nelson, and D. W. Thorn, A study of the mechanism
of edema associated with menstruation. *Endocrinology* 22:155-163 (1938).

91. R. L. Landau and K. Lugibihl, Catabolic and natriuretic effects of progesterone in man. *Recent Prog. Horm. Res.* 17:249-292 (1961).

92. B. Andersch, L. Hahn, M. Anderson, and B. Isaksson, Body water and
weight in patients with premenstrual tension. *Br. J. Obstet. Gynecol.* 85:
546-551 (1978).

93. W. G. Wong, R. I. Freedman, N. E. Levan, C. Hyman, and E. Quilligan,
Changes in the capillary filtration coefficient of cutaneous vessels in women with premenstrual tension. *Am. J. Obstet. Gynecol.* 114:950-953
(1972).

94. F. H. Netter, *The Endocrine System.* Ciba, New York, 1966.

95. G. W. DeMarchi and J. E. Tong, Menstrual, diurnal, and activation effects
on the resolution of temporally paired flashes. *Psychophysiology* 9:362-
367 (1972).

96. H. Kaulhausen, W. Oehm, and H. Breuer, Plasma renin activity during the
normal menstrual cycle. *Acta Endocrinol.* 173(Suppl.):160 (1973).

97. I. R. Johnson, Human endometrial renin levels during the menstrual cycle
(proceedings). *Br. J. Clin. Pharmacol.* 6:458P-459P (1978).

98. J. T. Fitzsimons, and B. J. Simons, The effect of drinking in the rat of intravenous infusion of angiotensin. *J. Physiol.* 203:45-57 (1969).

99. D. J. Paliac and P. A. Khairallah, Effect of angiotensin on uptake and release of norepinepnrine by brain. *Biochem. Pharmacol.* 16:2291-2298
(1967).

100. R. Capek, K. M. Masek, M. Sramka, M. Krsiak, and P. Svec, The similarities
of the angiotensin and bradykinin actions on the central nervous system.
Pharmacology 2:161-170 (1969).

101. J. M. Morgan and A. Routtenberg, Angiotensin injected into the neostriatum
after learning disrupts retention performance. *Science* 196:87-89 (1977).

102. W. B. Severs, A. E. Daniels, and J. P. Buckley, On the central hypertensive
effect of angiotensin II. *Int. J. Neuropharmacol.* 6:199-205 (1967).

103. W. B. Severs, J. Summy-Long, J. S. Taylor, and J. Connor, A central effect
of angiotensin: Release of pituitary pressor material. *J. Pharm. Ther.* 174:
27-34 (1970).

104. K. Fuxe, D. Ganten, T. Hökfelt, and P. Bolme, Immunohistochemical evidence for the existence of angiotensin II-containing nerve terminals in the brain and spinal cord in the rat. *Neurosci. Lett.* 2:229-234 (1976).

105. M. P. Printz and J. A. Lewicki, *Central Actions of Angiotensin and Related Hormones.* Pergamon Press, New York, 1977.

106. P. Ganten and G. Speck, The brain renin-angiotensin system: A model for the synthesis of peptides in the brain. *Biochem. Pharmacol.* 27:2379-2389 (1978).

107. D. J. Ramsay, The brain renin angiotensin systme: A re-evaluation. *Neuroscience* 4:313-321 (1979).

108. A. Vermeulen and L. Verdonck, Plasma androgen levels during the menstrual cycle. *Am. J. Obstet. Gynecol.* 125:491-494 (1976).

109. G. E. Abraham, Ovarian and adrenal contribution to peripheral androgens during the menstrual cycle. *J. Clin. Endocrinol. Metab.* 39:340-346 (1974).

110. W. O. Ribeiro, D. R. Mishell, and I. H. Thorneycroft, Comparison of the patterns of androstenedione, progesterone, and estradiol during the human menstrual cycle. *Am. J. Obstet. Gynecol.* 119:1026-1032 (1974).

111. M. S. Walker and S. McGilp, Excretory patterns of urinary free 11-hydroxy-corticosteroids and total oestrogens throughout the normal menstrual cycle. *Ann. Clin. Biochem.* 15:201-202 (1978).

112. A. R. Genazzani, T. Lemarchand-Beraud, M. L. Aubert, and J. Felber, Pattern of plasma ACTH, hGH and cortisol during the menstrual cycle. *J. Clin. Endocrinol. Metab.* 41:431-437 (1975).

113. M. L. Aubert, T. Lemarchand-Beraud, R. Peguillaume, and P. Desaulles, Cortisol secretion during the normal menstrual cycle. *Acta Endocrinol. (Copenh.)* 155:78 (1971).

114. B. N. Saxena, N. Dusitsin, and L. Lazarus, Human growth hormone, thyroid stimulating hormone and cortisol levels in the serum of menstruating Thai women. *J. Obstet. Gynaecol. Br. Commonw.* 81:563-567 (1974).

115. E. J. Sachar, Corticosteroids in depressive illness. *Arch. Gen. Psychiatry* 17:544-553 (1967).

116. W. F. Kelley, S. A. Checkley, and D. A. Bender, Cushing's syndrome, tryptophan and depression. *Br. J. Psychiatry* 136:125-132 (1980).

117. S. E. File and S. V. Vellucci, Studies on the role of ACTH and of 5-HT in anxiety, using an animal model. *J. Pharm. Pharmacol.* 30:105-110 (1977).

118. J. M. Abplanalp, L. Livingston, R. M. Rose, and D. Sandwich, Cortisol and growth hormone responses to psychological stress during the menstrual cycle. *Psychosom. Med.* 39:158-177 (1977).

119. A. Bertoli, R. DePerro, A. Fusco, A. Greco, R. Magnatto, and R. Lauro, Differences in insulin receptors between men and menstruating women

and influence of sex hormones on insulin binding during the menstrual cycle. *J. Clin. Endocrinol. Metab.* 50:246-250 (1980).

120. V. Halbreich, M. Ben-David, M. Assael, and R. Bronstein, Serum prolactin in women with premenstrual syndrome. *Lancet* 2:654-656 (1976).

121. A. N. Andersen, J. F. Larsen, O. R. Steenstrup, B. Svendstrup, and J. Nielsen, Effect of bromocriptine on the premenstrual syndrome. A double-blind clinical trial. *Br. J. Obstet. Gynecol.* 84:370-374 (1977).

122. J. J. Graham, P. E. Harding, P. H. Wise, and H. Berriman, Prolactin suppression in the treatment of premenstrual tension syndrome. *Med. J. Aust.* 2(3 Suppl.):18-20 (1978).

123. D. F. Horrobin, I. J. Lloyd, A. Lipton, P. Burstyn, N. Durkin, and K. Muiruri, Actions of prolactin on human renal function. *Lancet* 2:353-354 (1971).

124. S. Tamura and M. Igarashi, Serum prolactin levels during ovulatory menstrual cycle and menstrual disorders in women. *Endocrinol. Jpn.* 20:483-488 (1973).

125. M. Vekemans, P. Delvoye, M. L'Hermite, and C. Robyn, Serum prolactin levels during the menstrual cycle. *J. Endocrinol. Metab.* 44:989-993 (1977).

126. A. S. McNeilly, G. E. Evans, and T. Chard, Observations on prolactin levels during the menstrual cycle, in *Human Prolactin.* Excerpta Medica, Amsterdam, 1973.

127. G. Nattero, D. Bisbocci, and F. Ceresa, Sex hormone, prolactin levels, osmolarity and electrolyte patterns in menstrual migraine—relationship with fluid retention. *Headache* 19:25-30 (1979).

128. D. A. Adamopoulos, J. A. Loraine, S. F. Lunn, A. Coppen, and R. Daly, Endocrine profiles in premenstrual tension. *Clin. Endocrinol.* 283-292 (1972).

129. L. Wetterberg, J. Arendt, L. Paunier, P. Sizonenko, W. van Konselaar, and T. Hepden, Human serum melatonin changes during the menstrual cycle. *J. Clin. Endocrinol. Metab.* 42:185-188 (1976).

130. K. Hoffman, The action of melatonin on testis size and pelage color varies with season. *Int. J. Chronobiol.* 1:333 (1973).

131. D. C. Jimerson, H. J. Lynch, R. M. Post, P. Wurtman, and W. Bunney, Jr., Urinary melatonin rhythms during sleep deprivation in depressed patients and normals. *Life Sci.* 20:1501-1508 (1977).

132. F. Anton-Tay, Melatonin: Effects on brain function, in *Advances in Biochemical Psychopharmacology, Vol. II: Serotonin—New Vistas.* Raven Press, New York, 1979.

133. P. Patkai, G. Johannson, and B. Post, Mood, alertness, and sympathetic-adrenal medullary activity during the menstrual cycle. *Psychosom. Med.* 36:503-512 (1974).

134. H. Cramer, J. Rudolph, V. Consbruch, and K. Kendel, On the effects of melatonin on sleep and behavior in man, in *Advances in Biochemical Psychopharmacology, Vol. II: Serotonin–New Vistas* (E. Costa, G. L. Gessa, and M. Sandler, eds.). Raven Press, New York, 1974, pp. 187-191.

135. J. Carman, R. M. Post, R. Buswell, Negative effects of melatonin on depression. *Am. J. Psychiatry* 133:1181-1186 (1976).

136. J. D. Barchas, H. Akil, G. R. Elliot, R. Holman, and S. Watson, Behavioral neurochemistry: Neuroregulators and behavioral states. *Science* 200:964-978 (1978).

137. G. B. Colvin and C. H. Sawyer, Induction of running activity by intracerebral injections of estrogen in ovarectomized rats. *Neuroendocrinology* 4:309-320 (1969).

138. B. J. Meyerson and C. H. Sawyer, Monoamines and ovulation in the rat. *Endocrinology* 83:170-176 (1968).

139. A. Tagliamonte, P. Tagliamonte, and G. L. Gessa, Compulsive sexual activity induced by p-chlorophenylalanine in normal and pinealectomized male rats. *Science* 166:1433-1435 (1969).

140. C. Krodon, Effects of selective experimental changes in regional hypothalamic monoamine levels on superovulation in the immature rat. *Neuroendocrinology* 4:129-138 (1969).

141. M. M. Airaksinen and W. M. McIsaac, Estrus cycle in rats: The role of serotonin and norepinephrine. *Life Sci.* 7:471-476 (1968).

142. C. H. Sawyer, Stimulation of ovulation in the rabbit by intraventricular injection of epinephrine or norepinephrine. *Anat. Rec.* 112:385 (1952).

143. I. A. Kamberi, Effect of anterior pituitary perfusion and intraventricular injections of catecholamines and indoleamines on LH release. *Endocrinology* 87:1-12 (1970).

144. H. P. G. Schneider and S. M. McCann, Possible role of dopamine as transmitter to promote discharge of LH releasing factor. *Endocrinology* 85:121-132 (1969).

145. R. J. Wurtman and J. Axelrod, Sex steroids, cardiac, 3H-norepinephrine and tissue monoamine oxidase levels in the rat. *Biochem. Pharmacol.* 12:1417-1419 (1963).

146. G. G. S. Collins, J. Pryse-Davies, M. Sandler, and J. Southgate, Effect of pretreatment with oestradiol. Progesterone, and DOPA on monoamine oxidase activity in the rat. *Nature* 226:642-643 (1970).

147. E. L. Klaiber, Y. Kobayashi, D. M. Broverman, and F. Hall, Plasma monoamine oxidase activity in regularly menstruating women and in amenorrheic women receiving cyclic treatment with estrogens and a progesten. *J. Clin. Endocrinol.* 33:630-638 (1971).

148. E. C. G. Grant and J. Pryse-Davies, Effects of oral contraceptives on depressive mood changes and on endometrial monoamine oxidase and phosphatases. *Br. Med. J.* 111:777-780 (1968).

149. R. H. Belmaker, D. L. Murphy, R. J. Wyatt, and L. Loriaux, Human platelet monoamine oxidase changes during the menstrual cycle. *Arch. Gen. Psychiatry* 31:553-556 (1974).

150. A. Wirz-Justice, W. Pühringer, G. Hole, and R. Menzi, Monoamine oxidase and free tryptophan in human plasma. *Pharmakopsychiatr. Neuropsychopharmakol.* 8:310-317 (1975).

151. P. M. Greengrass and S. R. Toungue, Changes in brain monoamine concentrations during the oestrus cycle in the mouse: Possible pharmacologic implications. *J. Pharm. Pharmacol.* 23:897-898 (1971).

152. M. C. Boadle, J. Hughes, and R. H. Roth, Angiotensin accelerates catecholamine biosynthesis in sympathetically innervated tissues. *Nature* 222: 987-988 (1969).

153. S. A. Vogel, D. S. Janowsky, and J. M. Davis, Effect of estradiol stimulus-induced release of 3H-norepinephrine and 3H-serotonin from rat brain slices. *Res. Commun. Chem. Pathol. Pharmacol.* I:451-459 (1970).

154. D. S. Janowsky and J. M. Davis, Progesterone-estrogen effects of uptake and release of norepinephrine by synaptosomes. *Life Sci.* 9:525 (1970).

155. K. Fuxe, T. Hökfelt, and G. Jonsson, The effect of gonadal steroids on the tuberoinfundibular dopamine neurons, in *Hormonal Steroids.* Excerpta Medica, Hamburg, 1970.

156. S. Kalsner, Steroid potentiation of responses to sympathomimetic amines in aortic strips. *Br. J. Pharmacol.* 36:582-593 (1969).

157. M. M. Salseduc, I. I. Jofre, and J. A. Izquierdo, Monoamines oxidase and catechol-o-methyl transferase activity in cerebral structures and sexual organs of rats during their sexual cycle. *Med. Pharmacol. Exp.* 14:113-119 (1966).

158. F. Lamprecht, R. J. Matta, B. Little, and T. Zahn, Plasma DBH activity during the menstrual cycle. *Psychosom. Med.* 36:304-310 (1974).

159. J. S. Wiener, F. Elmadjian, Excretion of epinephrine and norepinephrine in premenstrual tension. *Fed. Proc.* 21:184 (1962).

160. F. A. DeLeon-Jones, J. Steinburg, H. Dekirmejian, and D. Garver, MHPG excretion during the menstrual cycle of women. *Commun. Psychopharmacol.* 2:267-274 (1978).

161. H. Beckman, F. K. Goodwin, Antidepressant response to tricyclics and urinary MHPG in unipolar patients. *Arch. Gen. Psychiatry* 32:17-21 (1975).

162. K. Ghose and P. Turner, The menstrual cycle and the tyramine pressor response test. *Br. J. Clin. Pharmacol.* 4:500-502 (1977).

163. E. Hackman, A. Wirz-Justice, and M. Lichtsteiner, The uptake of dopamine and serotonin in the rat brain during progesterone decline. *Psychopharmacologia* 32:183-191 (1973).

164. W. Ladisich, Influence of progesterone on serotonin metabolism: A possible causal factor for mood changes. *Psychoneuroendocrinology* 2:257-266 (1977).

165. F. Sicuteri, E. Del Bene, and C. Fonda, Sex, migraine and serotonin inter-relationships. *Monogr. Neural Sci.* 3:94-101 (1976).

166. P. M. Greengrass and S. R. Toungue, Brain monoamine metabolism in the mouse during the immediate post-partum period. *Br. J. Pharmacol.* 46: 533P-534P (1972).

167. A. Wirz-Justice and W. Pühringer, Seasonal incidence of an altered diurnal rhythm of platelet serotonin in unipolar depression. *J. Neural Transm.* 42:45-53 (1978).

168. J. Thomisto, E. Tukiainen, and U. G. Ahlfors, Decreased uptake of 5-hydroxytriptamine in blood platelets from patients with endogenous depression. *Psychopharmacology* 65:141-147 (1979).

169. A. Wirz-Justice and E. Chappius-Arntt, Sex specific differences in chlor-imipramine inhibition of serotonin uptake in human platelets. *Eur. J. Pharmacol.* 40:21-25 (1976).

170. B. D. Cox and D. P. Culame, Changes in plasma amino acid levels during the human menstrual cycle and in early pregnancy. A preliminary report. *Horm. Metabol. Res.* 10:428-433 (1978).

171. A. Lerdo de Tejada, Q. F. B. Ma. Estela Carreno, Q. F. I. Leonila Lopez, C. Wionczek, and S. Karchmen, Eliminacion urinaria de acido 5-hidroxi-indol acetico durante el ciclo menstrual humano. *Ginecol. Obstet. Mex.* 44:85-91 (1978).

172. W. A. Check, Old hormones reveal new surprises. *JAMA* 243:499-500 (1980).

173. F. Winston, Oral contraceptives, pyridoxine and depression. *Am. J. Psychiatry* 130:1217-1221 (1973).

174. N. Vijayan, V. K. Vijayan, and P. M. Dreyfus, Acetylcholinesterase activity and menstrual remissions in myasthenia gravis. *J. Neurol. Neurosurg. Psychiatry* 40:1060-1065 (1977).

175. D. S. Janowsky, M. K. El-Yousef, J. M. Davis, and H. J. Sekerke, A cholinergic-adrenergic hypothesis of mania and depression. *Lancet* 1:632-635 (1972).

176. K. Robinson, K. M. Huntington, and M. G. Wallace, Treatment of the premenstrual syndrome. *Br. J. Obstet. Gynecol.* 84:784-788 (1977).

Author Index

Aakvaag, A., 405(73), *421*

Abplanalp, J. M., 121(84), *127*, 181, 189, 190, *194*, 243(1), 244(1), *263*, 299(9), *315*, 351(40,41), *363*, 409(118), 410(118), *423*

Abraham, G. E., 370(31), *389*, 405 (77), 408(77), 409(109), *421*, *423*

Abrahamsson, L., 370(30), 374(30), 375(30), *389*

Abramson, M., 406(88), *422*

Abramson, P. R., 164, *173*

Abu-Fadil, S., 36(28), 38(32), *41*

Ach, N., 273, *283*

Adamopoulos, D. A., 410(128), *424*

Adams, D. B., 91, *94*, 132(13), 135 (20), 148(31), *152*, *153*, 168, 169, 170, *173*, *175*, 302, *316*, 349(17), *361*

Adams, P. W., 350(30), 353(30), *362*, 381(96), *393*

Addison, R. G., 101(7), 108(7), *123*

Addition, H., 101(7), 108(7), *123*

Adler, N. T., 44(1), 45(98), 48(2), *57*, *64*

Ahlfors, U. G., 414(168), *427*

Aijer, M. S., 67(61), *75*

Airaksinen, M. M., 411(141), *425*

Aitken, R. C. B., 229(21), *240*

Ajabor, L., 33(20), *41*

Åkerlund, M., 206(20), *215*

Akil, H., 411(136), *425*

Akiskal, H. S., 321, 325, 335, 336, *340*

Alagna, S., 381(89), *393*

Albala, A. A., 321, *340*

Alderete, M. R., 66(26), *73*

Al-Khouri, H., 236(34), *241*

Allen, W. M., 213, *216*

Alplanalp, J. M., 82, *94*

Altenhaus, A. L., 104, 116(47), 124 (47), *125*

Altschule, M., 352(80), *365*

Ambrosi, B., 293(18), *296*

Anastasi, H., 83, *94*

Andersch, B., 368(23), 369(23), 370 (30), 374(30), 375(30), *389,* 406 (92), *422*

Andersen, A. N., 374(62,63), 375 (63), 376(62), 377(68), *391, 392,* 410(121), *424*

Anderson, A. E., 293(17), *296*

Anderson, C. H., 402(58), *420*

Anderson, J. N., 18(44), *21*

Anderson, K. E., 206(20), *215*

Anderson, M., 406(92), *422*

Andersson, M., 368(23), 369(23), *389*

Ans, R., 293(21), *296*

Antebi, A., 202(6), *215*

Antonov, A. N., 149(35), *153*

Anton-Tay, F., 411(132), *424*

Antunes, J. L., 28(12), 29(9,11,12), 34(22,23), 35(23), *40, 41*

Aono, T., 27(8), *40*

Aparicio, N. J., 66(13), *73*

Apter, D., 150(38), *153,* 179, *194*

Araki, S., 32(16), *41*

Arendt, J., 411(129), *424*

Arezzini, C., 71(104), *76*

Arimura, A., 67(32), *74*

Armbruster, H., 406(82), *421*

Armitage, R., 91, *95*

Arnoff, M. S., 78, 82, 85, 89, *95*

Arnold, P. M., 104(36), 106(56), 108(56), 113(36), 116(36), 117 (56), 119(56), *124, 125,* 398(15), *418*

Aronoff, M. S., 327, 329, *341*

Arthur, M., 279, *287*

Asano, Y., 244(25), 245(25), *264,* 355(55), *364,* 397(4), *417*

Assael, M., 374(60), *391,* 410(120), *424*

Asso, D., 118(63,68), *126,* 222, *240,* 397(12), *417*

Atger, M., 19(46), *21*

Aubert, M. L., 409(112,113), 415(113), *423*

Auerbach, P., 44(3), *57*

Axelrod, J., 269, *289,* 412(145), *425*

Baccarini, I. M., 203(13), *215*

Bäckström, T., 371(40,41,42), *390,* 401(50), 402(50), 403(50,63), *419, 420*

Baird, D. T., 281, *283,* 402(57), *420*

Baker, A. H., 104, 115(44), *125*

Baker, M. A., 92, *94*

Baker, T. G., 7(4), *20*

Ball, P., 269, *283*

Ballinger, S., 355(54), *364*

Bancroft, J., 149(33), *153,* 349(20), *362*

Banks, M. H., 351(42), *363*

Barash, D., 112(26), *124*

Barchas, J. D., 411(136), *425*

Bardwick, J. M., 86, *95,* 163, *173, 174,* 328, *342,* 367(8), *388*

Barfield, M. A., 69(89), *76*

Barfield, R. J., 44(3,41), 46(45,89), 52(4,23), 55(85,89), *57, 59, 60, 63*

Baron, J., 90, *94*

Baron, M., 339, *341*

Barraclough, C. A., 67(56,57), *75*

Barron, A., 352(63), *364*

Barry, J., 71(105), *76*

Bartke, A., 71(98,99,101,102), *76*

Bates, P. E., 202(4), 206(4), *214*

Batho, K., 108, 119(73), *126,* 398(16), *418*

Baulieu, E.-E., 13(21), 17(39), 18(41), 19(46), *20, 21*

Baum, M. J., 46(5), *58,* 66(28), *73,* 140, *152*

Baumblatt, M. J., 353(81), *365*

Bauminger, S., 202(6), *215*

Bayard, F., 17(39), 18(41,43), *21*

Beach, F. A., 43(6), 44(9), 46(7,10), 48(10), *58*, 138(22), 139(22), 150(22), *152*

Beach, R. C., 348(2), *361*

Beardwood, C. J., 291(1), 292(12), 293(13), *295, 296*

Beattie, C. W., 268, 269, 270, *283*

Beaumont, P. J. V., 235(30), *241*, 323, *340*

Beck, A. T., 300(10,11), 310(10), 311(11), *315*

Beck, P., 406(83), *421*

Beck, R., 300(10), 310(10), *315*

Becker, D., 104(36), 106(56), 108 (56), 113(36), 116(36), 117(56), 119(56), *124, 125*, 398(15), *418*

Beckerhoff, R., 406(82), *421*

Beckman, H., 413(161), *426*

Beck-Peccoz, P., 293(18), *296*

Beech, H. R., 106, 118(63,65), *126*

Beery, R., 13(27), *20*

Behrman, H. R., 43(38), *60*

Behrman, S. J., 163, *173*

Beilby, J., 17(38), *21*

Belchetz, P. E., 33(17), 36(27), *41*

Bell, E. T., 292(11), *295*, 401(46), *419*

Belmaker, R. H., 381(90), *393*, 412 (149), *426*

Ben-David, M., 374(60), *391*, 410 (120), *424*

Bender, D. A., 409(116), *423*

Benedek, T., 86, 90, *94*, 131(12), *152*, 159, 160, 161, 162, 163, 172, *173, 174*, 299(2), 300, 302, 314, *315*, 328, 339, *340*, 399(24), 404(24), *418*

Benedek-Jaszmann, L. J., 234, *241*, 375(66), *391*

Benkert, O., 66(12), *73*

Bennett, S., 348(3), 351(3), 357(3), *361*

Berens, S. C., 370(32), *389*, 397(5), 407(5), 413(5), 415(5), *417*

Beresford, S. A., 351(42), *363*

Bergen, J., 351(44), *363*

Berger, G. S., 233(27), *241*, 348(15), *361*

Bergland, R. M., 8(8), *20*, 29(10), *40*

Bergman, E., 300(10), 310(10), *315*

Bergsjo, P., 177, *194*

Bernstein, B. E., 102, 112(31), 122 (31), *124*

Berriman, H., 375(65), 376(65), 377 (65), *391*, 410(122), *424*

Bertoli, A., 410(119), *423*

Besser, G. M., 66(11,14), *73*

Best, F. A., 202(12), *215*

Bex, F. J., 71(99), *76*

Beyer, C., 45(64), 46(47), 49(64), *60, 62*, 403(65), *420*

Bickers, W., 179, 184, *194*, 202(9), *215*

Biegon, A., 54(55), *61*

Billig, O., 352(78,79), *365*

Billings, J. J., 159, *174*

Billingsley, P. A., 92, *94*

Birnbaumer, L., 16(33), *21*

Birtchnell, J., 243(19), *264*

Bisbocci, D., 410(127), *424*

Bishop, W., 67(65), *75*

Biskind, M. S., 239(44), *242*

Black, I. B., 52(50), *61*, 268, *286*

Blake, C. A., 67(71), *75*

Blandau, R. J., 45(14), *58*

Blaustein, J. D., 46(12,13), 53(11,13), *58*

Bleuler, M., 404(72), *421*

Blüm, V., 69(93), *76*

Blumberg, A., 352(78), *365*

Blümel, A., 235(33), *241*

Boadle, M. C., 412(152), *426*

Bock, R., 352(56), 355(56), *364*

Bogdanove, E. M., 67(66), *75*

Bogumil, R. J., 7(6), *20,* 23(1), *40*
Bohnert, M., 300(11), 311(11), *315*
Bohnet, H. G., 293(14), *296*
Boling, J. L., 45(14), *58*
Bolme, P., 408(104), *423*
Bonsall, R. W., 140(24), *152,* 167, 173, *175*
Booth, J. E., 55(15,28), *58, 59*
Borghi, A., 295(35), *297*
Borison, R. L., 326, *341*
Bornstein, R., 374(60), *391*
Boss, A. M. B., 293(15), *296*
Bouffard, J. A., 397(10), *417*
Bower, W., 352(80), *365*
Boyar, R. J., 33(18), *41*
Boyar, R. M., 293(26), 294(28,30, 31), *297*
Bradley, J., 352(79), *365*
Brast, N., 158, *175,* 367(7), 380(7), 386(7), *388*
Brazeau, P., 67(38,40), *74*
Brenner, M. A., 15(30), *21*
Brett, E., 120(80), *127*
Breuer, H., 36(30), *41,* 269, *283,* 408(96), *422*
Brierre de Boisment, A., 320, *340*
Briggs, M., 268, *284*
Brightman, V. J., 108(11), 124(11), *123*
Brodie, H. K. H., 66(15), *73*
Bronstein, R., 410(120), *424*
Brooks, B., 317, 329, *340*
Brooks, J., 85, *94,* 305(35), 306(35), 309, *316*
Brooksbank, B. W. L., 150(40), *153*
Brooks-Gunn, J., 87, *98,* 121(82,86), *127,* 177, 178, 179, 180, 181, 182, 186, 190, 194, *194, 195, 196*
Broverman, D. M., 91, *94,* 106(42), 108(71,72), 114(42), 118(66), 119(66,71,72), *125, 126,* 268,

[Broverman]
   269, 270, 271, 272, 273, 274, 275, 276, 277, 278, 280, 282, *284, 286, 287, 288,* 351(33,43), 353(33,43), *362, 363,* 371(37,38), 381(38), *390,* 398(17), 412(147), *418, 425*
Brown, M., 38(34), *41,* 65(2), *72*
Brown, S., 380(84), *393*
Brown, S. E., 279, *287*
Brown, W. L., 348(7,8), 354(7), *361,* 379(81), *392*
Brown-Parlee, M., 243(2), *263*
Bruce, J., 368(22), *389,* 406(89), *422*
Bruns, M., 162, *174*
Brush, M. G., 229(18), 238(18), *240,* 371(44), 373(44), 374(56), 375 (44), 381(56), 387(56), *390, 391,* 401(49), *419*
Brut, A. D., 302(34), *316*
Bryan, W. L., 275, *284*
Buckley, J. P., 408(102), *422*
Budoff, P. W., 207(24), *216*
Bugat, R., 18(43), *21*
Bunney, W., Jr., 411(131), *424*
Burger, H. G., 67(62), *75*
Burrows, G., 243(3), 244(3), *263*
Burstyn, P., 410(123), *424*
Burt, A. D., 91, *94,* 148(31), *153,* 170, *173,* 349(17), *361*
Buswell, R., 411(135), *425*
Butler, W. R., 25(5), *40*
Butterstein, G. M., 56(16), *58*
Bychowski, G., 320, *340*

Calabresi, E., 295(35), *297*
Calamera, J. C., 66(13), *73*
Callaway, E., III, 274, *284*
Campbell, S., 235(32), *241,* 279, *284,* 372(49), *390*
Cancro, R., 325, *340*
Capek, R., 408(100), 413(100), *422*

Carett, B., 67(43), *74*

Carette, B., 71(106), *76*

Carlson, R. A., 13(26), *20*

Carman, J., 411(135), *425*

Carmel, P. W., 29(9,11), 32(16), 34 (22,23,24), 35(23), 38(33,36), *40, 41, 42*

Carminate, R., 71(104), *76*

Carney, A., 149(33), *153*

Carperntier, J., 13(18), *20*

Carr, W. J., 44(17), *58*

Carrer, H. F., 67(55), *75*

Carrol, B. J., 317, 324, 326, 330, *342*

Carroll, B. J., 177, 190, *195, 196,* 243(4), 254(35), *263, 265,* 299(6), 300(18), *315, 316,* 321, 325, *340, 344,* 374(58), 377(70), 378(75), 383(70), 385(58,109), *391, 392, 394,* 399(23), 402(23), 403(23), 408(23), 409(23), 414(23), *418*

Carstensen, H., 371(40,41), *390*

Carter, C. S., 56(36), *60*

Castaneda, T. A., 279, 283, *285*

Catt, K. J., 11(16), 13(19), *20*

Cattani, G., 295(35), *297*

Cavanagh, J. R., 132(15), *152*

Cavanaugh, J. R., 157, 158, *174*

Ceresa, F., 410(127), *424*

Cerutti, R., 230, *240*

Chan, W. Y., 202(10), 203(10), 204, 207(10,25), *215, 216,* 397(6), *417*

Chan, Y. W., 385(111,112,113), 386 (111), 387(112), *394*

Chang, H.-S., 91, *95,* 131(11), 132 (11), *152*

Chang, R. J., 27(7), *40*

Chappuis-Arndt, E., 54(46), *60,* 414 (169), *427*

Chaptal, C. V., 49(58), 55(24,58), *59, 61*

Chard, T., 410(126), *424*

Charney, N., 349(21), *362*

Chaussain, J. L., 293(22), *296*

Check, W. A., 415(172), *427*

Checkley, S. A., 409(116), *423*

Chen, J. J., 52(4), *57*

Cheng, M. F., 66(25), *73*

Cheng, R., 234(29), *241,* 325, *343,* 378(72), *392*

Chernovetz, M. E., 354(48), *363*

Chesney, M. A., 181, 182, *195,* 383 (107), *394*

Chiappa, S. A., 34(25), *41*

Christensen, L. W., 52(18), *58*

Chud, L., 66(29), 67(29), *73*

Cianchetti, C., 158, *174*

Clare, A. W., 243(9), *263,* 367(1), *388*

Clark, A., 131(6), *152,* 305(35), 306 (35), 309(35), *316*

Clark, J. H., 18(44), 19(45,48), *21,* 44(19), *58*

Clarke, A. E., 85, *94,* 120(78), 121 (86), *127,* 178, 180, 181, 187, *195, 196*

Clarkin, J., 78, 82, 85, 89, *95,* 327, 329, *341*

Clarkson, F., 275. *288*

Clayton, R. B., 79, 89, 91, 93, *96, 97,* 104(52), 106(52), 117(52), 118 (52), *125,* 157, *175*

Clemens, L. G., 52(18), 55(20), *58, 59*

Cobbin, D., 355(54), *364*

Cochi, D., 71(104), *76*

Cole, E. N., 374(57), *391*

Collins, G. G. S., 412(146), *425*

Collins, W. P., 235(32), *241,* 372(49), 386(116), 387(116), *390, 395*

Colquhoun, W. P., 91, *94*

Colvin, G. B., 403(64), 411(137), *420, 425*

Coniglio, L. P., 55(20), *59*

Conley, S. S., 406(86), *421*

Connor, J., 408(103), *422*

Conroy, R. W., 353(58), 355(58), *364*

Consbruch, V., 411(134), *425*

Coppen, A. J., 232, 238(40), *241,* 312(37), *316,* 319, 323, 324, 325, 326, 336, *340,* 354(47), *363,* 367(2), 369(27), 370(27), 375(64), 379(80), 380(27), 381 (97), *388, 389, 391, 392, 394,* 399(28), 410(128), *418, 424*

Coppen, W. R., 79, 83, *94*

Cormack, M., 398(13), *417*

Corner, G. W., 1, *20*

Corstensen, H., 401(50), 402(50), 403(50), *419*

Costin, A., 270, *284*

Coutinho, E. M., 201(1), 202(4,5), *214*

Cowchock, S., 25(3), 26(3), *40*

Cowley, J. J., 150(40), *153*

Cox, B. D., 414(170), *427*

Coy, D. H., 68(83), *75*

Cramer, H., 411(134), *425*

Cramer, O. M., 67(56), *75*

Crane, M. G., 405(78), 406(78), *421*

Craven, D., 239(43), *242,* 370(33), 372(33), 375(33), *390,* 401(51), 406(51), 407(51), *419*

Creasman, W. T., 279, 283, *285*

Creutzfeldt, O. D., 104(36), 106, 108, 113(36), 116(36), 117(56), 119(56), *124, 125,* 398(15), *418*

Crews, D., 66(26), *73*

Crisp, A. H., 292(8), *295*

Critchlow, B. V., 67(52), *74*

Croix, D., 71(105), *76*

Crowley, W. R., 54(22), 55(21), *59,* 269, 270, *284*

Csank, J., 274, *286*

Csapo, A. I., 204(16), *215,* 385(110, 114), 386(115), *394, 395*

Cuatrecasas, P., 13(17), *20*

Culame, D. P., 414(170), *427*

Cullberg, J., 245(26), 255(26), *264,* 323, 327, *340,* 348(16), 353(16), 360(16), *361,* 379(78), 380(78), 385(78), *392,* 402(62), *420*

Dahlen, H. G., 66(12), *73,* 293(14), *296*

Daiguji, M., 244(25), 245(25), *264,* 355(55), *364,* 397(4), *417*

Dally, P., 291(2), *295*

Dalterio, S., 71(98,99), *76*

Dalton, K., 79, 80, 81, *94, 95,* 101(9), 102, 108(12,13), 111(24,25), 112 (25,26), *123, 124,* 181, *195,* 217 (2), 219(3), 222(3), 223(3,5,6,7,8, 9,10,11,12), 226(3,16), 227(3), 228(16), 233(16,25), 237(2,16,37), *240, 241,* 243(12,13), *264,* 323, 324, 326, *340, 341,* 354(50), 359 (68), *363, 364,* 367(13), 370(13), 371(13), 372(13,47,48), 373(13, 48), 378(13), 383(13), 386(13), *388, 390,* 398(20), 399(20), 402 (20,60), 404(60), 405(20), 415 (20), *418, 420*

Dalton, M. E., 227(17), 236(17), *240*

Daly, C. D., 327, *340*

Daly, R. L., 118, *126,* 352(64), 358 (64), *364,* 410(128), *424*

Daly, V., 243(23), 244(23), *264,* 300 (16), *316,* 325, *343,* 400(33), *418*

Damilano, S., 17(39), 18(41), *21*

Dan, A. J., 90, *95,* 101(4), *123*

Daniels, A. E., 408(102), *422*

Daris, J. M., 269, *285*

DasGupta, P. K., 268, *288*

Davidson, D. W., 349(20), *362*

Davidson, J. M., 52(39), *60,* 251(31), 253(31), *265*

Davies, I. J., 49(67), *62*
Davies, T. F., 66(14), *73*
Davis, J., 359(70), *365*
Davis, J. M., 370(32), *389,* 397(2,5),
    403(2), 407(5), 408(2), 413(2,5,
    153,154), 415(5), 416(175), *417,*
    426, 427
Davis, K. B., 131, *152,* 156, *174*
Davis, P. G., 48(2), 52(23,25,56,77),
    55(24), *57, 59, 61, 63*
Dawood, M. Y., 202(10), 203(10),
    204, 207(10,25), *215, 216,* 385
    (112,113), 387(112), *394*
Day, J. B., 229(18), 238(18), *240,*
    374(55), 382(55), *391*
De Allende, I. L. C., 270, 274, *284*
deBruin, A. T., 108, 119(70), *126*
DeGrazia, C., 16(37), *21*
DeGroff, V., 54(55,78), *61, 63*
Dekirmejian, H., 413(160), *426*
Delaney, J., 177, *195*
Del Bene, E., 414(165), *427*
DeLeon-Jones, F. A., 413(160), *426*
Delitala, G., 381(89), *393*
Delvoye, P., 410(125), *424*
DeMarchi, G. W., 89, 93, *95,* 407
    (95), *422*
Demers, L. M., 203(14), *215*
Denef, C., 49(26), *59*
Dennerstein, L., 243(3), 244(3),
    263
DePerro, R., 410(119), *423*
Derewicz, H. J., 238(39), *241*
Desaulles, P., 409(113), 415(113),
    423
Desclin, J., 71(109), 72(109), *76*
DeSombre, E. R., 13(20), *20*
De Souza, V. F. A., 292(12), 293(13,
    15), *296*
Dessert, N., 66(15), *73*
Detre, T. P., 253(33), *265*
Deutsch, H., 320, 328, *341,* 399(25),
    418

de Vigne, J., 321, *340*
De Villa, L., 381(89), *393*
DeVoogd, T. J., 56(36), *60*
Devoto, M. C., 158, *174*
De Wardener, H. E., 239(42), *242*
Diakow, C., 67(80), *75*
Diamond, A. L., 93, *95,* 117(60), *126*
Diamond, B. I., 326, *341*
Diamond, M., 93, *95,* 117(60), *126*
Diamond, S. B., 243(22), 244(22),
    264, 312, *316,* 325, *341*
Dickey, R. P., 91, *96,* 104(40), 106
    (40), 114(40), *124,* 179, 184, *195*
Diczfalusy, E., 43(27), *59*
Diefenbach, W. P., 38(33), *41*
Dienstbier, R. A., 86, 91, *95,* 131(11),
    132(11), *152,* 178, *195*
Dierschke, D. J., 25(5), *40*
Dillman, W. H., 15(29), *21*
DiMarchi, G. W., 108, 117(58), 118
    (58), *125*
Di Mascio, A., 157, *175,* 351(32), *362*
Dissinger, M. L., 44(17), *58*
Distiller, L. A., 66(16), *73*
Djenderedjian, A. H., 321, 325, 335,
    336, *340*
Dlausner, E., 324, 329, *343*
Doering, C. H., 66(15,27), *73*
Doerr, P., 294(29), *297*
Doherty, P. C., 71(101,102,103), *76*
Donnelly, A. F., 121(84), *127,* 351
    (40,41), *363*
Dor-Shav, N. K., 104, 106, 115(45),
    125
Doty, R. L., 80, *95,* 101(2), *122,* 145
    (30), *153,* 167, 173, *174*
Doughty, C., 55(28), *59*
Douglas, V. I., 275, *284*
Downie, J., 202(8), *215*
Doyle, M. P., 82, *96,* 118(64), *126,*
    354(46), *363,* 400(38), 409(38),
    419
Drago, F., 71(100), *76*

Drake, D., 275, *284*

Draper, K. C., 381(87), *393*

Dravnicks, A., 151(42), *153*

Dreyfus, P. M., 415(174), *427*

Drye, R. C., 321, *341*

Dudley, C. A., 65(3,4), 66(9,10,29), 67(3,29,35,36,39,41,42,47), 68 (3,84), 69(3,41,84,85), 72(4,112), *72, 73, 74, 75, 76*

Dufau, M. L., 11(16), 13(19), *20*

Duffy, T., 348(6), *361*

Dunner, D. L., 243(22), 244(22), *264,* 312(38), *316,* 322, 325, *341,* 386(118), *395*

Durkin, N., 410(123), *424*

Dusitsin, N., 409(114), *423*

Dyball, R. E. J., 67(33), *74*

Dyer, R. G., 67(33), *74*

Dyk, R. B., 275, *289*

Dyrenfurth, I., 7(6), *20,* 23(1), 25(3), 26(3), 29(9), 34(22), *40, 41,* 293 (21), *296*

D'Zmura, T. L., 328, 339, *341*

Eagleson, H. E., 110(17), *123*

Eakin, S., 275, *284*

Edwards, D. A., 69(88), *76*

Ehrensing, R. H., 66(17), 72(110), *73, 76*

Ehrhardt, A. A., 350(27,28), *362*

Ehrlich, P., 10(14), *20*

Ekstein, R., 320, *341*

Elde, R., 67(30), *73*

Elliot, G. R., 411(136), *425*

Elmadjian, F., 413(159), *426*

El-Yousef, M. K., 416(175), *427*

Endicott, J., 243(6,7,8), 246(6), 248(6), 250(29,30), 259(6), *263, 265,* 300(20), 301, *316,* 317, 322, 330, 334, 336, *343, 344*

Endo, M., 244(25), 245(25), *264,*

[Endo] 355(55), *364,* 397(4), *417*

Engelund, A., 280, *285*

Engen, T., 397(10), *417*

Englander-Golden, P., 86, 91, *95,* 131 (11), 132(11), *152,* 178, *195*

Erickson, G. F., 10(13), 16(36), *20, 21*

Ernst, M. L., 279, *286,* 355(53), *364*

Eskay, R. L., 67(63), *75*

Eskildsen, P. C., 377(68), *392*

Esquirol, E., 320, *341*

Etgen, A. M., 52(29), *59*

Euller, E., 381(94), *393*

Evans, G. E., 410(126), *424*

Evans, I. M., 66(16), *73*

Evarts, E. V., 274, *286*

Evered, D., 374(57,59), 377(59), *391*

Everett, J. W., 67(53,54,59,69), *74, 75*

Everitt, B. J., 54(30), *59,* 140(23), *152*

Ewing, J., 352(64), 358(64), *364*

Facchinetti, F., 158, *174*

Faglia, G., 293(18), *296*

Faiman, C., 179, *197*

Fann, W. E., 397(2), 403(2), 408(2), 413(2), *417*

Faterson, H. F., 275, *289*

Fawcett, C. P., 67(65), *75*

Feder, H. H., 45(31), 46(32), 53(11), *58, 59*

Feichtinger, W., 381(94), *393*

Feighner, J. P., 325, 330, *341*

Feinberg, M., 321, *340*

Feinstein, A. R., 283, *285*

Felber, J., 409(112), *423*

Felice, M., 314, *316*

Felthous, A. R., 353(58), 355(58), *364*

Ferin, M., 2(3), 7(6), *20,* 23(1), 25(3), 26(3), 28(12), 29(9,11,12), 32(16), 34(22,23,24), 35(23), 38(33,36), *40, 41, 42,* 91, *95*

Ferrari, C., 293(18), *296*

Ferrero, G., 158, *174*

Fichter, M. M., 294(29), *297*

Field, P. M., 56(79,80), *63*

Fieve, R. R., 243(22), 244(22), *264,* 312(38), *316,* 322, 325, *341,* 386 (118), *395*

File, S. E., 409(117), *423*

Fink, G., 34(25), *41,* 67(58,61,62), 75

Finkelstein, H., 33(18), *41*

Finkelstein, J. W., 150(39), *153,* 293(26,27), *297*

Fioretti, P., 158, *174*

Firsch, R. E., 185, *195*

Fisher, R. A., 66(11), *73*

Fisher, S., 82, *97*

Fishman, J., 294(30), *297*

Fisk, N., 350(25), *362*

Fitzpatrick, C., 348(13), *361*

Fitzsimons, J. T., 408(98), *422*

Fleiss, J. L., 245(28), *264,* 322, *341*

Fleming, O., 348(9), *361*

Flerko, B., 67(32,67), *74, 75*

Flieder, K., 69(93), *76*

Floren, A., 352(63), *364*

Flores, F., 49(67), *62*

Florey, C. D., 274, *284*

Floru, R., 270, *284*

Flower, R. J., 386(119), 387(119), *395*

Floyd, S., 243(19), *264*

Flye, B., 322, 336, *344*

Flynn, W. E., 106(74), *126,* 351(39), *363*

Folkard, J., 350(30), 353(30), *362,* 381(96), *393*

Fonda, C., 414(165), *427*

Fontana, J., 203(14), *215*

Ford, A., 275, *285*

Ford, M., 167, 173, *174*

Foreman, M. M., 66(9,18,20), 67(36), 69(90), *73, 74, 76*

Forest, M. G., 46(40), *60*

Forte, G., 295(35), *297*

Fortin, J. N., 367(12), *388*

Foulkes, D., 161, *175*

Foulkes, P., 90, *99*

Fox, T. O., 51(91), *64*

Frank, R. T., 217, *239,* 299(1), *315,* 320, 323, 327, *341,* 371(34), *390,* 401(43), 403(43), *419*

Frantz, A. G., 29(9), 34(22), 38(33, 36), *40, 41, 42,* 69(91), *76*

Fraser, T. R., 292(10), *295*

Frasier, S. D., 179, *196*

Frazier, T. M., 80, *95*

Freed, S. C., 238, *241*

Freedman, R. I., 369(26), *389,* 406 (93), *422*

Freeman, H., 351(44), *363*

Freeman, S. K., 140(25), *152*

Freis, E. S., 56(16), *58*

Freud, S., 302(22), *316,* 399(26), *418*

Freund, A., 122(87), *127*

Freychet, P., 13(18), *20*

Friedman, E., 108(11), 124(11), *123*

Friedman, J., 108, 118(67), 119(67), *126*

Friedman, R. C., 78, 82, 85, 89, *95,* 327, 329, *341*

Friedman, S., 349(24), *362*

Friedrich, F., 381(94), *393*

Friend, J. N., 295(34), *297*

Fries, H., 349(23), *362,* 378(74), *392*

Frisk, M., 179, 185, *195, 196*

Frosch, J., 320, *341*

Fuchs, A.-R., 202(4,5), 206(4,21), *214, 216*

Fuchs, F., 202(4,10), 203(10), 204, 206(4,21), 207(10,25), *214, 215, 216,* 385(113), *394*
Fulmek, R., 381(94), *393*
Funk, I. C., 274, *287*
Fusco, A., 410(119), *423*
Fusi, S., 295(35), *297*
Fuxe, K., 54(30), *59,* 71(107), *76,* 408(104), 413(155), *423, 426*

Gallagher, J. R., 177, *195*
Gamberale, F., 104, 106, 116(49), 117(49), 118(49), *125*
Gambrell, R. D., 279, 283, *285*
Gammel, G., 66(12), *73*
Gannon, L., 182, *196*
Ganten, D., 408(104), *423*
Ganten, P., 408(106), *423*
Garfield, S. L., 274, *285*
Garnier, P. E., 293(22), *296*
Garver, D., 413(160), *426*
Garvin, J. E., 368(24), *389*
Gaston, J. B., 397(8), *417*
Gay, V. L., 9(10), *20*
Gebhard, P. H., 302(30,31), *316*
Geier, A., 13(27), *20*
Gelder, M. G., 323, *340*
Genazzani, A. R., 158, *174,* 409 (112), *423*
Gerall, A. A., 55(88), *63*
Gerkinds, V. R., 279, *287*
Gerlach, L., 34(24), *41*
Gershon, S., 325, 326, *343,* 378(73), *392*
Gershon, E. S., 339, *341*
Gessa, G. L., 71(100), *76,* 411(139), 412(139), *425*
Geyer, L. A., 44(3), *57*
Ghose, K., 238(40), *241,* 375(64), *391,* 414(162), *426*
Gibbon, M., 317, 322, 334, 336, *343*

Gibbs, F., 404(71), *421*
Gilbert, J., 274, *284*
Giles, P. F. H., 383(106), *394*
Gill, D. K., 235(32), *241,* 372(49), *390*
Gladue, B. A., 55(20), *59*
Glanville, E. V., 93, *95,* 397(11), 400 (11), *417*
Glass, G. S., 323, 324, *341*
Gleser, G. C., 328, 339, *341*
Glick, I. D., 346(77), 348(3), 351(3, 37), 353(37,49,57), 354(49), 355 (57), 357(3), 359(37), 360(49), *361, 363, 364, 365*
Glotfelthy, J. S., 270, *288*
Gold, A. R., 91, *94,* 132(13), 135(20), 148(31), *152, 153,* 168, 169, 170, *173, 175,* 302(34), *316,* 349(17), *361*
Gold, S., 314(39), *316*
Golder, M. G., 235(30), *241*
Goldfein, A., 353(49), 354(49), 360 (49), *363*
Goldfien, A., 349(24), *362*
Goldfoot, D. A., 140(25), *152*
Golub, L. I., 406(86), *421*
Golub, S., 102, 104, 106, 113(35), *124,* 377(71), *392*
Gomes-Pan, A., 66(14), *73*
Gomez-Mont, F., 291(4), *295*
Gonzaga, F. P., 367(11), *388*
Goodenough, D. R., 273, 275, *285, 289*
Goodwin, F. K., 413(161), *426*
Gordan, G. S., 283, *285*
Gordon, J. H., 56(34), *59,* 326, *341*
Gorden, P., 13(18), *20*
Gore, M. B. R., 293(15), *296*
Gorney, R., 79, *95,* 400(41), 406(84), 408(84), *419, 421*
Gorski, J., 13(26), *20*
Gorski, R. A., 48(33), 52(76), 56(34),

[Gorski]
   59, 63, 67(72,78,79), *75*
Gottschalk, L. A., 328, 339, *341*
Goy, R. W., 43(97), *64,* 140(25),
   152
Graff, H., 324, 329, *341*
Graham, J. J., 375(65), 376(65),
   377(65), *391,* 410(122), *424*
Grant, E. C. G., 326, 327, *341,* 401
   (48), 406(48), 412(148), *419,*
   425
Grant, J., 314(39), *316*
Grant, L. D., 67(50), *74*
Gray, H. E., 66(24), *73*
Gray, L. A., 226, *240,* 323, *341,*
   373(51), *391*
Gray, M. J., 405(75), *421*
Greco, A., 410(119), *423*
Greden, J. F., 321, *340*
Green, K., 204(17), 207(23), *215,*
   216
Green, R., 45(35), *60,* 217(2),
   237(2), *240*
Greenberg, S. G., 283, *285*
Greene, R., 323, 326, *341,* 367(15),
   388, 402(60), 404(60), *420*
Greengrass, P. M., 268, *285,* 412
   (151), 414(166), *426, 427*
Greenhill, J. D., 238, *241*
Greenough, W. T., 56(36), *60*
Greenstein, B. D., 236(34), *241*
Greenward, G. S., 402(58), *420*
Gren, R., 350(25), *362*
Griffith, M., 164, *174*
Grinker, R. R., 321, *341*
Grisanti, G. C., 350(27,28), *362*
Gross, H. A., 386(118), *395*
Grunebaum, H. U., 324, *342*
Gudelsky, G. A., 37(31), 38(31), *41*
Guevara, A., 402(57), *420*
Guillemin, R., 38(34), *41*
Gunderson, J. G., 321, 322, 336, *342*

Gurpide, E., 19(49,50,51), *21*
Gusberg, S. B., 19(50), *21,* 279, *285*
Guze, S. B., 325, 330, *341*

Hackman, E., 414(163), *426*
Haggard, M., 397(8), *417*
Hahn, L., 368(23), 369(23), 370(30),
   374(30), 375(30), *389,* 406(92),
   422
Hai, M. T. V., 17(40), *21*
Halasz, B., 34(21), 35(21), *41,* 67(68,
   72), *75*
Halberg, F., 2(3), *20*
Halbert, D. R., 203(14), *215*
Halbreich, U., 243(6,7,8), 246(6), 248
   (6), 259(6), *263,* 301(19), *316,* 374
   (60), *391,* 410(120), *424*
Hall, F., 108(71), 119(71), *126,* 268,
   269, 270, *286,* 371(37), *390,* 412
   (147), *425*
Hall, P. G., 400(40), *419*
Hall, R., 66(14), *73*
Hall, W. J., 202(12), *215*
Halmi, K. A., 293(16,19,20), *296*
Hamburg, D. A., 66(15,27), *73, 79,*
   97, 104(52), 106(52), 117(52),
   118(52), *125,* 157, *174, 175,* 359
   (69,74), *365,* 402(54), 414(54),
   420
Hamilton, G. V., 156, *174*
Hamilton, M., 276, *285*
Hammond, J., 233(27), *241*
Hammond, L. B., 279, 283, *285*
Hander, J. P., 66(14), *73*
Hansen, M. K., 206(19), *215*
Hansson, R. O., 354(48), *363*
Harding, P. E., 375(65), 376(65), 377
   (65), *391,* 410(122), *424*
Harding, S. S., 86, *98*
Harkness, R. A., 292(11), *295*
Harmatz, J. S., 157, *175,* 383(104), *394*

Harner, R., 398(18), 404(18), *418*

Harris, G. W., 43(37), *60*

Harris, J. J., 405(78), 406(78), *421*

Harrop, G. A., 406(79), *421*

Hart, R. D., 156, 157, *174*

Harter, N., 275, *284*

Hartley, L. R., 91, *95*

Haskett, R. F., 181, 189, 190, *194,
    195,* 243(1), 244(1), 254(35),
    263, 265, 299(9), 300(18), *315,
    316,* 317, 321, 324, 325, 326,
    330, *340, 342, 344,* 377(70),
    378(75), 383(70), *392*

Haupt, M., 269, *283*

Hauptman, B., 351(37), 353(37),
    359(37), *363*

Haynes, R. C., Jr., 381(88), *393*

Heald, F. P., 177, *195,* 314(39),
    316

Hearn-Sturtevant, M. D., 234, *241,*
    375(66), *391*

Heiman, J. R., 158, 165, *174*

Held, B., 18(42), *21*

Hellman, L., 33(18), *41,* 293(26,27),
    294(30), *297*

Helmer, O. M., 402(53), 406(80),
    414(53), *420, 421*

Helper, M. M., 274, *285*

Henderson, B. E., 279, *287*

Hendricks, C. H., 201(3), *214*

Heninger, G. R., 323, 324, *341*

Henkin, R. I., 92, *95,* 118, *126*

Henzl, M. R., 204(16), *215,* 385
    (114), *395*

Hepden, T., 411(129), *424*

Herbert, J., 92, *96,* 140(23), *152*

Heritage, A. S., 67(50), *74*

Herrman, G., 243(23), 244(23), *264,*
    300(16), *316,* 325, *343,* 400(33),
    418

Herrmann, W. L., 279, *288*

Herrmann, W. M., 348(2), *361*

Hertz, D. G., 90, *95*

Herzberg, B. N., 354(47), *363,* 379
    (80), 380(84), 381(87), *392, 393*

Hill, J. C., 385(111), 386(111), *394*

Hineman, S., 300(16), *316,* 325, *343,*
    400(33), *418*

Hoch, P. H., 320, *342*

Hoff, J. D., 293(23), *296*

Hoffman, K., 411(130), *424*

Hökfelt, T., 54(30), *59,* 67(30), 71
    (107), *73, 76,* 408(104), 413(155),
    423, 426

Holberg, F., 91, *95*

Holderg, I., 243(16), *264*

Holding, T. A., 300(17), *316*

Hole, G., 412(150), 413(150), 414
    (150), *426*

Hollenberg, M. D., 13(17), *20*

Hollingworth, H. L., 274, *285*

Hollingworth, L. S., 110(16), *123*

Holman, R., 411(136), *425*

Hoon, E. F., 158, *176*

Hoon, P. W., 158, *176*

Hopson, J. L., 173, *174*

Horney, J., 243(18), *264*

Horney, K., 302, *316*

Horowitz, R. I., 283, *285*

Horrobin, D. F., 69(95), *76,* 374(57,
    59), 377(59), *391,* 410(123), *424*

Hortling, H., 179, 185, *195, 196*

Horton, R., 281, *283*

Hostetter, G., 68(81), 69(81), *75*

Hotchkiss, J., 25(5), *40*

Hrbek, J., 383(103), *394*

Hseuh, A. J. W., 10(13), 13(19), 16
    (36), 19(45,48), *20, 21*

Huang, S., 29(11), *41*

Hudgens, G. A., 92, *94*

Huffman, J., 179, 184, *195*

Huggins, G. R., 167, 173, *174, 175*

Hughes, A., 13(28), *21*

Hughes, J., 412(152), *426*

Humphrey, G., 275, *285*
Humphries, O., 274, *286*
Hunt, L., 101(7), 108(7), *123*
Huntington, K. M., 383(108), *394*,
    416(176), *427*
Hunzicker-Dunn, M., 16(33), *21*
Hurt, S. W., 78, 82, 85, 89, *95*, 327,
    329, *341*
Hutt, C., 112(27), *124*
Hyman, C., 369(26), *389*, 406(93),
    422

Igarashi, M., 410(124), *424*
Inaba, M., 269, 280, *285*
Ingermarsson, I., 206(20), *215*
Inman, W. H. W., 280, *285*
Ireland, J. J., 16(35), *21*
Irit Gil-Ad, 71(104), *76*
Isaksson, B., 368(23), 369(23), *389*,
    406(92), *422*
Israel, S. L., 226, *240*, 371(35), *390*,
    402(59), *420*
Ivey, M. E., 86, *95*, 163, *174*, 328,
    342, 367(8), *388*
Izquierdo, J. A., 413(157), *426*

Jacobowitz, D. M., 39(37), *42*, 55
    (21), *59*, 269, 270, *284*
Jacobsen, H. I., 10, *20*
Jacobson, E., 320, *342*
Jacubowicz, D., 387(121), *395*
Jaffe, B. M., 43(38), *60*
Jaffe, R. B., 25(4), 27(7), *40*
Jakubowicz, D., 224, *240*
James, C. E., 367(16), 370(16), 374
    (16), 382(16), *389*
James, N., 321, *340*
James, W. H., 132(14), *152*, 168,
    169, 172, *174*
Jamieson, M. G., 67(58), *75*

Jamison, T. S., 70(96), *76*
Janowsky, D. S., 79, *95*, 269, *285*,
    359(70), *365*, 370(32), *389*, 397
    (2,5), 400(41), 403(2), 406(84),
    407(5), 408(2,84), 413(2,5,153,
    154), 415(5), 416(175), *417, 419,
    421, 426, 427*
Jarath, B., 351(35), *363*
Jarreh-Zadeh, A., 402(52), 414(52),
    419
Jelovsek, F. R., 279, 283, *285*
Jenner, F. A., 229, *240*
Jensen, E. V., 10, 13(20), *20*
Jensen, M. R., 90, *95*
Jewelewicz, R., 7(6), *20*, 23(1), *40*,
    293(21), *296*
Jimerson, D. C., 411(131), *424*
Job, J. C., 293(22), *296*
Jofre, I. I., 413(157), *426*
Joh, T., 52(51), *61*
Johannson, G., 90, *97*, 411(133), 413
    (133), *424*
Johanssen, E. D. B., 237(35,36), 238
    (35), *241*
Johansson, E. D. B., 373(50), 378(77),
    390, 392
Johansson, G., 381(92), *393*
Johnson, A. L., 150(40), *153*, 380(84),
    381(87), *393*
Johnson, I. R., 408(97), *422*
Johnson, J. H., 120(76), *127*
Johnson, V. E., 302, *316*
Johnston, P., 52(39), *60*
Jonassen, J. J., 16(32), *21*
Jones, D. E., 203(14), *215*
Jones, G. S., 203(15), *215*
Jones, J. C., 239(42), *242*
Jones, W. H., 354(48), *363*
Jonsson, G., 54(30), *59*, 413(155),
    426
Jordan, R., 66(12), *73*
Jordheim, O., 380(85), *393*

Jorgensen, R. S., 270, *285*
Josso, N., 46(40), *60*
Judson, W. E., 402(53), 406(80),
    414(53), *420, 421*
Jungblut, P. W., 13(28), *21*

Kafiez, A. A., 71(99), *76*
Kahn, E., 322, 336, *344*
Kalra, P. S., 67(60,65,70), *75*
Kalsner, S., 413(156), *426*
Kalz, F., 367(12), *388*
Kamata, K., 269, 280, *285*
Kamberi, I. A., 412(143), *425*
Kane, F. J., 348(10), 352(64), 355
    (51), 356(59), 358(64), 359(71),
    361, 364, 365, 402(52), 414(52),
    419
Kane, R. E., 369(29), 370(29), 385
    (29), *389*
Kantero, R. L., 179, 183, 184, 185,
    187, 191, *195, 196*
Kantor, H. I., 279, *286*
Kantor, H. J., 355(53), *364*
Kapen, S., 33(18), *41,* 293(26,27),
    297
Kaplan, A. P., 397(11), 400(11), *417*
Kapland, H. R., 93, *95*
Karchmen, S., 415(171), *427*
Karen, L. M., 44(41), *60*
Karp, S. A., 273, 275, *285, 289*
Karsch, F. J., 25(5), *40*
Kashiwagi, J., 243(20), 244(20), 250
    (20), *264*
Kashiwagi, T., 300(15), 304, 305,
    309, 312, *316,* 325, 336, *342*
Kastin, A. J., 66(17), 72(110), *73,
    76*
Kastin, A. K., 68(83), *75*
Katcher, A. H., 108(11), 124(11),
    123
Kato, J., 268, *286*

Katz, F. H., 405(76), 406(83), 408
    (76), *421*
Katz, J. L., 293(27), 294(28), *297*
Katz, S. I., 13(19), *20*
Kaulhausen, H., 408(96), *422*
Kawakami, K., 67(34), *74*
Keeler, M., 352(64), 355(51), 358
    (64), *364*
Kehrer, E., 209, *216*
Keiner, M., 49(71), *62,* 67(51), *74*
Keith, L., 151(42), *153*
Kelley, B., 79, *95,* 400(41), *419*
Kelley, D. B., 48(66), 52(66), *62,*
    67(49), *74*
Kelley, W. F., 409(116), *423*
Kellie, A. E., 17(38), *21*
Kelly, M. J., 67(35,36,39,42), 69(85),
    74, 75
Kemeter, P., 381(94), *393*
Kendall, D. A., 268, *286*
Kendel, K., 411(134), *425*
Kennedy, G. C., 69(87), *76*
Keogh, E. G., 33(17), 36(27), *41*
Kephart, W. M., 131(7), *152*
Kernberg, O. F., 321, 330, 336, *342*
Kerr, G. D., 229, 238, *240,* 382(99),
    385(99), *394*
Kerr, M. D., 279, *286*
Kersey, K., 16(32), *21*
Kessel, N., 79, 83, *94,* 232, *241,* 319,
    323, 324, *340,* 367(2), *388,* 399
    (28), *418*
Keverne, E. B., 140(23), *152,* 167,
    175, 400(42), *419*
Keyes, P. L., 16(34), *21*
Khairallah, P. A., 408(99), 412(99),
    422
Khalaf, S., 293(21), *296*
Khani, M. K., 321, 325, 335, 336,
    340
Khylchevskaya, R. I., 268, *286*
Killam, E. K., 270, *286*

Killam, K. F., 270, *286*
Kinch, R. A., 383(105), *394*
Kingstone, D., 293(15), *296*
Kinsey, A. C., 302, *316*
Kinugasa, T., 27(8), *40*
Kistner, R. W., 279, *286*
Kizer, J. S., 39(37), *42*
Klaiber, E. L., 91, *94*, 106, 108, 114
  (42), 118(66), 119(66,71,72),
  125, 126, 268, 269, 270, 271,
  272, 274, 275, 276, 277, 278,
  280, 282, *284, 286, 287, 288*,
  351(33,43), 353(33,43), *362*,
  363, 371(37,38), 381(38), *390*,
  398(17), 412(147), *418, 425*
Klein, D. F., 253(32), *265*, 323, 335,
  342, 351(37), 353(37), 359(37),
  363
Klein, F., 91, *95*
Kleitman, N., 91, *95*
Klerman, G. L., 321, 324, *342, 343*,
  350(31), 351(32), *362*
Kligman, A., 145(30), *153*
Kline, N., 352(61,62), 357(61,62),
  358(62), *364*
Kluge, H., 352(56), 355(56), *364*
Knight, R. P., 320, *342*
Knobil, E., 25(5), 27(6), 29(13), 31
  (6,13), 32(6), 33(13,17,19), 34
  (13), 35(13), 36(27), *40, 41*
Knoth, M., 377(68), *392*
Knuppen, R., 269, *283*
Kobayashi, R. M., 39(37), *42*
Kobayashi, T., 268, *286*
Kobayashi, Y., 91, *94*, 106(42), 108
  (71,72), 114(42), 119(71,72),
  125, 126, 268, 269, 270, 272,
  274, 275, 276, 277, 278, 282,
  284, 286, 288, 351(33,43), 353
  (33,43), *362, 363*, 371(37,38),
  381(38), *390*, 412(147), *425*
Koch, Y., 202(6), *215*

Koerner, D., 15(29), *21*
Koeske, G. F., 84, *96*, 121(81), *127*
Koeske, R. K. D., 82, 84, 85, *96*, 121
  (81), *127*
Kolb, J. E., 322, *342*
Komisaruk, B. R., 48(2), *57*, 66(22),
  69(86), *73, 75*
Komnenich, P., 91, *96*, 102, 104, 106,
  113(39), 114(40), *124*
Kopell, B. S., 79, 89, 91, 93, *96, 97*,
  104, 106, 117(52), 118(52), *125*,
  157, *175*, 358(65), 359(65), *364*
Kopen, I. J., 39(37), *42*
Korn, A., 381(94), *393*
Kornetsky, C., 274, *286*
Kostin, I. W., 104, 115(44), *125*
Koullapis, E. N., 386(116), 387(116),
  395
Kow, L.-M., 44(42), 45(43), *60*, 67
  (80), *75*
Kozlowski, G. P., 68(81), 69(81), *75*
Kraemer, G. W., 66(27), *73*
Kraemer, H. C., 66(15), *73*
Kraepelin, E., 334, *342*
Kramp, J. L., 308(36), *316*, 323, *342*,
  367(14), *388*, 400(36), *419*
Kravetz, M. A., 140(25), *152*
Kreiger, D. T., 8(9), *20*
Kreitmann, B., 18(43), *21*
Krey, L. C., 25(5), *40*, 45(62), 49(58),
  52(62), 53(63,68), 54(57), 55(58),
  61, 62, 67(59), *75*
Krieger, M. S., 46(45), 55(85), *60, 63*,
  67(48), *74*
Krivanek, J., 355(54), *364*
Krodon, C., 411(140), *425*
Krotoszynski, B. K., 151(42), *153*
Krsiak, M., 408(100), 413(100), *422*
Krulich, L., 67(65), *75*
Krus, D. N., 351(44), *363*
Kueng, W., 54(46), *60*
Kuhl, H., 10(12), *20*

Kuhn, M., 49(67), *62*
Kuhn, T. S., 78, *96*
Kullander, S., 374(61), 376(61), *391*
Kuo, H. S., 18(42), *21*
Kupfer, D. J., 253(33), *265*
Kurachi, K., 27(8), *40*
Kursrok, R., 267, *288*
Kuster, G., 36(30), *41*
Kutner, J., 348(6), *361*
Kutner, M., 167, 173, *175*
Kutner, S. J., 348(7,8), 354(7), *361,*
    379(81), *392*
Kyger, K., 358(66), *364*

Lachelin, G. C. L., 36(28), 38(32),
    41
Ladisich, W., 348(4), *361,* 414(164),
    426
Ladosky, W., 36(30), *41*
Lafleur, D., 386(118), *395*
Laguna, J., 291(4), *295*
Laidlaw, J., 398(19), *418*
Lake, C. R., 381(93), *393*
Lamont, A., 93, *97*
Lamprecht, F., 381(91), *393,* 413
    (158), *426*
Lamprecht, S. A., 202(6), *215*
Landau, R. L., 406(91), *422*
Landauer, A. A., 106, 117(50), *125*
Lane, D. M., 91, *96,* 104(40), 106
    (40), 114(40), *124*
Langenstein, S., 104(36), 106(56), 108
    (56), 113(36), 116(36), 117(56),
    119(56), *124, 125,* 398(15), *418*
Lansky, M., 323, 324, *341*
LaPietra, O., 158, *174*
Larsen, J. F., 374(62,63), 375(63),
    376(62), 377(68), *391, 392,* 410
    (121), *424*
Larsen, L., 367(6), 379(83), 383
    (83), *388, 392*

Larsson, K., 45(64), 46(47), 49(64),
    60, 62
Lasley, B. L., 30(15), *41,* 293(23),
    296
Laude Wiele, R. S., 91, *95*
Lauro, R., 410(119), *423*
Law, O. T., 67(74,75), *75*
Lazarus, L., 409(114), *423*
Lazerus, J. H., 15(30), *21*
Leary, P. M., 108, 119(73), *126,* 398
    (16), *418*
Leblanc, H., 36(28), *41*
Leckman, F., 339, *341*
Lederman, M., 104, 115(43), *125*
Lee, K. L., 279, 283, *285*
Lee, P., 179, *195*
Leeton, J., 349(19), *362*
Lehfeldt, H., 209(26), *216*
Lehmann, H. E., 274, *286*
Lein, A., 30(15), *41*
LeMagnen, J., 151(41), *153*
Lemarchand-Beraud, T., 409(112,113),
    415(113), *423*
Lennane, M. B., 188, *195*
Lennane, R. J., 188, *195*
Leonila Lopez, Q. F. I., 415(171), *427*
Lerdo de Tejada, A., 415(171), *427*
Leshner, A. I., 82, *96,* 118(64), *126,*
    354(46), *363,* 400(38), 409(38),
    419
Less, V. W. K., 67(62), *75*
Leuba, C., 131(5), *152*
Levan, N. E., 369(26), *389,* 406(93),
    422
Levran, D., 13(27), *20*
Lewicki, J. A., 408(105), *423*
Lewin, K., 122(87), *127*
Lewis, S. A., 162, *174*
Leyden, J. L., 145(30), *153*
L'Hermite, M., 410(125), *424*
Lichtsteiner, M., 414(163), *426*
Lidz, R. W., 348(14), *361*

Lieberburg, I., 43(48), 49(48,58), 50(48,52), 51(48,52), 54(48,52), 55(58), *60, 61*
Liebowitz, M. R., 253(32), *265*
Lief, H. I., 92, *98,* 149(32), *153,* 171, *175,* 349(21), *362*
Lindner, H. R., 202(6), 207(22), *215, 216*
Ling, N., 38(34), *41*
Linkie, D. M., 13(24,25), *20*
Liotta, A. S., 8(9), *20*
Lipsett, M. B., 279, *286*
Lipton, A., 410(123), *424*
Lipton, M. A., 351(34), 353(34), *362,* 402(52), 414(52), *419*
Lisk, R. D., 69(89), *76*
Liskey, N. E., 101(10), *123*
Lisky, N., 243(17), *264*
Liss, J. L., 330, *344*
Little, B. C., 90, *96,* 104, 106, 108, 117(54), 118(54), 119(54), *125,* 354(45), *363,* 381(91), *393,* 413 (158), *426*
Little, M., 13(28), *21*
Livingston, L., 82, *94,* 409(118), 410(118), *423*
Livingston-Vaughan, L., 351(40), *363*
Lloyd, I. J., 410(123), *424*
Lloyd, T. S., 233, *241*
Locatelli, V., 71(104), *76*
Lockhart, A., 106, 117(51), *125*
Loeb, L. S., 44(17), *58*
Logothetis, J., 398(18), 404(18), *418*
Lohr, N., 321, *340*
Longcope, C., 281, *283*
Loraine, J. A., 292(11), *295,* 401 (46), 410(128), *419, 424*
Loriaux, D. L., 293(17), *296,* 381 (90), *393*

Loriaux, L., 412(149), *426*
Loucks, J., 106, 117(55), *125*
Lough, O. M., 102, 116(20), 122(20), *123*
Louis, K. M., 29(11), *41*
Luce, G. G., 91, *96*
Luetscher, J., 406(82), *421*
Luff, M. C., 131(10), 132(10), *152,* 165, 168, 171, *175*
Lugibihl, K., 406(91), *422*
Luine, V. N., 52(49,50,51), 54(57,78), *61, 63,* 268, *286*
Lumbers, E. R., 406(81), *421*
Lund, R., 294(29), *297*
Lunde, D. T., 79, 89, 91, 93, *96, 97,* 104(52), 106(52), 117(52), 118 (52), *125,* 157, *175,* 359(74), *365*
Lundström, V., 204(17), 207(23), *215, 216*
Lunenfeld, B., 13(27), *20*
Lunn, S. F., 410(128), *424*
Luschen, M. E., 164, *174*
Luttge, W. G., 45(35), *60,* 66(23,24), *73*
Lynch, H. J., 411(131), *424*

McAdoo, B. C., 66(15), *73*
McCance, R. A., 131(10), 132(10), *152,* 165, 168, 171, *175*
McCann, S. M., 65(6,8), 66(6,8,9,29), 67(29,60,64,65), *73, 75,* 150(37), *153,* 412(144), *425*
McClintock, M. K., 82, *96*
McClure, J. J., 243(20), 244(20), 250 (20), *264*
McClure, J. M., 243(21), 244(21), *264*
McClure, J. N., 243(24), 244(24), *264,* 300(13,14,15), 304(15), 305(15), 309(15), 312(15), *316,* 324, 325, 336, *342, 344*

McClure, J. N., Jr., 325, *342,* 400
   (31,32), *418*
McCullagh, E. P., 292(9), *295*
McDonald, P. A., 55(28), *59*
McDonald, P. G., 403(65), *420*
McElin, T. W., 368(24), *389*
McEwen, B. S., 34(24), *41,* 43(48),
   45(62,74), 47(74), 48(59,60,61),
   49(26,48,58,81), 50(48,52,53),
   51(48,52,54), 52(25,49,50,51,
   56,77), 53(53,63,68), 54(48,52,
   55,57,78), 55(24,58), *59, 60, 61,
   62, 63,* 268, *286*
Macfarlane Smith, I., 276, *287*
McGilp, S., 409(111), *423*
McGinnis, M. Y., 45(62), 52(62),
   53(63), *62*
McGinnis, P. R., 66(27), *73*
Macgregor, G. A., 239, *242*
McIntosh, T. K., 44(3), 46(89), 55
   (89), *57, 63*
McIsaac, W. M., 411(141), *425*
Mack, T. M., 279, *287*
Mackenberg, E. J., 276, *287*
MacKinnon, I. L., 79, *96,* 325, *342,*
   367(17), *389*
MacKinnon, P. C. B., 79, *96,* 325,
   342, 367(17), *389*
MacLusky, N. J., 45(62), 50(52,53),
   51(52), 52(62), 53(53,68), 54
   (52), *61, 62*
McMaster, R., 349(19), *362*
McNatty, K. P., 16(37), *21*
McNeill, T. H., 36(29), 37(29), *41*
McNeilly, A. S., 66(11), 71(97), *73,
   76,* 410(126), *424*
McQueen, J., 279, *284*
Ma. Estela Carreno, Q.F.B., 415(171),
   427
Magliocco, E. B., 328, 339, *341*
Magnatto, R., 410(119), *423*
Magnus, C., 49(26), *59*

Mair, R. G., 397(10), *417*
Majcher, D., 271, 274, 275, 282, *284*
Makris, A., 16(37), *21*
Mallin, R., 324, 329, *341*
Mancini, J. F., 66(13), *73*
Mandell, A. J., 300(12), *316,* 406(84),
   408(84), *421*
Mandell, H., 79, *96*
Mandell, M., 79, *96*
Mandell, M. P., 300(12), *316*
Mangoni, A., 158, *174*
Manku, M. S., 374(57,59), 377(59),
   391
Marcus, D., 300(11), 311(11), *315*
Marinari, K. T., 82, *96,* 118(64), *126,*
   354(46), *363,* 400(38), 409(38),
   419
Markanda, N. D., 239(42), *242*
Marrone, B. L., 45(31), *59*
Marshall, G., 33(19), *41*
Marshall, J. C., 292(10), 293(13), *295,
   296*
Martin, C. E., 302(30,31), *316*
Martin, H. J., 182, *196*
Martin, J. B., 67(37,38,40), *74*
Masala, A., 381(89), *393*
Masek, K. M., 408(100), 413(100),
   422
Maslow, A. H., 131(4), *152*
Mason, I., 71(102), *76*
Massey, F. M., 279, 283, *285*
Mast, M., 93, *95,* 117(60), *126*
Masters, W. H., 213, *216,* 302, *316*
Mathews, A., 149(33), *153*
Mathews, D., 69(88), *76*
Matsenbaugh, A., 179, *195*
Matsumoto, S., 80, *96*
Matta, R. J., 354(45), *363,* 381(91),
   393, 413(158), *426*
Mattsson, B., 369(28), 371(42), 377
   (28), *389, 390,* 403(63), *420*
Maxwell, A. E., 245(27), *264*

May, R. R., 86, *96,* 323, *342*
Mead, R., 318, *342*
Meagher, W., 67(75), *75*
Meares, R. A., 108, 118(67), 119 (67), *126*
Mecklenburg, R. S., 293(17), *296*
Mefferd, R. B., Jr., 112(33), *124*
Mehrotra, P. K., 268, *288*
Meites, J., 9(11), *20*
Melges, F. T., 79, *97,* 157, *175*
Melody, G. F., 191, *196*
Meltzer, H. L., 386(118), *395*
Menczer, J., 13(27), *20*
Mendels, J., 382(100), *394*
Menduke, H., 406(86), *421*
Menon, K. M. J., 16(34), *21*
Menzi, R., 54(46), *60,* 412(150), 413(150), 414(150), *426*
Merrill, L. R., 164, *173*
Messent, P. R., 275, *287*
Mester, J., 17(38), *21*
Meyer-Bahlburg, H. F., 350(27,28), *362*
Meyerson, B. J., 411(138), 412 (138), *425*
Michael, C., 279, *286*
Michael, R. P., 92, *96,* 129(2), 130 (2,3), 138(21), 140(21,24), 143 (21), *152,* 167, 173, *175,* 401 (44,47), 403(67), *419, 420*
Michael, S. D., 71(98,102,103), *76*
Micic, S., 377(68), *392*
Midgley, A. R., 9(10), 15(31), 16 (34), *20, 21,* 25(4), *40*
Mikhail, G., 7(6), *20,* 23(1), *40*
Milch, P. O., 15(30), *21*
Milgrom, E., 17(40), 19(46), *21*
Milhaud, G., 293(22), *296*
Miller, R., 251(31), 253(31), *265*
Miller, W. R., 92, *98,* 149(32), *153,* 171, *175,* 349(21), *362*
Millodot, M., 93, *97*

Milne, H. B., 369(27), 370(27), 380 (27), *389*
Milton, L. J., 279, *286,* 355(53), *364*
Minaguchi, H., 268, *286*
Minardi, J., 279, *284*
Minkoff, K., 300(10), 310(10), *315*
Mirsky, A. F., 274, *287*
Mishara, B. L., 104, 115(44), *125*
Mishell, D. R., 409(110), *423*
Mishler, E. G., 88, *97*
Misurec, J., 270, *287*
Mitra, J., 69(87), *76*
Miyake, A., 27(8), *40*
Modianos, D., 66(21), *73*
Moncada, S., 386(119), 387(119), *395*
Monroe, S., 25(4), *40*
Montgomery, M. O., 44(42), *60*
Moos, R. H., 79, 83, 89, 91, 93, *96, 97,* 101(8), 104(52), 106(52), 117(52), 118(52), *123, 125,* 157, *174, 175,* 185, 192, *196,* 229(19), *240,* 299 (7), *315,* 323, *343,* 359(72,74), *365,* 367(3), 368(3), 379(79), *388, 392,* 397(1), *417*
Morali, G., 45(64), 49(64), *62*
Moran, L. J., 112(33), *124*
Morgan, H. G., 292(7), *295*
Morgan, J. M., 408(101), *422*
Moriarty, D., 108(72), 119(72), *126,* 268, 272, *286,* 351(33), 353(33), *362,* 371(38), 381(38), *390*
Morin, L. P., (65), *62*
Morrell, F., 398(18), 404(18), *418*
Morrell, J. I., 48(66), 52(66), *62,* 67 (48), *74*
Morris, N. M., 8(7), *20,* 91, *99,* 101(5), *123,* 129(1), 130(1), 132(1), 133 (16,17,18), 134(17,19), 135(19), 136(19), 137(19), 140(27), 141 (16), 142(16), 143(28), 146(17), 147(17), *152,* 166, 167, 168, 169,

[Morris]
170, 172, 173, *175,* 345(1), 359
(73), *360, 365,* 380(86), *393,*
401(45), *419*
Morriss, G. M., 400(42), *419*
Mortimer, C. H., 66(11), *73*
Morton, J. H., 101(7), 108(7), *123,*
371(36), *390,* 402(56), *420*
Morton, T., 397(10), *417*
Moss, R. L., 65(3,4,5,6,8), 66(6,8,9,
10,18,19,20,29), 67(3,5,19,29,35,
36,39,41,42,44,45,46,47,74), 68
(3,84), 69(3,41,84,85,90), 70(96),
72(4,5,112), *72, 73, 74, 75, 76,*
150(37), *153*
Mountjoy, C. Q., 66(14), *73*
Mtabji, J. B., 374(57), *391*
Mueller, L. M., 381(95), *393*
Muhlbauer, H. L., 386(118), *395*
Muiruri, K., 410(123), *424*
Mukai, T., 400(35), *419*
Müller, E. E., 35(26), *41,* 71(104),   ˙
76
Munchel, M. E., 102, 104, 106, 116
(48), 124(48), *125,* 275, *287*
Munday, M. R., 229(18), 238(18),
240, 371(44), 372(45), 373(44),
375(44), *390,* 401(49), *419*
Munoz, R., 325, 330, *341*
Murad, F., 381(88), *393*
Murphy, D. L., 381(90), *393,* 412
(149), *426*
Murray, M. A. F., 66(11), *73*
Musland, R. P., 177, *195*
Myers, B. M., 66(28), *73*
Myers, C. S., 110(8), *123*

Naftolin, F., 33(20), *41,* 46(32), 49
(67), *59, 62*
Nahanek, K., 270, *287*
Nakai, Y., 33(17), 36(27), *41*

Nance, D. M., 67(79), *75*
Naor, S., 207(22), *216*
Napoli, A., 67(73), *75*
Naquet, R., 270, *286*
Narayana, K., 268, *286*
Nassar, B. A., 374(57,59), 377(59),
391
Nattero, G., 410(127), *424*
Navratil, J., 382(101), 383(103), *394*
Nee, J., 243(6,8), 246(6), 248(6), 259
(6), *263*
Nelson, K. R., 406(90), 408(90), *422*
Nesheim, B. I., 206(18), *215*
Nestianu, V., 270, *284*
Netter, F. H., 407(94), *422*
Nicol, G. C., 381(87), *393*
Nielsen, J., 374(62), 376(62), 377
(68), *391, 392,* 410(121), *424*
Nies, A., 253(34), *265*
Nillius, S. J., 237(35), 238(35), *241,*
293(24,25), *297,* 349(23), *362,*
373(50), *390*
Nistico, G., 35(26), *41*
Niswender, G. D., 9(10), *20*
Noble, E. P., 158, *175,* 367(7), 380
(7), 386(7), *388*
Noble, R. G., 46(10), 48(10), *58*
Nogami, Y., 80, *96*
Norman, R. L., 67(71), *75*

O'Brien, C. P., 92, *98,* 149(32), *153,*
171, *175,* 349(21), *362*
O'Brien, P. M. S., 235, 239(43), *241,*
242, 368(25), 370(33), 371(25),
372(25,33), 375(33), 379(25),
384(25), *389, 390,* 401(51), 406
(51), 407(51), *419*
O'Brien, S., 372(46), *390*
O'Conner, J. F., 78, 79, *97,* 299(5),
300(5), 303(5), *315,* 317, 323,
343

O'Donohue, T. L., 55(21), *59,* 269, 270, *284*

Oehm, W., 408(96), *422*

Oelkers, W., 235, *241*

Oestberg, B., 317, 322, 323, *344*

Ohkuri, S., 80, *96*

Ohman, R., 370(30), 374(30), 375 (30), *389*

Olambiwonnu, N. O., 179, *196*

O'Malley, B. W., 19(47), *21*

OOms, M. P., 55(87), *63*

Oppenheimer, J. H., 15(29), *21*

Orci, L., 13(18), *20*

Orndoff, R. K., 46(10), 48(10), *58*

Orndorff, M. M., 145(30), *153*

Osathanondh, R., 16(37), *21*

Osmun, J. D., 377(70), 378(75), 383(70), *392*

Osmun, J. N., 190, *195,* 300(18), *316,* 317, 324, 325, 326, 330, *342, 344*

Osofsky, J. J., 82, *97*

Ota, J., 400(35), *419*

Outram, D. H., 369(27), 370(27), 380(27), *389*

Paden, C., 54(55), *61*

Page, R. B., 8(8), *20,* 29, *40*

Paige, K. E., 86, *97,* 178, *196,* 326, 327, *343,* 351(38), *363*

Paliac, D. J., 408(99), 412(99), *422*

Palkovits, M., 39(37), *42*

Pallis, D. J., 243(16), *264,* 300(17), *316*

Paloutzian, R. F., 67(74), *75*

Papanicolaou, G. N., 267, *287*

Paracchi, A., 293(18), *296*

Park, D., 52(51), *61*

Parker, C. W., 386(120), *395*

Parker, L., 104, 115(44), *125*

Parker, R. T., 279, 283, *285*

Parlee, M. B., 78, 79, 80, 82, 84, 86, 87, 89, 91, 92, *97,* 101(3), 104, 106, 108, 113(34), 117(34), 120 (77), *123, 124, 127,* 178, 181, 182, 190, *196,* 299(4), 303, 304, *315,* 318, *343,* 368(19), 386(19), *389,* 398(21), 399(21), *418*

Parlow, A. F., 179, *196*

Parmentier, M., 71(109), 72(109), *76*

Parrott, R. F., 55(28), *59*

Parry, B. L., 348(12), 350(12), *361*

Parsons, B., 52(56), 53(63,68), *61, 62*

Pasteels, J. L., 71(109), 72(109), *76*

Paterson, M. E., 279, *287*

Patkai, P., 90, *97,* 381(92), *393,* 411 (133), 413(133), *424*

Pattie, F., 318, *343*

Paul, V., 271, 274, 275, 282, *284*

Paunier, L., 411(129), *424*

Paykel, E. S., 351(32), *362*

Peach, M. J., 377(69), *392*

Peck, E. J., 18(44), 19(45,48), *21*

Peck, E. J., Jr., 44(19), *58*

Peguillaume, R., 409(113), 415(113), *423*

Pellegrini-Quarantotti, B., 71(100), *76*

Pennington, V. M., 243(10), *264*

Penny, R., 179, *196*

Peron, F. G., 71(98), *76*

Perr, I. N., 323, 324, *343*

Perrini, N., 406(85), *421*

Perry, J. C., 321, *343*

Persky, H., 78, 92, *98,* 149(32), *153,* 171, *175,* 349(21), *362*

Petro, Z., 49(67), *62*

Pfaff, D. W., 34(24), *41,* 44(42), 45 (43), 46(70), 48(59,60,61,66), 49 (71), 52(25,56,66,72,73), 53(68), 56(69), *59, 60, 61, 62,* 65(7), 66 (7,21), 67(48,49,51,80), 68(82), 69 (82), *73, 74, 75*

Pfeffer, R. I., 279, *287*
Philipp, E., 376(67), *391*
Phillips, L., 273, *287*
Phoenix, C. H., 43(97), *64*
Picard, J. Y., 46(40), *60*
Pickles, V. R. A., 202(7,11,12), *215,*
    397(7), *417*
Pierce, D. M., 164, *174*
Pierson, W. R., 106, 117(51), *125*
Pike, M. C., 279, *287*
Piliego, N., 406(85), *421*
Pinel, P., 318, *343*
Pintor, C., 158, *174*
Pintos-Dantas, C. R., 201(2), *214*
Pirke, K. M., 294(29), *297*
Plant, T. M., 33(17), 36(27), *41*
Plapinger, L., 45(74), 47(74), *62*
Podell, J. E., 273, *287*
Polatin, P., 320, *342*
Pollack, E. I., 55(85), *63*
Pomeroy, W. B., 302(30,31), *316*
Porter, J. C., 37(31), 38(31), *41*
Porteus, S. D., 273, *287*
Post, B., 90, *97,* 381(92), *393,* 411
    (133), 413(133), *424*
Post, R. M., 411(131,135), *424, 425*
Poulain, P., 67(43), 71(105,106),
    74, 76
Powers, B. J., 67(77), *75*
Powers, J. B., (75), *63,* 67(73), *75*
Poyser, N. L., 202(8), *215*
Prange, A., Jr., 150(36), *153*
Prange, A. J., 351(34), 353(34), *362*
Prentice, R., 279, *288*
Presser, H. B., 80, *98*
Preti, G., 167, 173, *174, 175*
Price, J. M., 381(95), *393*
Prichard, J. C., 319, *343*
Primac, D. W., 274, *287*
Printz, M. P., 408(105), *423*
Procope, B.-J., 382(102), *394*
Prusoff, B., 351(32), *362*

Pryse-Davies, J., 326, 327, *341,* 401
    (48), 406(48), 412(146,148), *419,*
    425
Pugh, T., 351(35), *363*
Pühringer, W., 412(150), 413(150),
    414(150,167), *426, 427*
Pulkkinen, M. O., 204(16), *215,* 385
    (110,114), 386(115), *394, 395*
Pupp, L., 67(68), *75*

Quadagno, D. M., 52(76), *63*
Quigley, M. E., 16(36), *21,* 38(35),
    40(35), *42*
Quilligan, E. J., 369(26), *389,* 406
    (93), *422*

Raboch, J., 209(28), *216*
Rabon, A., 351(34), 353(34), *362*
Rack, P. H., 79, *99*
Radford, H. M., 67(53), *74*
Radinger, N., 352(61), 357(61), *364*
Rado, S., 320, *343*
Radwanska, E., 233, *241*
Rainbow, T. C., 52(77), 53(63), 54
    (55,78), *61, 62, 63*
Raisman, G., 56(79,80), *63*
Rakoff, J. S., 295(33), *297*
Ramsay, D. J., 408(107), *423*
Rebar, R. W., 16(36), *21,* 24(2), 25(2),
    40
Reddy, V. V., 49(67), *62*
Redgrove, J. A., 78, 89, *98,* 122(88),
    127
Reed, R., 351(35), *363*
Rees, L., 243(11), *264,* 326, *343,* 399
    (29), 402(61), 410(61), *418, 420*
Reeves, B. D., 368(24), *389*
Regestein, Q., 279, *287*
Reich, D., 404(71), *421*
Reich, M., 405(74), 407(74), *421*

Reich, T., 243(21,24), 244(21,24), *264,* 300(14), *316,* 324, 325, *342, 344,* 400(31,32), *418*

Reichert, L. E., 9(10), 15(31), 16 (32,34), *20, 21*

Reinisch, J. M., 350(26), *362*

Reis, D., 52(51), *61*

Renaer, M., 212(29), *216*

Renaud, L. P., 67(37,38,40), *74*

Repczynski, C. A., 164, *173*

Reynolds, B., 314(39), *316*

Rezek, D. L., 55(95), *64*

Ribeiro, W. O., 409(110), *423*

Ricci, C. A., 279, 283, *285*

Richard, D. H., 235(30), *241*

Richards, D. H., 323, *340*

Richards, J. S., 16(32,35), *21*

Richardson, G., 359(67), *364*

Richart, R. M., 2(3), *20,* 91, *95*

Riddle, O., 69(92), *76*

Rigg, L. A., 295(33), *297*

Rinzler, C., 324, 329, *343*

Ripley, H. S., 267, *287*

Riskind, P., 65(4), 66(19), 67(19, 47), 72(4), *72, 73, 74*

Rivier, C., 38(34), *41*

Rivier, J., 65(2), *72*

Rizkallah, T., 7(6), *20,* 23(1), *40*

Robel, P., 17(39), 18(41), *21*

Robertson, D. M., 17(38), *21*

Robins, E., 250(29,30), *265,* 300 (20), *316,* 325, 330, *341, 344*

Robinson, A., 34(22), *41*

Robinson, D., 253(34), *265*

Robinson, D. B., 353(58), 355(58), *364*

Robinson, K., 383(108), *394,* 416 (176), *427*

Robinson, M., 406(87), *422*

Robyn, C., 410(125), *424*

Rochlin, D., 352(61,62), 357(61, 62), 358(62), *364*

Rockmore, L., 274, *287*

Rodgers, C. H., 268, 269, 270, *283*

Rodier, W. I., III, 270, *287*

Rodin, J., 85, *98,* 115(46), 116(46), *125*

Rodrigue, E. M., 328, *343*

Rodriquez-Sierra, J. F., 66(22), *73*

Roffe, B. D., 238(39), *241*

Roffwarg, H., 33(18), *41,* 293(26), 294(28), *297*

Rogel, M. J., 140(26), *152*

Rogers, M. L., 86, *98*

Rolfes, A. I., 16(32), *21*

Romth, P., 405(76), 408(76), *421*

Rondell, P., 7(5), *20*

Rose, D. P., 350(30), 353(30), *362,* 381(96), *393*

Rose, M. J., 79, *99*

Rose, R. M., 82, *94,* 121(84), *127,* 181, 189, 190, *194,* 243(1), 244(1), *263,* 299(9), *315,* 351(40,41), *363,* 409(118), 410(118), *423*

Rosenberg, A., 351(36), *363*

Rosenblatt, H., 34(23), 35(23), *41*

Rosenblatt, S., 69(94), *76*

Rosenthal, R. H., 321, 325, 335, 336, *340*

Rosenthal, R. J., 85, *98,* 324, 329, *343*

Rosniatowski, C., 10(12), *20*

Rosnow, R. L., 85, *98*

Ross, G. T., 1, *20*

Rosseinsky, D. R., 400(40), *419*

Rosvold, H. E., 274, *287*

Roth, R. H., 412(152), *426*

Roulston, J. E., 239(42), *242*

Rouse, P., 379(82), *392*

Routtenberg, A., 408(101), *422*

Roy, E. J., 49(81), 52(82), *63*

Rubenstein, B. B., 86, 90, *94,* 159, 160, 161, 162, 163, 172, *173, 174,* 299(2), 300, 302, 314, *315*

Rubin, B. S., 54, (84), *63*
Rubenstein, B. B., 328, 339, *340*
Rubinstein, A. A., 243(22), 244(22),
    264, 312(38), *316,* 325, *341*
Ruble, D. N., 85, 87, *94, 98,* 120
    (78), 121(82,83,86), *127,* 177,
    178, 179, 180, 181, 182, 186,
    187, 190, 194, *194, 195, 196,*
    305(35), 306(35), 309(35), *316,*
    399(27), *418*
Rudolph, J., 411(134), *425*
Rush, A. J., 348(12), 350(12), *361*
Russell, G. F. M., 82, *98,* 120(75),
    127, 291(1), 292(5,7,11), 293
    (13), *295, 296,* 368(22), *389,*
    406(89), *422*
Russell, M. J., 145(29), *153*
Ryan, K. J., 16(37), *21,* 46(32), 49
    (67), *59, 62,* 279, *287,* 371(43),
    390

Saayman, G. S., 401(47), 403(67),
    419, 420
Sabur, M., 293(15), *296*
Sachar, E. J., 409(115), *423*
Sachs, B. D., 55(85), *63*
Sakuma, Y., 52(72,73), *62,* 67(34),
    68(82), 69(82), *74, 75*
Salseduc, M. M., 413(157), *426*
Salzer, H., 381(94), *393*
Sampson, G. A., 229, 230, 238, *240,*
    327, *343,* 367(9), 373(9), 386(9),
    388
Samson, W., 66(29), 67(29), *73*
Sanborn, B. M., 18(42), *21*
Sanders, J. L., 101(6), *123*
Sandler, M., 412(146), *425*
Sandman, C. A., 72(110), *76,* 93, *99,*
    108(57), 117(57), *125,* 397(9),
    417
Sandwich, D., 82, *94,* 409(118),

[Sandwich]
    410(118), *423*
Santen, R. J., 295(34), *297*
Sar, M., 50(86), *63,* 67(50), *74*
Sarason, I. G., 82, *98,* 120(76), *127*
Sarkar, D. K., 34(25), *41*
Saunders, D., 355(54), *364*
Sawyer, C. H., 67(70,71), *75,* 403(64),
    411(137,138), 412(138,142), *420,*
    425
Saxena, B. N., 409(114), *423*
Scapagnini, U., 35(26), *41,* 71(100),
    76
Scapo, A. I., 201(2), *214*
Schacht, S., 243(6,8), 246(6), 248(6),
    259(6), *263,* 301(19), *316*
Schacter, S., 85, *98*
Schader, R. I., 383(104), *394*
Schally, A. V., 66(13), 67(32), 68(83),
    72(110), *73, 74, 75, 76*
Schatzoff, M., 185, *197*
Scheffler, I., 78, *98*
Schiff, I., 16(37), *21,* 279, *287,* 371
    (43), *390*
Schildkraut, J. J., 276, 282, *287*
Schilling, K. M., 86, *98,* 121(85), *127*
Schmitt, W., 351(35), *363*
Schnall, M., 275, *284*
Schneider, H. P. G., 66(12), *73,* 412
    (144), *425*
Schneider, H. T., 36(30), *41*
Schöneshöfer, 235(33), *241*
Schou, M., 234(29), *241,* 325, *343,*
    378(72), *392*
Schrader, S. L., 82, *99*
Schuckit, M. A., 243(23), 244(23),
    264, 300(16), *316,* 325, *343,*
    400(33), *418*
Schwank, J., 106, 117(53), *125*
Schwartz, A., 202(6), 207(22), *215,*
    216
Schwartz, H. L., 15(29), *21*

Schwartz, W. D., 370(31), *389*
Schwarz, U. D., 405(77), 408(77), *421*
Schwarzstein, L., 66(13), *73*
Seager, C. P., 348(9), *361*
Secher, N. J., 206(19), *215*
Seed, M., 350(30), 353(30), *362*, 381(96), *393*
Sekerke, H. J., 416(175), *427*
Selby, C., 235(31), *241*, 368(25), 371(25), 372(25), 379(25), 384 (25), *389*, 401(51), 406(51), 407(51), *419*
Selby, D., 370(33), 372(33), 375 (33), *390*
Selby, S., 239(43), *242*
Selye, H., 403(66), 404(70), 411 (66), 415(66), *420, 421*
Serif, C. W., 259(36), *265*
Setalo, G., 67(32), *74*
Severgnini, A., 293(18), *296*
Severs, W. B., 408(102,103), *422*
Sevringhaus, E. L., 267, *287*
Seward, G. H., 110(19), 111(21), 122(19), *123*
Shader, R. I., 157, *175*, 323, *342*
Shah, J., 151(42), *153*
Shainess, N., 359(75), *365*
Shapre, R. M., 71(97), *76*
Shatin, L., 274, *287*
Shaw, D. M., 326, *340*
Shea, D., 271, 274, 275, 282, *284*
Sheets, C. S., 66(23), *73*
Sheldrake, P., 398(13), *417*
Shelley, E. M., 317, 323, *343*
Shelly, E. M., 78, 79, *97*, 299(5), 300(5), 303(5), *315*
Sherfey, M. J., 302, *316*
Sheridan, P. J., 13(23), *20*, 50(86), *63*
Sherif, C. W., 82, *99*
Sherman, B. M., 293(16,19,20), *296*

Sherwood, N. M., 34(25), *41*
Shetty, T., 270, *288*
Shirley, E., 91, *95*
Shore, H., 279, *286*
Shorr, E., 267, *287*
Shryne, J. E., 52(76), 56(34), *59, 63*, 67(79), *75*
Sicuteri, F., 414(165), *427*
Siegel, J. M., 120(76), *127*
Siegenthaler, W., 406(82), *421*
Siiteri, P. K., 13(24), *20*
Silbergeld, S., 158, *175*, 367(7), 380 (7), 386(7), *388*
Silver, E., 351(36), *363*
Silver, M. A., 300(11), 311(11), *315*
Silverman, A. J., 28(12), 29(12), *41*, 67(31), *74*
Silverman, E.-M., 102, 113(37,38), *124*
Silverthorne, C., 80, *95,* 101(2), *122*
Simon, B., 318, 319, *343*
Simons, B. J., 408(98), *422*
Simpson, G., 352(61,62), 357(61,62), 358(62), *364*
Sims, E. A. H., 405(75), *421*
Singer, J. E., 85, *98*
Singer, J. J., 67(76), *75*
Singer, K., 234(29), *241*, 325, *343*, 378(72), *392*
Singer, M. T., 321, 322, 336, *342*
Singh, E. J., 203(13), *215*
Sizonenko, P., 411(129), *424*
Skinner, S. L., 406(81), *421*
Slaby, A. E., 356(60), *364*
Sladek, J. R., 36(29), 37(29), *41*
Sletten, I. W., 325, 326, *343*
Sletten, J. W., 378(73), *392*
Slob, A. K., 55(87), *63*
Smith, A. J., 111(22), *123*
Smith, C. A., 149(34), *153*
Smith, D. C., 279, *288*
Smith, D. M., 16(37), *21*

Smith, G. N., 202(12), *215*
Smith, J., 352(63), *364*
Smith, M. S., 71(98,101,102), *76*
Smith, S. L., 78, *98, 177, 196,* 238, *241,* 299(3), *315,* 323, 326, 327, *343,* 368(18), 370(18), 371(18), 372(18), 373(52), 383(52), *389, 391,* 397(3), 400(30), 401(3), 402(3), 407(3), *417, 418*
Snider, D. E., 386(120), *395*
Snyder, D. B., 106, 114(41), *124*
Snyder, L., 54(55), *61*
Sodergard, R., 371(41), *390*
Sodersten, P., 46(47), *60*
Solomon, S., 405(75), *421*
Somerville, B. W., 373(53), *391*
Sommer, B., 90, *98,* 101(1), 102, 104, 106, 108(15), 112(30,32), 120(1), 121(32), 124(15), *122, 123, 124,* 181, *196,* 275, *288,* 299(8), *315,* 368(20), 384(20), *389,* 398(14,22), *417, 418*
Southam, A. L., 367(11), *388*
Southam, A. M., 56(34), *59*
Southgate, J., 412(146), *425*
Sowton, S. C. M., 110(18), *123*
Soyka, L. F., 268, 269, 270, *283*
Spada, A., 293(18), *296*
Speck, G., 408(106), *423*
Spielberger, C. D., 82, *98*
Spitz, C. J., 132(13), 135(20), *152,* 168, 169, *175*
Spitzer, R. L., 250(29,30), *265,* 300 (20), *316,* 317, 322, 330, 334, 336, *343, 344*
Spurzheim, G., 319, *344*
Sramka, M., 408(100), 413(100), *422*
Srivastava, K., 268, *288*
Steele, S. J., 17(38), *21*
Steenstrup, O. R., 374(62), 376(62), *391,* 410(121), *424*

Steerman, C., 56(36), *60*
Steinburg, J., 413(160), *426*
Steiner, M., 177, 190, *195, 196,* 243 (4), 254(35), *263, 265,* 299(6), 300 (18), *315, 316,* 317, 321, 324, 325, 326, 330, *340, 342, 344,* 355(52), *364,* 374(58), 377(70), 378(75), 383(70), 385(58,109), *391, 392, 394,* 399(23), 402(23), 403(23), 408(23), 409(23), 414(23), *418*
Sterescu-Volanschi, M., 270, *284*
Sterling, K., 15(30), *21*
Stern, A., 320, *344*
Stern, L. O., 78, 79, *97,* 299(5), 300 (5), 303(5), *315,* 317, 323, *343*
Stewart, D., 353(57), 355(57), *364*
Stewart, I., 83, *98,* 243(15), *264,* 367 (4), *388*
Stokes, J., 382(100), *394*
Stone, G., 274, *284*
Stone, M. H., 317, 321, 322, 323, 327, 329, 334, 336, 339, *340, 344*
Stone, S. C., 91, 93, *96, 99,* 104(40), 106(40), 108(57), 114(40), 117 (57), *124, 125,* 397(9), *417*
Stonehill, E., 292(8), *295*
Stopes, M., 156, *175*
Strausfeld, K. S., 405(75), *421*
Strauss, D., 92, *98,* 149(32), *153,* 171, *175,* 349(21), *362*
Strindberg, L., 104(49), 106(49), 116 (49), 117(49), 118(49), *125*
Stromberg, P., 151(42), *153*
Strong, R., 350(30), 353(30), *362,* 381(96), *393*
Studd, J. W. W., 279, *287,* 378(76), *392*
Stumpf, W. E., 50(86), *63,* 67(50), *74*
Sturdee, D. W., 279, *287*
Sturgis, S. H., 177, 179, 184, *195, 196*
Sugarman, A. A., 108, 119(70), *126*
Sullivan, J. J., 101(7), 108(7), *123.*

[Sullivan]
251(31), 253(31), *265*
Summy-Long, J., 408(103), *422*
Sundsfjord, J. A., 405(73), *421*
Supton, M. J., 177, *195*
Surks, M. I., 15(29), *21*
Sutherland, H., 83, *98,* 243(15), *264,* 367(4), *388*
Svanberg, L., 374(61), 376(61), *391*
Svanborg, K., 207(23), *216*
Svare, B. B., 71(102,103), *76*
Svec, P., 408(100), 413(100), *422*
Svendstrup, B., 374(62), 376(62), 377(68), *391, 392,* 410(121), *424*
Swandby, J. R., 86, *98*
Swanson, D., 352(63), *364*
Swanson, E. M., 90, *99,* 161, *175*
Symonds, E. H., 235(31), *241*
Symonds, E. M., 239(43), *242,* 368 (25), 370(33), 371(25), 372(25, 33), 375(33), 379(25), 384(25), *389, 390,* 401(51), 406(51,81), 407(51), *419, 421*
Szego, C. M., 13(22), *20*
Szendro, P., 13(28), *21*

Tagliamonte, A., 411(139), 412 (139), *425*
Tagliamonte, P., 411(139), 412(139), *425*
Tait, J. F., 281, *283*
Takahashi, S., 244(25), 245(25), *264,* 355(55), *364,* 397(4), *417*
Takaoka, Y., 49(67), *62*
Talan, K., 323, 324, *341*
Taleisnk, S., 67(55,64), *75*
Talwar, P. P., 348(15), *361*
Tamura, S., 410(124), *424*
Tanizawa, O., 27(8), *40*
Tarika, J., 321, *340*
Tasto, D. L., 181, 182, *195,* 383(107), *394*

Taubert, H.-D., 10(12), *20*
Taylor, J. S., 408(103), *422*
Taylor, J. W., 367(10), 371(39), *388, 390*
Taylor, R. W., 229(18), 238(18), *240,* 367(16), 370(16), 371(44), 373(44, 54), 374(16), 375(44), 382(16), *389, 390, 391,* 401(49), 402(55), *419, 420*
Tedford, W. H., 106, *126*
Tedford, W. H., Jr., 351(39), *363*
Tejasen, T., 67(69), *75*
Tenhunen, T., 179, *196*
Teran, C., 13(28), *21*
Terkel, J., 69(94), *76*
Terman, L. M., 131, *152,* 156, *175*
Theander, S., 291(3), *295*
Thi, M. T. L., 19(46), *21*
Thom, M. H., 279, *287*
Thomas, C. N., 55(88), *63*
Thomas, D. A., 46(89), 55(89), *63*
Thomisto, J., 414(168), *427*
Thompson, C., 302, *316*
Thompson, D. J., 279, *288*
Thompson, H., 106, 117(55), *125*
Thomson, A. D., 325, *342*
Thorn, D. W., 406(90), 408(90), *422*
Thorn, G. W., 406(79,90), 408(90), *421, 422*
Thorneycroft, I. H., 409(110), *423*
Thornton, M. J., 381(95), *393*
Thurstone, L. L., 273, *288*
Tiger, L., 112(28,29), *124*
Timeras, P. S., 404(68,69), *420, 421*
Timonen, S., 382(102), *394*
Tirsch, W., 104(36), 106(56), 108(56), 113(36), 116(36), 117(56), 119 (56), *124, 125,* 398(15), *418*
Toft, D. O., 19(47), *21*
Tokarz, R. R., 66(26), *73*
Tolis, G., 39(38), *42*
Tong, J. E., 89, 93, *95, 99,* 108, 117 (58), 118(58), *125,* 407(95), *422*

Tong, T. E., 108, 117, *126*
Tonge, S. R., 268, *285*
Tonks, C. M., 79, *99,* 243(5), *263,*
   324, *344,* 368(21), 382(21), *389*
Tonzetich, J., 173, *175*
Toran-Allerand, C. D., 56(90), *64*
Torghele, J. R., 323, 336, *344,* 406
   (88), *422*
Torres, F., 398(18), 404(18), *418*
Tose, R. M., 349(18), *361*
Toth, E., 177, *195*
Toubeau, G., 71(109), 72(109), *76*
Toungue, S. R., 412(151), 414(166),
   426, 427
Townsend, P. T., 235(32), *241,* 372
   (49), *390*
Travaglini, P., 293(18), *296*
Treadway, R. C., 402(52), 414(52),
   419
Trey, L., 67(59), *75*
Trojanowski, D., 295(34), *297*
Tsafriri, A., 202(6), *215*
Tsai, C. C., 24(2), 25(2), 33(20),
   40, 41
Tseng, L., 19(50,51), *21*
Tuch, R. H., 79, *99,* 108(14), *123,*
   243(14), *264*
Tukiainen, E., 414(168), *427*
Tulchinsky, D., 16(37), *21,* 279,
   287
Tupper, W. R., 292(9), *295*
Turgeon, J., 67(57), *75*
Turnbull, C., 251(31), 253(31), *265*
Turner, D., 66(13), *73*
Turner, P., 414(162), *426*
Tyrer, G., 349(20), *362*
Tyson, J. E., 381(93), *393*

Uchalich, D., 182, *196*
Udry, J. R., 8(7), *20,* 91, *99,* 101(5),
   123, 129(1), 130(1), 132(1), 133

[Udry]
   (16,17,18), 134(17,19), 135(19),
   136(19), 137(19), 140(27), 141(16),
   142(16), 143(28), 146(17), 147(17),
   152, 166, 167, 169, 170, 172, 173,
   175, 345(1), 359(73), *360, 365,*
   380(86), *393,* 401(45), *419*
Ugenas, A. J., 279, 283, *285*
Underwood, L. E., 133(18), *152,* 169,
   175
Uno, T., 108, 119(69), *126*

Vaitukaitais, J. L., 293(17), *296*
Vale, W., 38(34), *41,* 65(2,3), 67(3),
   68(3,84), 69(3,84), *72, 75*
Valenstein, E. S., 67(73,77), *75*
Vandeberg, G., 33(20), *41*
Vandenberg, G., 24(2), 25(2), *40*
van der Schoot, P., 55(92), *64*
van der Vaart, P. D. M., 55(92), *64*
Vande Wiele, R. L., 1, 2(3), 7(6), *20,*
   23(1), 25(3), 26(3), 34(23), 35(23),
   40(39), *40, 41, 42,* 293(21), *296*
Vane, J. R., 386(119), 387(119), *395*
Van Emde Boas, C., 156, 171, *176*
van Konselaar, W., 411(129), *424*
Vaughan, L., 29(9), *40*
Vekemans, M., 410(125), *424*
Vellucci, S. V., 409(117), *423*
Verdonck, L., 409(108), *423*
Verghese, A., 400(34), *419*
Vermeulen, A., 409(108), *423*
Vessey, M. P., 280, *285*
Vetter, W., 406(82), *421*
Vidal, N., 403(65), *420*
Vigersky, R. A., 293(17), *296*
Vigiani, C., 295(35), *297*
Vihko, R., 150(38), *153,* 179, *194*
Viinikka, L., 150(38), *153*
Vijayan, N., 415(174), *427*
Vijayan, V. K., 415(174), *427*

Vila, J., 106, 118(65), *126*
Vito, C. C., 51(91), *64*
Vogel, S. A., 413(153), *426*
Vogel, W., 91, *94,* 106(42), 108(72), 114(42), 118(66), 119(66,72), *125, 126,* 268, 270, 271, 272, 274, 275, 276, 277, 278, 280, 282, *284, 286, 287, 288,* 351(33, 43), 353(33,43), *362, 363,* 398 (17), *418*
Voisin, F., 319, *344*
Vollman, R. F., 179, 193, *196*
von Schoultz, B., 369(28), 377(28), *389*
Vreeburg, J. T. M., 46(5), 55(87,92), *58, 63, 64*

Wachelicht, H., 269, 270, *284*
Wachslicht, H., 55(21), *59*
Wade, G. N., 46(12,13), 52(82), 53 (13), *58, 63*
Wade-Evans, T., 279, *287*
Wahlberg, I., 104(49), 106(49), 116 (49), 117(49), 118(49), *125*
Wakeling, A., 292(12), 293(13,15), *296*
Wald, I., 243(21), 244(21), *264*
Wald, J. A., 300(14), *316,* 400(31), *418*
Walker, C. E., 164, *174*
Walker, M. S., 409(111), *423*
Wallace, M. G., 383(108), *394,* 416 (176), *427*
Waller, L., 143(28), *152,* 167, *175*
Wallin, P., 131(6), *152*
Walløe, L., 206(18), *215*
Wallsh, R., 324, 329, *343*
Wang, C. F., 10(13), *20,* 30(14,15), 31(14), *41,* 293(23), *296*
Wantanabe, M., 405(75), *421*
Wapner, S., 351(44), *363*

Ward, I. L., 55(93), *64*
Ward, M. M., 93, *99,* 108, 117(57), *125,* 397(9), *417*
Wardlaw, S. L., 38(36), *42*
Warembourg, M., 53(94), *64*
Warner, P., 349(20), *362*
Warnes, H., 348(13), *361*
Warren, D. E., 106(74), *126,* 351(39), *363*
Warren, M. P., 7(6), *20,* 23(1), 25(3), 26(3), *40,* 293(21), *296*
Watson, M. J., 66(14), *73,* 229(18), 238(18), *240*
Watson, P. E., 406(87), *422*
Watson, S., 411(136), *425*
Webb, W. W., 358(66), *364*
Weber, J. C. P., 369(27), 370(27), 380 (27), *389*
Webster, S. K., 182, *196*
Wechsler, D., 273, *288*
Weekes, L. R., 324, *344,* 400(37), *419*
Wehrenberg, W. B., 38(36), *42*
Weick, R. F., 25(5), *40*
Weiner, H., 293(27), *297*
Weiss, G., 25(5), *40*
Weiss, N. S., 283, *288*
Weissman, M. M., 350(31), 351(32), 356(60), *362, 364*
Weitzman, E. D., 33(18), *41*
Weitzman, E. L., 293(26,27), *297*
Welner, A., 330, *344*
Wendestam, C., 370(30), 374(30), 375(30), *389*
Wentz, A. C., 203(15), *215*
Werble, B., 321, *341*
Werch, A., 369(29), 370(29), 385(29), *389*
Westerholm, B., 280, *285*
Wetterberg, L., 411(129), *424*
Wetzel, R. D., 243(20,21,24), 244(20, 21,24), 250(20), *264,* 300(13,14, 15), 304(15), 305(15), 309(15),

[Wetzel]
312(15), *316,* 324, 325, 336,
342, 344, 400(31,32), *418*
Whalen, R. E., 45(35), 55(95), *60,*
64, 360(76), *365*
While, R. J., 49(67), *62*
Whisnant, L., 120(79,80), *127*
Whitehead, M. I., 279, *284,* 372(49),
390
Whithead, M. I., 235(32), *241*
Whitmore, M. R., 86, 91, *95,* 131
(11), 132(11), *152,* 178, *195*
Wickham, M., 102, 104, 111(23),
124, 275, *288*
Widdowson, E. E., 131(10), 132(10),
152, 165, 168, 171, *175*
Wide, L., 293(24,25), *297,* 371(41),
390
Widholm, O., 179, 183, 184, 185,
187, 191, 192, *195, 196,* 367(5),
388
Wieczarek, V., 352(56), 355(56), *364*
Wiener, J. S., 413(159), *426*
Wiesbader, H., 267, *288*
Wilcott, R. C., 274, *285*
Wilcoxon, L. H., 82, *99*
Wildt, L., 33(19), *41*
Wilhelm, H., 106(56), 108(56), 117
(56), 119(56), *125,* 398(15), *418*
Wilks, J. W., 203(15), *215*
Williams, E. Y., 324, *344,* 400(37),
419
Williams, R., 379(83), 367(6), 383(83),
388, 392
Wilson, E. O., 400(39), *419*
Wilson, I., 351(34), 353(34), *362*
Wilson, J. D., 349(22), *362*
Wilson, W. P., 270, *288*
Wincze, J. P., 158, *176*
Wineman, E. W., 118(62), *126*
Winer, J., 179, *195*
Winokur, G., 325, 330, *341*

Winston, F., 348(11), 349(11), 353
(81), 354(11), *361, 365,* 381(98),
394, 415(173), *427*
Winter, J. S. D., 179, *197*
Wionczek, C., 415(171), *427*
Wiqvist, N., 204(17), *215*
Wirz-Justice, A., 54(46), *60,* 412(150),
413(150), 414(150,163,167,169),
426, 427
Wise, P. H., 375(65), 376(65), 377(65),
391, 410(122), *424*
Wiseman, S., 243(23), 244(23), *264*
Witkin, H. A., 273, 274, 275, *288, 289*
Wittkower, E. D., 367(12), *388*
Wolin, I., 49(67), *62*
Wong, S., 93, *99,* 108, 117, *126*
Wong, W. G., 406(93), *422*
Wong, W. H., 369(26), *389*
Wood, C., 224, *240,* 367(6), 379(83),
383(83), 387(121), *388, 392, 395*
Woodruff, R. A., 325, 330, *341*
Woolley, D. E., 404(68), *420*
Worsley, A., 348(5), 349(19), 351(5),
361, 362
Wulff, M. H., 270, *285*
Wunderlich, M., 202(8), *215*
Wurtman, P., 411(131), *424*
Wurtman, R. J., 185, *197,* 269, *289,*
412(145), *425*
Wuttke, W., 104, 106(56), 108(56), 113
(36), 116(36), 117(56), 119(56), *124,*
125, 293(14), *296,* 398(15), *418*
Wyatt, M., 314(39), *316*
Wyatt, R. J., 381(90), *393,* 412(149),
426
Wynn, V. T., 92, *99,* 350(29,30), 353
(30), *362,* 381(96), *393*

Xavier, R., 202(4), 206(4),
214
Xenakis, T., 179, *195*

Yalom, I. L. D., 79, *97,* 157, *174,*
    175, 350(25), 359(74), *362, 365*
Yamada, Y., 71(108), *76*
Yamaji, T., 25(5), *40*
Yamashita, I., 244(25), 245(25),
    264, 355(55), *364,* 397(4), *417*
Yarbrough, G. G., 72(111), *76*
Yen, S. S. C., 16(36), *21,* 24(2), 25
    (2), 30(14,15), 31(14), 33(20),
    36(28), 38(32,35), 40(35), *40, 41,*
    42, 65(1), *72,* 293(23), 294(32),
    295(33), *296, 297*
Young, W. C., 43(96,97), *64*
Yusoff Dawood, M., 397(6), *417*

Zacharias, L., 185, *197*
Zacur, H. A., 381(93), *393*
Zadina, J. E., 68(83), *75*
Zahn, T. P., 104, 106, 108, 117(54),
    118(54), 119(54), *125,* 354(45),

[Zahn]
    363, 381(91), *393,* 413(158), *426*
Zamudio, R., 293(19), *296*
Zegans, L., 120(79,80), *127*
Zelesnik, A. J., 15(31), 16(34), *21*
Zemlan, F. P., 45(98), 54(22), *59, 64*
Ziegler, M. G., 381(93), *393*
Zigmond, R. E., 48(60,61), *61,* 67(80),
    75
Zilboorg, G., 320, *344*
Zimmer, C. H., 102, 113(37,38), *124*
Zimmer, R. A., 238(39), *241*
Zimmerman, E. A., 28(12), 29(11,12),
    34(22,24), *41,* 67(31), *74,* 104,
    106, 108, 113(34), 117(34), *124*
Zohn, T. P., 90, *96*
Zor, U., 202(6), 207(22), *215, 216*
Zubiran, S., 291(4), *295*
Zumpe, D., 129(2), 130(2), *152,* 401
    (47), 403(67), *419, 420*
Zuspan, F. P., 203(13), *215*

Subject Index

Acetylcholine, 38
  premenstrual tension and, 415-
    416
Adenohypophysis, 8
Adolescence, menstrual distress in,
    177-197
  developmental analyses of, 178-
    181
  dysmenorrhea, 181-189
  premenstrual tension, 189-194
Adrenergic neurotransmitters, ef-
    fects of estrogen on syn-
    thesis of, 268
Adrenocorticotropin (ACTH), 8,
    39, 71
Ambulatory schizophrenia, 320
Amenorrhea, 39, 40, 120
  manipulations of EEG photic
    driving response by estro-
    gen administration for,
    271-273

[Amenorrhea]
  oral contraceptives and, 349-351
γ-Aminobutyric acid (GABA), 38
Amphetamine, 274
Androgen hypothesis, 409
Anorexia nervosa, 40, 120, 291-297
Anovulation, 39
As-if personality, 320
ATD (1,4,6-androstatriene-3, 17-
    dione), 55

Basal body temperature (BBT), 133,
    134
Bellergal for premenstrual syndrome
    treatment, 382
Betamimetic drugs, 206
Biochemical aspects of the men-
    strual cycle, 11-19
Bromocriptine, 238
  for premenstrual syndrome

[Bromocriptine]
    treatment, 374-377

Caffeine, 274
Catechol-o-methyltransferase, 269,
    294, 413
Central nervous system, effect of
    menstrual cycle on, 116-
    119
Chlomiphene, 292-293
Chlorpromazine, 274
Cognitive behavior and the men-
    strual cycle, 101-127
    effect of cognitive factors on
      menstrual events, 119-121
    effect of menstrual cycle on cog-
      nitive performance, 110-
      119
      cognitive function, perceptual-
        motor performance and
        cognitive style, 112-116
      intellectual performance, 110-
        112
      sensory-motor function and cen-
        tral nervous system corre-
        lates, 116-119
Cognitive task performances, estro-
    gen and, 273-276
Corticosteroid binding globulin
    (CBG), 11
Cyclic AMP, 2-3, 16

Depression
    estrogens and, 276-279
    hormonal characteristics of, 280-
      282
    manipulation of EEG photic
      driving responses by estro-
      gen administration for,
      271-273

[Depression]
    oral contraceptives and, 350-354
    postpartum, oral contraceptives
      and, 355
    puerperal, 233
    vitamin levels and, 350
Diethylstilbestrol (DES), 26
5α-Dihydrotestosterone, 51
Diuretic therapy for premenstrual
    syndrome treatment, 368-
    371
Diuretics, 238-239
DNA (deoxyribonucleic acid), 12, 44
Dopamine, 36, 37
Dysmenorrhea, 181-189, 199-208,
    220
Dyspareunia, 209-214

EEG photic driving responses
    cyclic changes across menstrual
      cycle of, 270-271
    effects of estrogen and progesterone
      on, 269-270
    manipulations in amenorrheic and
      depressed women of, 271-273
Endocervical gland activities, vaginal
    cytology and, 4-5
Endocrine function, hypothalamus and,
    27-33
Endometrial MAO, 327
Endometriosis, 220-222
Estradiol, 11
Estradiol negative feedback loop, 24
Estradiol positive feedback loop, 24-
    26
17β-Estradiol, 16, 19, 23, 24, 26, 35,
    50
Estrogen
    action of, 48-57
      functional concommitants of
        estrogen binding in neural

[Estrogen]
    tissue, 52-57
    topography and cellular aspects
      of, 48-52
  depression and, 276-279
  effects on neurotransmitter up-
    take and degradation, 268-
    269
  positive feedback loop of, 26
Estrogen and central nervous system
    (CNS) function, 267-289
  action on adrenergic functioning,
    268
  adverse effects of high dose
    therapy, 279-280
  cyclic changes of EEG photic
    driving responses across
    menstrual cycle, 270-271
  effects on cognitive task perfor-
    mances, 273-276
  effects on the EEG photic driving
    index, 269-270
  effects on mental depression, 276-
    279
  effects on neurotransmitter de-
    gradation, 268-269
  effects on neurotransmitter up-
    take, 269
  effects on synthesis of adrenergic
    neurotransmitters, 268
  hormonal characteristics of de-
    pressed women, 280-282
  interactions with progesterone
    and testosterone, 269
  manipulations of EEG photic
    driving responses in amenor-
    rheic and depressed women,
    271-273
Estrone, 19
Etiology of premenstrual tension,
    236, 397-426
  biologic hypotheses, 401-416

[Etiology of premenstrual tension]
  psychological hypotheses, 399-400
  sociobiologic hypothesis, 400
External dyspareunia, 209-210

Fenoterol, 206
Follicle-stimulating hormone (FSH),
    3, 8, 9, 15, 16, 23-27, 30-34,
    40, 65, 412
  anorexia nervosa and, 293

Glucocorticoid hypothesis, premen-
    strual tension and, 409
Gonadotropin-releasing hormone
    (GnRH), 10, 16, 28-40
  anorexia nervosa and, 293
Growth hormone (GH), 8, 29

Hamilton depression ratings, before
    and after three months of
    estrogen or placebo treat-
    ment, 277, 278
High dose estrogen therapy, adverse
    effects of, 279-280
Histamine, 38
Human chorionic gonadotrophin
    (HCG), 7
Hypothalamic peptides and sexual be-
    havior, 65-76
  analogs of LHRH and sexual be-
    havior, 68-69
  brain LHRH and mating behavior,
    66-67
  interaction of LHRH prolactin,
    and sexual behavior, 69-
    71
Hypothalamus, 8-10
  endocrine function and, 27-
    33

Insulin hypothesis, premenstrual
    tension and, 410
Intellectual performance, 110-112
Internal dyspareunia, 211-213
Intrauterine contraceptive device
    (IUD), 208
Involutional psychiatric illness,
    oral contraceptives and,
    355

Latent psychosis, 320
β-Lipotropin, 8
Lithium salts for premenstrual syn-
    drome treatment, 377-378
Luteinizing hormone (LH), 3, 8, 9,
    11-17, 23-27, 30-34, 45,
    65, 133, 134
  anorexia nervosa and, 292-295
Luteinizing hormone/follicle-
    stimulating hormone-
    releasing factor (LH/
    FSH-RF), 9
Luteinizing hormone-releasing
    hormone (LHRH), 9, 65-
    72, 150

Males, postnatal sexual develop-
    ment, oral contraceptives
    and, 350
Melatonin, premenstrual tension
    and, 411
Menstrual attitude questionnaire,
    311
Menstrual distress, 219-220
Menstrual distress in adolescence,
    177-197
  developmental analysis of, 178-
    181
  dysmenorrhea, 181-189
  premenstrual tension, 189-194

Mineralocorticoid hypothesis, premen-
    strual tension and, 405-409
Monoamine neurotransmitters, pre-
    menstrual tension and, 411-
    415
Monoamine oxidase (MAO) inhibitors,
    268, 269, 327, 411-412
Moos Menstrual Distress Question-
    naire (MMDQ), 229

Neuroendocrine regulation of sexual
    behavior, 43-64
  estrogen action and, 48-57
    functional concomitants of
      estrogen binding in neural
      tissues, 52-57
    topography and cellular aspects
      of action, 48-52
    hormone regulation of reproduc-
      tion in rats, 44-48
Neuroendocrinologic control of the
    menstrual cycle, 23-42
  dysfunction of the menstrual cycle,
    38-40
  feedback loops, 24-27
  hypothalamus and endocrine func-
    tion, 27-33
  ovarian-hypothalamic-hypophyseal
    functional integration, 34-38
Neuroleptic agents for premenstrual
    syndrome treatment, 382
Neurotransmitter degradation, effects
    of estrogen on, 268-269
Neurotransmitter uptake, effects of
    estrogen on, 269

Oral contraceptives (OCs), 345-365
  mood and behavioral changes and,
    346-371
  progesterone as a psychopharmaco-

[Oral contraceptives (OCs)]
  logic agent, 357-358
 psychotropic actions of, 352-353
 side effects of, 356-357
 used in patients without psychiatric illness, 345-350
 used as psychotropic hormones,
  350-355
Ovarian hormone hypothesis, premenstrual tension and,
  401-405
Oviducts, 6-7

Paramenstruum, 222
Passive accidents, 80-81
Perceptual-motor performance,
  112-116
Physical activity for premenstrual
  syndrome treatment, 382-
  383
Physiology of the menstrual cycle,
  1-21
 hormone receptors, 11-15
 hypothalamus, 8-10
 menstruation, 3
 ovaries and ovulation, 7-8
 oviducts and gamete transport,
  6-7
 pituitary gland, 8-10
 receptor regulation, 15-19
  ovary, 15-16
  uterus, 16-19
 reproductive system, 2-3
 uterus and its morphologic
  changes, 5-6
 vaginal cytology and endocervical gland activities,
  4-5
Pinozide, 36
Pituitary gland, 8-10
Postnatal depression, 226

Postnatal sexual development in
  males, oral contraceptives
  and, 350
Postpartum depression, oral contraceptives and, 355
Preeclampsia, 226, 233
Premenstrual affective syndrome
  (PAS), 300-314
 criteria for, 305
  in inpatient and outpatient
   psychiatric samples, 310
  psychiatric depression and, 307
Premenstrual Assessment Form (PAF),
  246-262
Premenstrual syndromes, 78-84, 243-
  265
 bromocriptine, 374-377
 diuretic therapy, 368-371
 lithium salts, 377-378
 methodologic considerations, 368
 oral contraceptives and, 354
 progesterone, 371-374
 progestins and oral contraceptive
  combinations, 378-381
 pyridoxine, 381-382
 treatment of, 367-395
Premenstrual tension (PMT), 217-242,
  299, 317-344
 borderline syndromes, 320-323
 case histories, 330-336
 definition, 219-222
 diagnosis of, 222-229
 diagnosis of menstrual distress, 229-
  230
 differences between progesterone
  and progestogens, 236-237
 distress in adolescence, 189-194
 etiology of, 236, 397-426
  biologic hypotheses, 401-416
  psychological hypotheses, 399-
   400
  sociobiologic hypothesis, 400

[Premenstrual tension (PMT)]
  extrapolation of survey results,
    235
  history of, 318-320
  problems encountered in surveys,
    232-235
  progesterone treatment, 237-238
  psychiatric syndromes related to
    menstrual cycle, 323-327
  psychodynamic considerations,
    327-329
  severity of symptoms, 230-232
  sociologic surveys, 222
  timing of symptoms, 230
Premenstruum, 222
Primary dysmenorrhea, 200-207
Progesterone, 16, 19, 203
  effects on EEG photic driving
    response of, 269-270
  interactions of estrogen with,
    269
  for premenstrual syndrome treat-
    ment, 371-374
  progestogens and, 236-237
  as a psychopharmacologic agent,
    oral contraceptives and,
    357-358
  for treatment of premenstrual
    tension, 237-238
Progesterone feedback loop, 26-27
Progestins and oral contraceptive
    combinations for premen-
    strual syndrome treatment,
    378-381
Progestogens, progesterone and,
    236-237
Prolactin (PRL), 69-71, 374-377
  premenstrual tension and, 410-
    411
Prostaglandins (PGs), 202-204
Pseudoneurotic schizophrenia,
    320

Psychology of the menstrual cycle,
    77-99
  correlation studies, 79-83
  longitudinal research, 88-94
  retrospective questionnaires, 83-88
Psychopathology, 299-316
Psychotherapy for premenstrual syn-
    drome treatment, 382
Puerperal depression, 233
Pyridoxine, 239
  for treatment of premenstrual syn-
    drome, 381-382

Recurrent menstrual psychosis, oral
    contraceptives and, 355
Reproductive system, 2-3
Research Diagnostic Criteria (RDC),
    250, 252, 262
RNA (Ribonucleic acid), 44, 52

Schizophrenia, 320-323
Secondary (acquired) dysmenorrhea,
    208
Sensory-motor function, 116-119
Serotonin, 37, 414-415
Sex hormone binding globulin
    (SHBG), 227-228
Sexual behavior and the menstrual
    cycle, 155-176
  sexuality, 156-171
    daily reports, 165-171
    dream analysis, 159-163
    erotic stimulation, 163-165
    retrospective questionnaire, 156-
      159
  summary and implications, 171-
    173
Sexual behavior in the menstrual cycle,
    129-153
  future research, 148-151

[Sexual behavior in the menstrual
       cycle]
   implications of nonsocial influ-
       ences on human behavior,
       131
   mammalian/nonhuman primate
       patterns, 129-131
   present research, 147-148
       daily testosterone measure,
       147
   development of adolescent
       heterosexual behavior, 148
   female-initiated behavior, 147
   questions pursued, 131-147
       existence of a pattern, 131-
       138
       how pattern is produced, 138-
       147
Sexuality, oral contraceptives and,
       349
Short feedback loop, 27
Spasmodic dysmenorrhea, 220

Spironolactone, 239

Terbutaline, 206
Testosterone, 11
   interactions of estrogen with, 269
Testosterone metabolism, 280-281
Thyrotropin-releasing hormone (TRH),
       29, 65
Thyroid-stimulating hormone (TSH),
       8, 9
Trichomonas vaginalis, 210

Uterus, morphologic changes of,
       5-6

Vaginal cytology, endocervical gland
       activities and, 4-5
Vitamin B, 239
Vitamin levels, depression and, 350